From Basic Research to New Tools and Challenges for the Genotoxicity Testing of Nanomaterials

From Basic Research to New Tools and Challenges for the Genotoxicity Testing of Nanomaterials

Editors

Valérie Fessard
Fabrice Nesslany

MDPI • Basel • Beijing • Wuhan • Barcelona • Belgrade • Manchester • Tokyo • Cluj • Tianjin

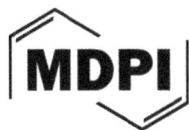

Editors
Valérie Fessard
Anses, Unité de Toxicologie
France

Fabrice Nesslany
Institut Pasteur de Lille, Service Toxicologie
France

Editorial Office
MDPI
St. Alban-Anlage 66
4052 Basel, Switzerland

This is a reprint of articles from the Special Issue published online in the open access journal *Nanomaterials* (ISSN 2079-4991) (available at: https://www.mdpi.com/journal/nanomaterials/special_issues/genotoxic_test_nano).

For citation purposes, cite each article independently as indicated on the article page online and as indicated below:

LastName, A.A.; LastName, B.B.; LastName, C.C. Article Title. *Journal Name* **Year**, *Volume Number*, Page Range.

ISBN 978-3-0365-0112-3 (Hbk)
ISBN 978-3-0365-0113-0 (PDF)

Cover image courtesy of Burel Agnès.

© 2021 by the authors. Articles in this book are Open Access and distributed under the Creative Commons Attribution (CC BY) license, which allows users to download, copy and build upon published articles, as long as the author and publisher are properly credited, which ensures maximum dissemination and a wider impact of our publications.

The book as a whole is distributed by MDPI under the terms and conditions of the Creative Commons license CC BY-NC-ND.

Contents

About the Editors vii

Valérie Fessard and Fabrice Nesslany
From Basic Research to New Tools and Challenges for the Genotoxicity Testing of Nanomaterials
Reprinted from: *Nanomaterials* **2020**, *10*, 2073, doi:10.3390/nano10102073 1

Alba García-Rodríguez, Laura Rubio, Laura Vila, Noel Xamena, Antonia Velázquez, Ricard Marcos and Alba Hernández
The Comet Assay as a Tool to Detect the Genotoxic Potential of Nanomaterials
Reprinted from: *Nanomaterials* **2019**, *9*, 1385, doi:10.3390/nano9101385 5

Elisabeth Elje, Espen Mariussen, Oscar H. Moriones, Neus G. Bastús, Victor Puntes, Yvonne Kohl, Maria Dusinska and Elise Rundén-Pran
Hepato(Geno)Toxicity Assessment of Nanoparticles in a HepG2 Liver Spheroid Model
Reprinted from: *Nanomaterials* **2020**, *10*, 545, doi:10.3390/nano10030545 25

Anna Poma, Giulia Vecchiotti, Sabrina Colafarina, Osvaldo Zarivi, Massimo Aloisi, Lorenzo Arrizza, Giuseppe Chichiriccò and Piero Di Carlo
In Vitro Genotoxicity of Polystyrene Nanoparticles on the Human Fibroblast Hs27 Cell Line
Reprinted from: *Nanomaterials* **2019**, *9*, 1299, doi:10.3390/nano9091299 47

Alena Kazimirova, Naouale El Yamani, Laura Rubio, Alba García-Rodríguez, Magdalena Barancokova, Ricard Marcos and Maria Dusinska
Effects of Titanium Dioxide Nanoparticles on the *Hprt* Gene Mutations in V79 Hamster Cells
Reprinted from: *Nanomaterials* **2020**, *10*, 465, doi:10.3390/nano10030465 61

Filomena Mottola, Concetta Iovine, Marianna Santonastaso, Maria Luisa Romeo, Severina Pacifico, Luigi Cobellis and Lucia Rocco
NPs-TiO$_2$ and Lincomycin Coexposure Induces DNA Damage in Cultured Human Amniotic Cells
Reprinted from: *Nanomaterials* **2019**, *9*, 1511, doi:10.3390/nano9111511 73

Chiara Uboldi, Marcos Sanles Sobrido, Elodie Bernard, Virginie Tassistro, Nathalie Herlin-Boime, Dominique Vrel, Sébastien Garcia-Argote, Stéphane Roche, Fréderique Magdinier, Gheorghe Dinescu, Véronique Malard, Laurence Lebaron-Jacobs, Jerome Rose, Bernard Rousseau, Philippe Delaporte, Christian Grisolia and Thierry Orsière
In Vitro Analysis of the Effects of ITER-Like Tungsten Nanoparticles: Cytotoxicity and Epigenotoxicity in BEAS-2B Cells
Reprinted from: *Nanomaterials* **2019**, *9*, 1233, doi:10.3390/nano9091233 89

Pégah Jalili, Sylvie Huet, Rachelle Lanceleur, Gérard Jarry, Ludovic Le Hegarat, Fabrice Nesslany, Kevin Hogeveen and Valérie Fessard
Genotoxicity of Aluminum and Aluminum Oxide Nanomaterials in Rats Following Oral Exposure
Reprinted from: *Nanomaterials* **2020**, *10*, 305, doi:10.3390/nano10020305 107

Francisco Casillas-Figueroa, María Evarista Arellano-García, Claudia Leyva-Aguilera, Balam Ruíz-Ruíz, Roberto Luna Vázquez-Gómez, Patricia Radilla-Chávez, Rocío Alejandra Chávez-Santoscoy, Alexey Pestryakov, Yanis Toledano-Magaña, Juan Carlos García-Ramos and Nina Bogdanchikova
Argovit™ Silver Nanoparticles Effects on *Allium cepa*: Plant Growth Promotion without Cyto Genotoxic Damage
Reprinted from: *Nanomaterials* **2020**, *10*, 1386, doi:10.3390/nano10071386 . . . . **121**

Lauris Evariste, Laura Lagier, Patrice Gonzalez, Antoine Mottier, Florence Mouchet, Stéphanie Cadarsi, Pierre Lonchambon, Guillemine Daffe, George Chimowa, Cyril Sarrieu, Elise Ompraret, Anne-Marie Galibert, Camélia Matei Ghimbeu, Eric Pinelli, Emmanuel Flahaut and Laury Gauthier
Thermal Reduction of Graphene Oxide Mitigates Its In Vivo Genotoxicity Toward *Xenopus laevis* Tadpoles
Reprinted from: *Nanomaterials* **2019**, *9*, 584, doi:10.3390/nano9040584 . . . . **141**

Sarah McCarrick, Francesca Cappellini, Amanda Kessler, Nynke Moelijker, Remco Derr, Jonas Hedberg, Susanna Wold, Eva Blomberg, Inger Odnevall Wallinder, Giel Hendriks and Hanna L. Karlsson
ToxTracker Reporter Cell Lines as a Tool for Mechanism-Based (Geno)Toxicity Screening of Nanoparticles—Metals, Oxides and Quantum Dots
Reprinted from: *Nanomaterials* **2020**, *10*, 110, doi:10.3390/nano10010110 . . . . **157**

About the Editors

Valérie Fessard (Dr.) is a toxicologist with longstanding expertise in food contaminant toxicology, especially genotoxicity, intestinal and hepatic human cell models and high-content screening for multi-parametric toxic effects. After earning a Ph.D. and a post-doctorate in ecotoxicology, she moved to human toxicology and dedicated her research to public health and hazard assessment. She has been working on engineered nanomaterials for nearly 10 years. In this context, she coordinated the French/German project SolNanoTox (2013–2017) and is/was involved in several European projects (Nanogenotox, NanoReg, Riskgone). She has been the head of the Toxicology of Contaminants unit in the French Agency for Food, Environmental and Occupational Health & Safety for 12 years.

Fabrice Nesslany (Dr.) is a toxicologist with longstanding expertise in regulatory genotoxicology testing. He was involved in several European projects aiming to assess the hazards and risks of nanomaterials (Nanogenotox, NanoReg1, 2). He has been the Head of the Toxicology Laboratory of Institut Pasteur de Lille for 10 years. He has numerous appointments as an expert toxicologist in French safety agencies (Agency for Food, Environmental and Occupational Health & Safety; French Agency of Human Health Products, High Council of Public Health) and participates in several specialized expert committees. He is also a French expert for OECD.

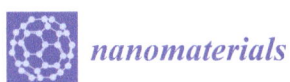

Editorial

From Basic Research to New Tools and Challenges for the Genotoxicity Testing of Nanomaterials

Valérie Fessard [1],* and Fabrice Nesslany [2],*

[1] Unit of Toxicology of Contaminants, Fougères Laboratory, French Agency for Food, Environmental and Occupational Health & Safety, 10B rue C. Bourgelat, 35306 Fougères, France
[2] Genotoxicology Department, Institut Pasteur de Lille, 1, Rue du Professeur Calmette, 59000 Lille, France
* Correspondence: valerie.fessard@anses.fr (V.F.); fabrice.nesslany@pasteur-lille.fr (F.N.)

Received: 8 October 2020; Accepted: 15 October 2020; Published: 20 October 2020

Genotoxicity is one of the key endpoints investigated as early as possible before marketing a product. Several assays can be performed to evaluate the genotoxicity and mutagenicity of compounds, covering the detection of DNA lesions and of DNA repair activities as well as the quantification of the three types of mutations at the gene, chromosome and genome levels. Most of these tests have an established or draft guideline from the Organization for Economic Co-operation and Development (OECD). Nevertheless, if these assays have been developed for chemicals, they are not fully suitable for testing the genotoxicity/mutagenicity of nanomaterials, and the adaptation of the experimental conditions for such compounds is still debated. This Special Issue "From Basic Research to New Tools and Challenges for the Genotoxicity Testing of Nanomaterials" aimed to provide new results on a large range of nanomaterials using a broad panel of genotoxicity assays and to solve some of the numerous issues faced on this topic.

Researchers from various institutes have contributed to the success of this Special Issue, with a total of 10 articles that were selected for publication. The content of these 10 papers covers different topics that were proposed in the text of the Special Issue. However, the topics concerning interferences with *in vitro* genotoxicity assays and proposals for nanomaterial reference controls have not been addressed as well as the approaches based on grouping, ranking, and read-across. This issue contains mostly data from *in vitro* studies. In addition to classical cell lines such as hamster and human fibroblasts [1,2] or human lung cells [3,4], new models have been also used for investigating nanomaterials genotoxicity: ToxTracker reporter cell lines [5], human amniotic cells [6] and 3D HepG2 spheroids [7]. In this issue, three papers also deal with *in vivo* studies: on the plant *Allium cepa* [8], on the tadpoles of *Xenopus laevis* [9] and on rats [10]. Moreover, a broad range of nanomaterials have been tested, including plastic particles [2] that recently became of increasing concern for environmental and public health.

Among the various assays available for investigating genotoxicity and mutagenicity, most of the papers used the comet assay to visualize the DNA fragmentation both in *in vitro* [3,4,6,7] and *in vivo* [10] studies. The micronucleus assay to detect chromosome and genome mutations was also largely performed in cell lines [2,4] as well as in whole organisms [8–10]. In contrast, only one article deals with the gene mutation Hprt assay [1].

Concerning the role of the physico-chemical characteristics, it was reported that the surface area is one of the dose metrics showing a better correlation with the genotoxicity of quantum dots [5], while the metal/coating agent ratio is a key parameter for the toxicity observed with the commercially available AgNPs formulation Argovit™ [8]. Similarly, the thermal reduction of graphene oxides generates a material that was no longer genotoxic at low concentrations [9]. In contrast, the type of synthesis used for producing tungstene particles did not significantly affect the toxicity [4]. The impact of size was investigated on the toxic responses either using two protocols of dispersion with TiO_2 nanoparticles leading to different size distribution [1] or by testing similar nanomaterials with different primary sizes [5]. Such results are integrated into a "safe by design" approach by investigating solutions to decrease the genotoxicity of the nanomaterials through specific coatings, production processes or treatments as examples.

As already reported in the literature, oxidative stress was suggested as one mechanism involved in the genotoxic responses observed [2–4,9]. Co-exposure to nanomaterials and other compounds can affect the genotoxicity [2,6].

It has been suggested that the genotoxic effects generated by nanomaterials can be due to the dissolution and formation of ions. Nevertheless, although when ions are formed, it does not preclude that nanoforms per se can also induce some genotoxicity. In this issue, the comparison of nanoforms with an ionic counterpart has been done for aluminum after gavage to rats [10] and for silver in *Allium cepa* [8]. In both cases, the genotoxic effects observed could not be solely explained by the formation of ions from the nanoforms tested.

The testing of genotoxicity faces the tremendous number of nanomaterials that can theoretically differ for only one parameter. Therefore, high throughput methodologies can facilitate the screening. A high throughput methodology applied to the comet assay has been used in the European project NanoReg [3]. ToxTracker reporter cell lines [5] can be also a way to quickly assess the activation of cellular stress response pathways.

In conclusion, the papers presented in this Special Issue show how the evaluation of the genotoxicity remains challenging for nanomaterials. Nevertheless, this Special Issue highlights steps forward that have been investigated to overcome some of the concerns. Still, a reliable evaluation of the genotoxic hazard of nanomaterials will support the attempt to protect the health of the populations without strangling innovation.

Author Contributions: V.F. and F.N. wrote and reviewed this Editorial Letter. All authors have read and agreed to the published version of the manuscript.

Funding: This research received no external funding.

Acknowledgments: We would like warmly to acknowledge all authors who submitted their research work to this Special Issue "From Basic Research to New Tools and Challenges for the Genotoxicity Testing of Nanomaterials". Great thanks to the reviewers who contributed to the peer-review of the submitted manuscripts in order to get high-quality papers. We also wish to address a special thanks to the Assistant Editor, Mirabelle Wang, for her patience, her kindness and her help to manage with this special issue.

Conflicts of Interest: The authors declare no conflict of interest.

References

1. Kazimirova, A.; El Yamani, N.; Rubio, L.; García-Rodríguez, A.; Barancokova, M.; Marcos, R.; Dusinska, M. Effects of Titanium Dioxide Nanoparticles on the *Hprt* Gene Mutations in V79 Hamster Cells. *Nanomaterials* **2020**, *10*, 465. [CrossRef]
2. Poma, A.; Vecchiotti, G.; Colafarina, S.; Zarivi, O.; Aloisi, M.; Arrizza, L.; Chichiricco, G.; Di Carlo, P. In Vitro Genotoxicity of Polystyrene Nanoparticles on the Human Fibroblast Hs27 Cell Line. *Nanomaterials* **2019**, *9*, 1299. [CrossRef] [PubMed]
3. García-Rodríguez, A.; Rubio, L.; Vila, L.; Xamena, N.; Velázquez, A.; Marcos, R.; Hernández, A. The Comet Assay as a Tool to Detect the Genotoxic Potential of Nanomaterials. *Nanomaterials* **2019**, *9*, 1385. [CrossRef]
4. Uboldi, C.; Sanles Sobrido, M.; Bernard, E.; Tassistro, V.; Herlin-Boime, N.; Vrel, D.; Garcia-Argote, S.; Roche, S.; Magdinier, F.; Dinescu, G.; et al. In Vitro Analysis of the Effects of ITER-Like Tungsten Nanoparticles: Cytotoxicity and Epigenotoxicity in BEAS-2B Cells. *Nanomaterials* **2019**, *9*, 1233. [CrossRef] [PubMed]
5. McCarrick, S.; Cappellini, F.; Kessler, A.; Moelijker, N.; Derr, R.; Hedberg, J.; Wold, S.; Blomberg, E.; Odnevall Wallinder, I.; Hendriks, G.; et al. ToxTracker Reporter Cell Lines as a Tool for Mechanism-Based (Geno)Toxicity Screening of Nanoparticles—Metals, Oxides and Quantum Dots. *Nanomaterials* **2020**, *10*, 110. [CrossRef] [PubMed]
6. Mottola, F.; Iovine, C.; Santonastaso, M.; Romeo, M.L.; Pacifico, S.; Cobellis, L.; Rocco, L. NPs-TiO$_2$ and Lincomycin Coexposure Induces DNA Damage in Cultured Human Amniotic Cells. *Nanomaterials* **2019**, *9*, 1511. [CrossRef] [PubMed]

7. Elje, E.; Mariussen, E.; Moriones, O.H.; Bastús, N.G.; Puntes, V.; Kohl, Y.; Dusinska, M.; Rundén-Pran, E. Hepato(Geno)Toxicity Assessment of Nanoparticles in a HepG2 Liver Spheroid Model. *Nanomaterials* **2020**, *10*, 545. [CrossRef] [PubMed]
8. Casillas-Figueroa, F.; Arellano-García, M.E.; Leyva-Aguilera, C.; Ruíz-Ruíz, B.; Luna Vázquez-Gómez, R.; Radilla-Chávez, P.; Chávez-Santoscoy, R.A.; Pestryakov, A.; Toledano-Magaña, Y.; García-Ramos, J.C.; et al. Argovit™ Silver Nanoparticles Effects on *Allium cepa*: Plant Growth Promotion without Cyto Genotoxic Damage. *Nanomaterials* **2020**, *10*, 1386. [CrossRef] [PubMed]
9. Evariste, L.; Lagier, L.; Gonzalez, P.; Mottier, A.; Mouchet, F.; Cadarsi, S.; Lonchambon, P.; Daffe, G.; Chimowa, G.; Sarrieu, C.; et al. Thermal Reduction of Graphene Oxide Mitigates Its In Vivo Genotoxicity Toward *Xenopus laevis* Tadpoles. *Nanomaterials* **2019**, *9*, 584. [CrossRef] [PubMed]
10. Jalili, P.; Huet, S.; Lanceleur, R.; Jarry, G.; Hegarat, L.L.; Nesslany, F.; Hogeveen, K.; Fessard, V. Genotoxicity of Aluminum and Aluminum Oxide Nanomaterials in Rats Following Oral Exposure. *Nanomaterials* **2020**, *10*, 305. [CrossRef] [PubMed]

Publisher's Note: MDPI stays neutral with regard to jurisdictional claims in published maps and institutional affiliations.

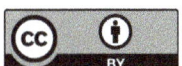 © 2020 by the authors. Licensee MDPI, Basel, Switzerland. This article is an open access article distributed under the terms and conditions of the Creative Commons Attribution (CC BY) license (http://creativecommons.org/licenses/by/4.0/).

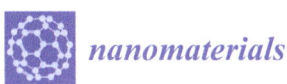

Article

The Comet Assay as a Tool to Detect the Genotoxic Potential of Nanomaterials

Alba García-Rodríguez [1], Laura Rubio [2], Laura Vila [1], Noel Xamena [1,3], Antonia Velázquez [1,3], Ricard Marcos [1,3,*] and Alba Hernández [1,3,*]

[1] Department of Genetics and Microbiology, Faculty of Biosciences, Universitat Autònoma de Barcelona, 08193 Cerdanyola del Vallès (Barcelona), Spain; albagr.garcia@gmail.com (A.G.-R.); lauravilavecilla@hotmail.com (L.V.); noel.xamena@uab.cat (N.X.); antonia.velazquez@uab.cat (A.V.)
[2] Nanobiology Laboratory, Department of Natural and Exact Sciences, Pontificia Universidad Católica Madre y Maestra, PUCMM, Santiago de los Caballeros 50000, Dominican Republic; l.rubio@ce.pucmm.edu.do
[3] Consortium for Biomedical Research in Epidemiology and Public Health (CIBERESP), Carlos III Institute of Health, 28029 Madrid, Spain
* Correspondence: ricard.marcos@uab.es (R.M.); alba.hernandez@uab.es (A.H.); Tel.: +34-93-581-2052 (R.M.); +34-93-581-8048 (A.H.); Fax: +34-93-581-2387 (R.M & A.H)

Received: 6 August 2019; Accepted: 18 September 2019; Published: 27 September 2019

Abstract: The interesting physicochemical characteristics of nanomaterials (NMs) has brought about their increasing use and, consequently, their increasing presence in the environment. As emergent contaminants, there is an urgent need for new data about their potential side-effects on human health. Among their potential effects, the potential for DNA damage is of paramount relevance. Thus, in the context of the EU project NANoREG, the establishment of common robust protocols for detecting genotoxicity of NMs became an important aim. One of the developed protocols refers to the use of the comet assay, as a tool to detect the induction of DNA strand breaks. In this study, eight different NMs—TiO_2NP (2), SiO_2NP (2), ZnONP, CeO_2NP, AgNP, and multi-walled carbon nanotubes (MWCNT)—were tested using two different human lung epithelial cell lines (A549 and BEAS-2B). The comet assay was carried out with and without the use of the formamidopyrimidine glycosylase (FPG) enzyme to detect the induction of oxidatively damaged DNA bases. As a high throughput approach, we have used GelBond films (GBF) instead of glass slides, allowing the fitting of 48 microgels on the same GBF. The results confirmed the suitability of the comet assay as a powerful tool to detect the genotoxic potential of NMs. Specifically, our results indicate that most of the selected nanomaterials showed mild to significant genotoxic effects, at least in the A549 cell line, reflecting the relevance of the cell line used to determine the genotoxic ability of a defined NM.

Keywords: comet assay; FPG enzyme; TiO_2NP; SiO_2NP; ZnONP; CeO_2NP; AgNP; multi-walled carbon nanotubes (MWCNT)

1. Introduction

Nanomaterials (NMs) are being increasingly used in many fields, due to their new physicochemical properties at the nanometric scale [1]. In this context, the evidence seems to indicate that the use of such NMs will continue experiencing an exponential increase. This opens a new scenario where people will certainly be exposed to such NMs. Since human health risks associated with such exposures are uncertain, new information on their potentially harmful effects is urgently required.

Among the different health effects that NMs can cause, those related to their potential interaction with DNA requires special attention. Thus, the detection of the genotoxic effects induced by NMs is emerging as a specific research field covering such demands [2,3]. Since different NMs can react with

DNA following different mechanisms, a wide range of tools have been proposed to detect and quantify different genotoxic effects; among them, the comet assay stands out.

The comet assay measures the induction of DNA breaks as well as oxidatively damaged DNA bases by using single-cell gel electrophoresis [4,5]. The simplicity of the assay and its potential use in any type of eukaryotic cell has expanded its use in many fields, and this assay is successfully used in in vitro and in vivo testing, including human biomonitoring studies [6]. The comet assay has already been used to test different NMs as it has been summarized in different reviews [7–9]. Several criticisms have been raised about the use of the comet assay to test NMs arguing that their presence in the head, or in the tail of the comet, can interfere with the scoring [7]. This means that the scoring of NMs using the comet assay is under discussion. At present, there is no official guideline for using the comet assay in in vitro studies. In this frame, the EU project NANoREG has aimed to establish strong protocols to be used in the testing of NMs, mainly from a regulatory point of view. According to its simplicity, sensitivity, and speed, the comet assay was one of the proposed test protocols. To reach that objective, we here present the results obtained with the comet assay testing eight different NMs namely NM100 and NM101 (TiO_2NPs), NM110 ($ZnONPs$), NM200 and NM203 (SiO_2NPs), NM212 (CeO_2NPs), NM300K (AgNPs), and NM401 (MWCNT, multiwalled carbon nanotubes). Taking into account that inhalation is one of the main routes of exposure to NMs, two different human cell lines (A549 and BEAS-2B) have been used as a model of human bronchial epithelial cells. To cover one of the aims of the NANoREG project a high throughput approach was used. Thus, GelBond films (GBF) instead of glass slides were used, allowing the fitting of 48 microgels on the same GBF, in comparison with the 1–2 samples contained in a glass slide.

2. Material and Methods

2.1. Selected NMs

The tested NMs were: 100 and 6 nm anatase TiO_2NPs (NM100 and NM101), 18.3 and 24.7 nm amorphous SiO_2NPs (NM200 and NM203), 147 nm ZnONPs (NM110), 33 nm CeO_2NPs (NM212), AgNPs (NM300K), and 64.2 nm MWCNT (NM401). All eight NMs were supplied by the NANoREG Consortium, and the EU Joint Research Centre at Ispra (Italy) prepared and sent aliquots to all the participants. Although these NMs were well characterized in the frame of the project, we confirmed nanoparticle size and morphology by transmission electron microscopy (TEM) using a JEOL 1400 instrument (JEOL Ltd., Tokyo, Japan). In addition, the hydrodynamic size in whole-cell culture medium was measured by using dynamic light scattering (DLS). This analysis was performed on a Malvern Zetasizer Nano-ZS zen3600 (Malvern Panalytical, Malvern, UK) instrument.

2.2. Cell Culture

The transformed human bronchial epithelial BEAS-2B cell line was kindly provided by Dr. H. Karlson, from the Swedish Karolinska Institute (Stockholm, Sweden). The adenocarcinomic human alveolar basal epithelial A540 cell line was kindly provided by Dr. G. Linsel, from the Federal Institute for Occupational Safety and Health of Germany (BAuA, Berlin, Germany), BEAS-2B cells were cultured as a monolayer in 75 cm^2 culture flasks coated with 0.03% collagen in serum-free bronchial epithelial cell growth medium (BEGM, Lonza, CA, USA) and passaged weekly. A549 cells were also cultured in 75 cm^2 culture flasks with DMEM high glucose (Life Technologies, Carlsbad, CA, USA) supplemented with 10% fetal bovine serum (FBS; PAA, Pasching, Austria), 1% of non-essential amino acids (NEAA; PAA, Pasching, Austria) and 2.5 µg/mL Plasmocin™ (InvivoGen, San Diego, CA, USA). Log-phase cells were grown on 12 well plates without 0.03% collagen coating, to determine, cytotoxicity and DNA damage levels. Cells were maintained in a humidified atmosphere of 5% CO_2 and 95% air at 37 °C.

We selected epithelial lung cells because inhalation is considered one of the most relevant exposure routes for humans. In addition, both BEAS-2B cells have been extensively used in the testing of nanomaterials.

2.3. Cell Viability

BEAS-2B and A549 cells were exposed to different concentrations of the selected NMs, according to previous toxicity data, and exposures lasting for 24 h. The highest tested dose ranged from 10 µg/mL, for the most toxic NMs (ZnONP), to 200 µg/mL for the least toxic NMs. According to the obtained toxicities, up to 4 different concentrations were selected to determine cell viability. The 4 appropriate subtoxic concentrations were chosen to work with the comet assay enabling the establishment of dose/response relationships. Untreated cells, just with cell culture medium, were used as a negative control.

Toxicity was measured directly counting the number of cells surviving the 24 h exposure treatments. The procedure was as follows: after exposure, cells were washed three times with 0.5 mL of PBS (1%), to eliminate dead cells, and incubated 3 min at 37 °C with 0.25 mL of trypsin-EDTA (Ethylenediaminetetraacetic acid) (1%) to detach and individualize them. After these initial steps, cells were diluted (1/10) in ISOTON™ (isotonic buffer) and counted with a ZTM Series colter-counter (Beckman Coulter Inc., Brea, CA, USA) [10].

The final viability values were determined by averaging three independent viability experiments, each containing three replicates per each concentration.

2.4. The Comet Assay

The alkaline comet assay facilitates the determining of the levels of both the genotoxic (DNA breaks) and the oxidative DNA damage (ODD). The detection of ODD can be easily detected when the comet assay is complemented with the use of formamidopyrimidine DNA glycosylase (FPG) enzyme. This enzyme detects oxidized DNA bases, cut them and, consequently, transient DNA breaks are generated. The net oxidative effect is determined by subtracting the breaks induced in normal conditions from those obtained when FPG enzyme is used. The used protocol is as follows: exposed/control cells were washed with PBS 1X thrice, detached with trypsin-EDTA 1%, incubated at 37 °C for 5 min, and centrifuged at 130 g for 8 min. After that, cells were resuspended in PBS 1X to obtain the concentration of 1×10^6 cells/mL. The obtained cells were mixed 1:10 with 0.75% low melting point agarose at 37 °C, dropped on GelBond® films (GBF) (Life Sciences, Vilnius, Lithuania) in triplicates, and lysed in cold lysis buffer overnight at 4 °C. As a high throughput approach, the use of GBF instead of glass slides allowed for the fitting of 48 microgels on the same GBF.

After that, the GBF were gently washed twice with enzyme buffer for 5 and 50 min respectively at 4 °C. Then, the GBF were incubated with enzyme buffer containing, or not, FPG enzyme 1:25,000 for 30 min at 37 °C, followed by a washing step with electrophoresis buffer for 5 min. A second incubation in electrophoresis buffer was followed, to allow DNA unwinding and expression of alkali-labile sites, for 25 min at 4 °C. Subsequently, electrophoresis was carried out at 20 V and 300 mA at 4 °C. GBF were washed twice with cold PBS 1X for 5 and 10 min respectively, cells were fixed in absolute ethanol for at least 1 h and air-dried overnight at room temperature. Cells were stained with 1:10,000 SYBR Gold in TE buffer for 20 min at room temperature. GBF were mounted and visualized in an epifluorescent microscope (Olympus BX50, Hamburg, Germany) at 20× magnification. The DNA damage was quantified with the Komet 5.5 Image analysis system (Kinetic Imaging Ltd, Liverpool, UK) as the percentage of DNA in the tail. A total of 100 comet images randomly selected were analyzed per sample. Two different samples were analyzed for each condition, in each one of the three experiments performed.

2.5. Statistical Analysis

All measurements were made in triplicate, at least for two separate experiments. Results are expressed in mean ± standard error. The one-way ANOVA with Tukey's post-test and an unpaired Student's *t*-test were used to compare differences between means. Data were analyzed with GraphPad Prism version 5.00 for Windows (GraphPad Software, San Diego, CA, USA, http://graphpad.com). Differences between means were considered significant at $p < 0.05$.

3. Results and Discussion

3.1. Nanoparticles Characterization

First of all, we wish to point out that the nanomaterials used were supplied by the UE JRC at Ispra, and are considered as reference nanomaterials, and used in many different EU projects. This means that they have been extensively characterized. To gather sound genotoxicity data, it is necessary to ensure that nanoparticles are well dispersed [11]. In our case, we have used the dispersion protocol generated in the frame of the NanoGenotox EU project [12]. As observed in Figure 1, TEM images show that each NMs is dispersed distinctly, depending on its primary structure. For example, AgNPs and TiO$_2$NPs (NM101) are clearly not or less agglomerated than the rest of the NPs. Then, by selecting over 100 particles in random fields of view, we determined the TEM diameters in dry conditions, and the obtained results are indicated in Table 1. The same table also shows the DLS results, that measured the average of the NPs hydrodynamic size when were dispersed and suspended in a liquid. As expected, the average of the hydrodynamic sizes, once dispersed in the culture medium, are higher than those reported by TEM in the dried form, due to their interactions with the proteins. Since exposures last for 24 h, we aimed to detect if time has important effects on dispersion by inducing NMs aggregation. Thus, our results summarized in Table 1 do not seem to indicate that the incubation time has a direct effect on the NMs agglomeration. Concretely, only NM200, NM203, and NM300K showed apparent increases in the hydrodynamic size after 24 h, regarding the values observed just after the dispersion procedure (0 h). It should be indicated that, due to the fibrillary characteristics of MWCNT NM401, we do not report DLS values for this NM (ND). Nevertheless, we indicated their average length and thickness, as evaluated by TEM. Although some of the values, observed mainly after 48 h, were difficult to interpret, these discrepancies over-time are not important, because only exposures lasting for 24 h were used in the comet assay.

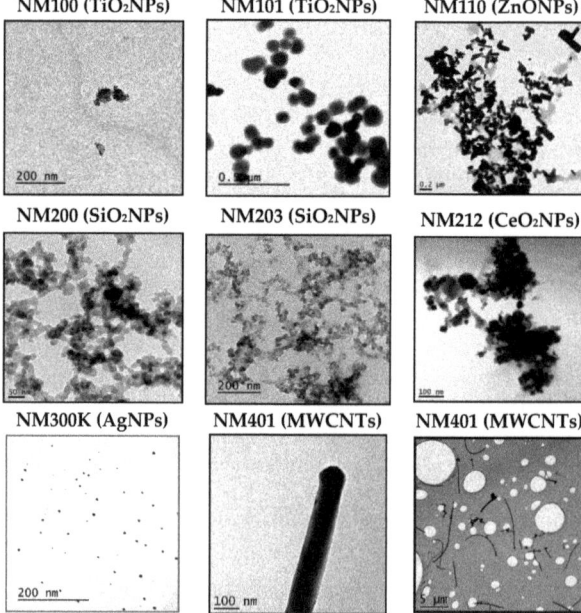

Figure 1. Representative TEM images of the eight used nanoparticles (NPs). Figures correspond to TiO$_2$NPs (NM100), TiO$_2$NPs (NM101), ZnONPs (NM110), SiO$_2$NPs (NM200), SiO$_2$NPs (NM203), CeO$_2$NPs (NM212), AgNPs (NM300K), and MWCNT (NM401). For NM401 two images are include to visualize their length and thickness.

Table 1. Comparison of pristine sizes (transmission electron microscopy, TEM) and 10 and 100 µL dispersions (dynamic light scattering, DLS). Sizes were evaluated just after the dispersion procedure and 24 h later.

		NM100 (TiO$_2$NPs)				NM101 (TiO$_2$NPs)	
TEM		104.01 ± 39.42 nm		TEM		54.69 ± 35.39 nm	
DLS	0 h	10 µg/mL	194.6 ± 8.49	DLS	0 h	10 µg/mL	152,2 ± 62.47
		100 µg/mL	166.2 ± 1.01			100 µg/mL	166.1 ± 12.55
	24 h	10 µg/mL	151.6 ± 6.30		24 h	10 µg/mL	265.1 ± 10.50
		100 µg/mL	141.2 ± 2.23			100 µg/mL	141.5 ± 84.88
		NM110 (ZnONPs)				NM200 (SiO$_2$NPs)	
TEM		132.37 ± 69.53 nm		TEM		16.5 ± 4.18 nm	
DLS	0 h	10 µg/mL	260.3 ± 88.63	DLS	0 h	10 µg/mL	67.76 ± 0.10
		100 µg/mL	213.9 ± 92.48			100 µg/mL	70.59 ± 1.43
	24 h	10 µg/mL	117.2 ± 37.71		24 h	10 µg/mL	75.84 ± 3.62
		100 µg/mL	114.7 ± 0.86			100 µg/mL	147.8 ± 13.70
		NM203 (SiO$_2$NPs)				NM212 (CeO$_2$NPs)	
TEM		24.26 ± 9.38 nm		TEM		70.33 ± 49.61 nm	
DLS	0 h	10 µg/mL	69.56 ± 9.50	DLS	0 h	10 µg/mL	229.9 ± 10.13
		100 µg/mL	86.86 ± 68.08			100 µg/mL	230.5 ± 4.05
	24 h	10 µg/mL	121.4 ± 10.02		24 h	10 µg/mL	117.1 ± 4.70
		100 µg/mL	342 ± 76.05			100 µg/mL	124.0 ± 1.51
		NM300K (AgNPs)				NM401 (MWCNTs)	
TEM		7.75 ± 2.48 nm		TEM		4.23 ± 1.01 (diameter), 6012.09 ± 4091.45 (length)	
DLS	0 h	10 µg/mL	28.71 ± 17.67	DLS	0 h	10 µg/mL	ND
		100 µg/mL	38.46 ± 16.31			100 µg/mL	ND
	24 h	10 µg/mL	81.37 ± 4.63		24 h	10 µg/mL	ND
		100 µg/mL	97.23 ± 6.22			100 µg/mL	ND

3.2. Toxic/Genotoxic Effects of NM100 and NM101 (TiO$_2$NPs)

TiO$_2$NPs are one of the most produced NMs. They are included in many products, such as paints, coatings, plastics, papers, inks, medicines, pharmaceuticals, food products, cosmetics, sunscreens, and toothpaste [13]. This extensive use makes it necessary to evaluate their potential risk for human health.

Toxicity data are required to determine the range of concentrations to be used in genotoxicity studies. In our case, we have not detected relevant toxic effects for the two selected TiO$_2$NPs (Figures 2A and 3A). Although TiO$_2$NPs have largely been evaluated from the genotoxic point of view, the already reported results are not sufficiently clear to reach a convincing conclusion [14]. Nevertheless, in our study, we have demonstrated that both TiO$_2$NPs (NM100 and NM101) are able to induce direct DNA strand breaks, as detected by the comet assay (Figures 2 and 3), although no oxidative DNA damage induction was detected on the DNA bases. Overall, we can say that A540 cells are more sensitive than BEAS-2B cells and, consequently, exposures induced higher levels of damage in that cell line. Furthermore, NM100 showed to be slightly more genotoxic than NM101. From the literature, positive DNA damage induction for both used cell lines has been reported. Nevertheless, some studies failed to detect DNA damage induction. Thus, negative results in BEAS-2B cells were obtained under different exposure scenarios [15–17]. In addition, negative findings in the comet assay were also reported in the A549 cells [18]. From the different positive reports in BEAS-2B cells, nanosized anatase and fine rutile produced a concentration and time-dependent effect in exposures lasting up to 72 h [19]. On the other hand, using the NM100 and NM101 nanomaterials (as in our study) Di Bucchiano et al. demonstrated a weak but positive induction of genotoxic effects, NM100 being the most dangerous [20]. A recent study in BEAS-2B indicated that the induced effects were associated with the shape. In this way, only those forms that were clearly internalized (food grade, P25, and platelets) were able to induce genotoxicity [21]. As in our case, A549 cells showed a higher sensitivity to TiO$_2$NPs and, consequently, positive effects were reported for both small and spherical anatase and rutile forms after short-term exposures [22], and also after long-term exposures lasting up to two months [23]. In addition, the positive induction of DNA damage was reported at non-toxic concentrations, but induced DNA damage decreased when exposures extended from 3 to 24 h [24]. Interestingly, there is one study comparing the effects of TiO$_2$NPs in BEAS-2B and A549 cells. In that study, direct and oxidative DNA damage was only observed in A549 cells [16], confirming the highest sensitivity of this cell line.

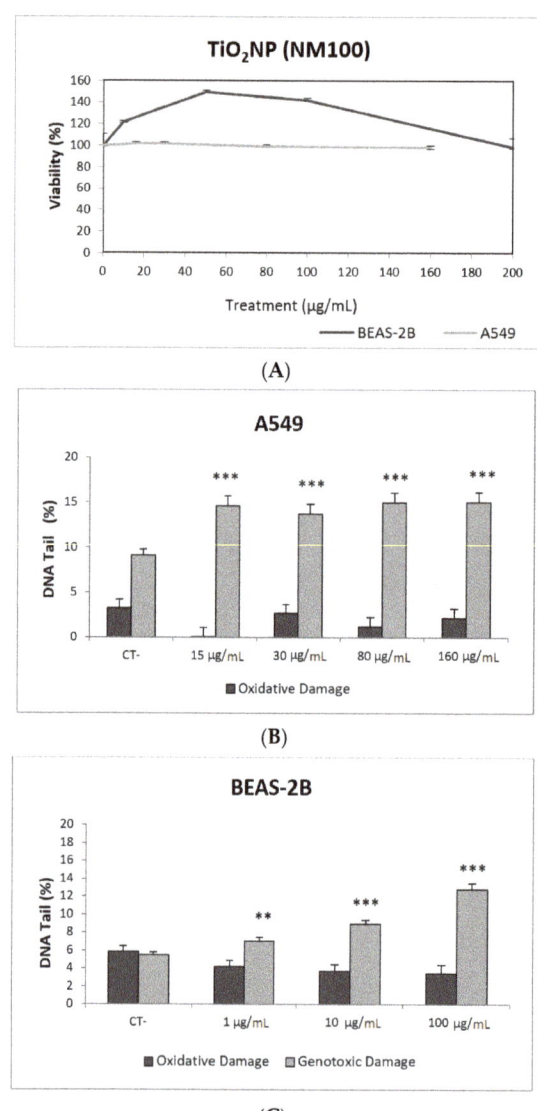

Figure 2. Results from the TiO$_2$NPs (NM100) on A549 and BEAS-2B cells. (**A**) Toxicity curves for both cell lines. (**B**) Genotoxicity results obtained in A549 cells. (**C**) Genotoxicity results obtained in BEAS-2B cells. Genotoxicity data are plotted as mean ± SEM of two independent experiments. ** $p \leq 0.01$, *** $p \leq 0.001$ (one way-ANOVA). CT, control.

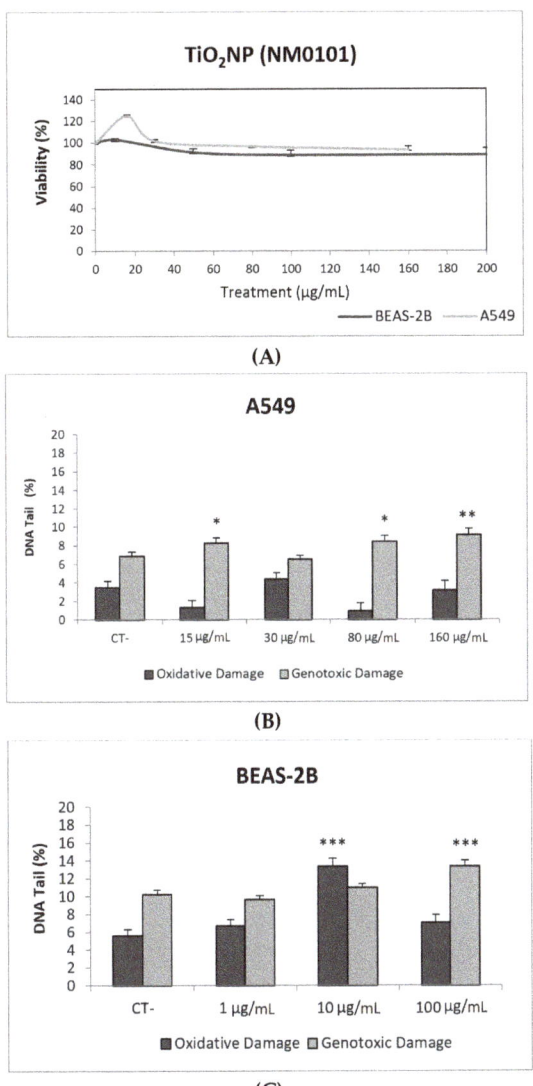

Figure 3. Results from the TiO$_2$NPs (NM101) on A549 and BEAS-2B cells. (**A**) Toxicity curves for both cell lines. (**B**) Genotoxicity results obtained in A549 cells. (**C**) Genotoxicity results obtained in BEAS-2B cells. Genotoxicity data are plotted as mean ± SEM of two independent experiments. * $p \leq 0.05$, ** $p \leq 0.01$, *** $p \leq 0.001$ (one way-ANOVA). CT, control.

ZnONPs, together with TiO$_2$NPs, are among the most produced NMs. ZnONPs are widely used in personal care products, sensors, antibacterial creams, and biomedical applications. Their broad range of applications raises concerns regarding their potential health effects [25]. In our study, ZnONPs (NM110) exerted a very important toxic effect in both cell lines, with the concentration of 10 µg/mL being completely toxic to BEAS-2B cells. However, ZnONPs were unable to cause direct DNA damage in A549 and BEAS-2B cells. It should be indicated that some genotoxic effects were observed in A549 cells when the FPG enzyme was used. Thus, significant increases in the levels of oxidative DNA damage were observed in cells exposed to 0.2 and 6 µg/mL, as indicated in Figure 4.

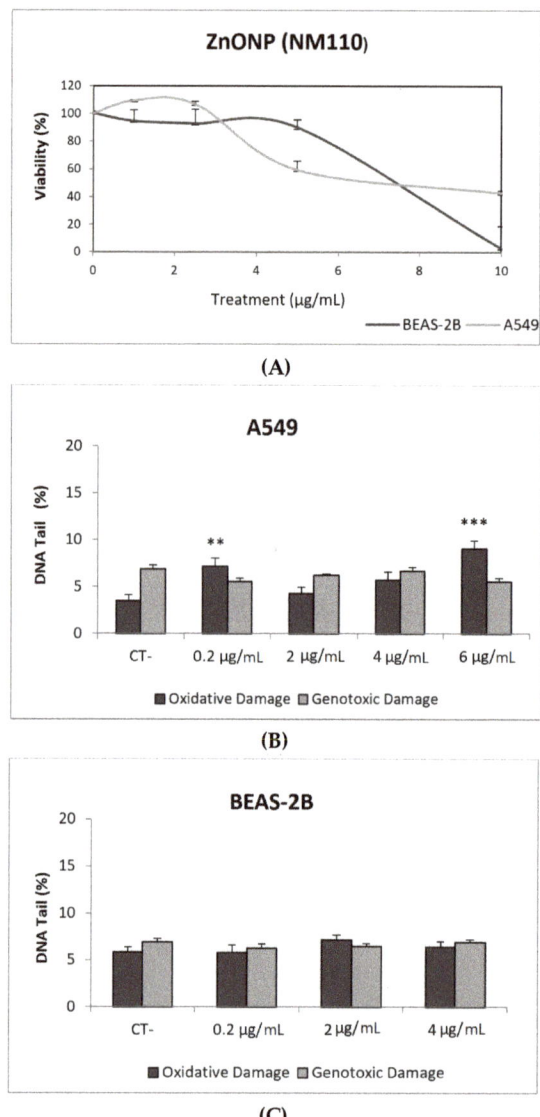

Figure 4. Results from the ZnONPs (NM110) on A549 and BEAS-2B cells. (**A**) Toxicity curves for both cell lines. (**B**) Genotoxicity results obtained in A549 cells. (**C**) Genotoxicity results obtained in BEAS-2B cells. Genotoxicity data are plotted as mean ± SEM of two independent experiments. ** $p \leq 0.01$, *** $p \leq 0.001$ (one way-ANOVA). CT, control.

ZnONPs are easily taken up by cells, and quickly dissolved intracellularly to their ionic form, which can cause the strongly observed toxicity. The use of ICP-MS techniques demonstrated that, after 48 h in culture media, more than 80% of the initial ZnONPs dissolved to their ionic form [26]. In that study, although the authors found that exposures lasting for 24 h induced significant levels of DNA damage in mouse fibroblast cells, this DNA damage induction was not evident when cells were exposed long-term (up 12 weeks). Similar effects were observed in BEAS-2B cells, where short-term exposures lasting for 3–6 h were able to induce DNA damage in the absence of BSA [27]. Positive genotoxic effects were also obtained in A549 cells at short exposure times (4 h). Nevertheless, this genotoxicity was not associated with oxidative DNA damage, nor the induction of intracellular Reactive Oxygen Species (ROS) levels [28]. More recently, ZnONPs were also evaluated in A549 cells affecting cell survival, and inducing high levels of DNA damage at cytotoxic concentrations. Lower concentrations also were able to induce a genotoxic response and the induced damage persisted over 24 h [24]. The disparity of reported data, mainly related to the exposure times, reflects the relevance of the intracellular solubility as a modulator of the observed effects.

Due to their appealing properties, SiO_2NPs are extensive and increasingly used in agriculture, food, and consumer products including cosmetics. Accordingly, large amounts are placed in the global market and, consequently, into the environment. Many products containing SiO_2NPs are listed in a consumer product inventory and placed in the third position among the most produced NMs worldwide [20]. Although many studies have been carried out, to identify the toxicological mechanisms of action of SiO_2NPs, no conclusive positions have been established linking their physicochemical properties to toxicity, bioavailability, or human health effects [29]. In a similar way, although potential biomarkers of genotoxicity have been suggested, the obtained experimental results are not conclusive enough, due to a variety of factors [30]. Our findings showed similar results for both evaluated SiO_2NPs, with BEAS-2B being more sensitive than A549 cells to their toxic effects. Regarding their genotoxic potential, both SiO_2NPs were able to induce direct genotoxicity in both cell lines. Nevertheless, in A549 cells both SiO_2NPs were able to induce oxidative DNA damage at the concentrations of 15 and 30 µg/mL (Figures 5 and 6).

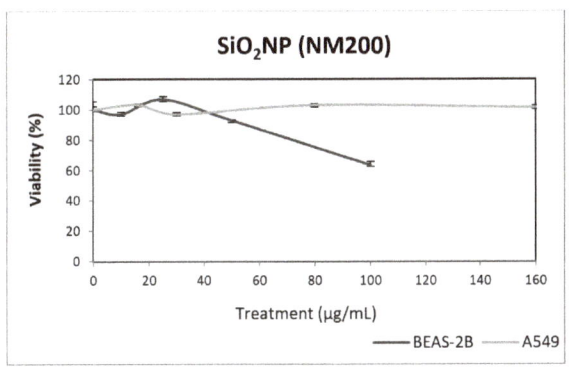

(A)

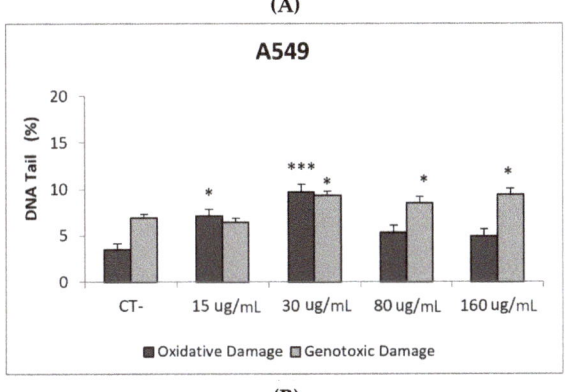

(B)

Figure 5. *Cont.*

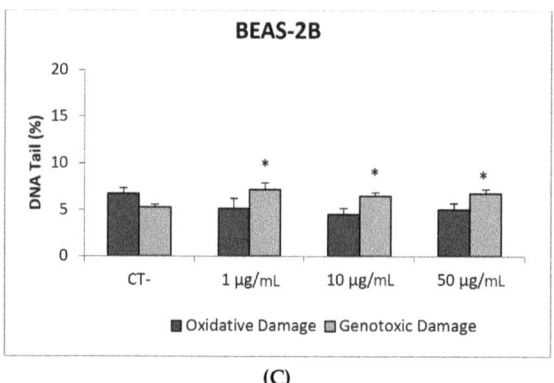

(C)

Figure 5. Results from the SiO$_2$NPs (NM200), on A549 and BEAS-2B cells. (**A**) Toxicity curves for both cell lines. (**B**) Genotoxicity results obtained in A549 cells. (**C**) Genotoxicity results obtained in BEAS-2B cells. Genotoxicity data are plotted as mean ± SEM of two independent experiments. * $p \leq 0.05$, *** $p \leq 0.001$ (one way-ANOVA). CT, control.

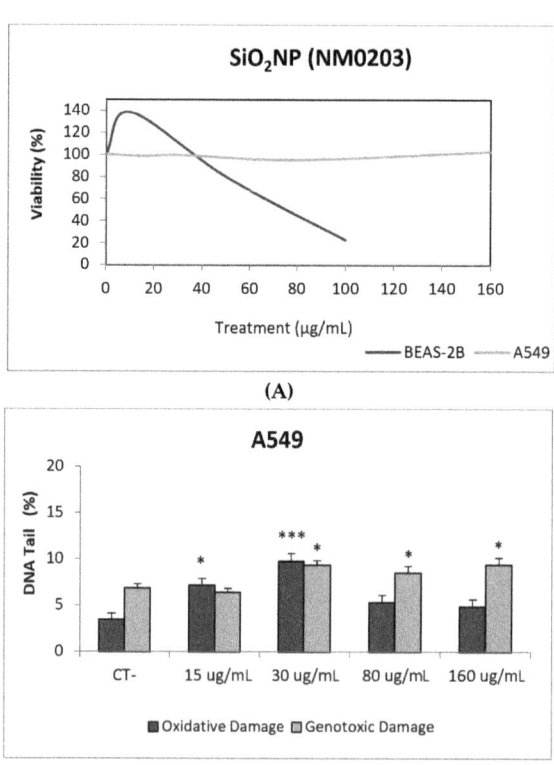

Figure 6. *Cont.*

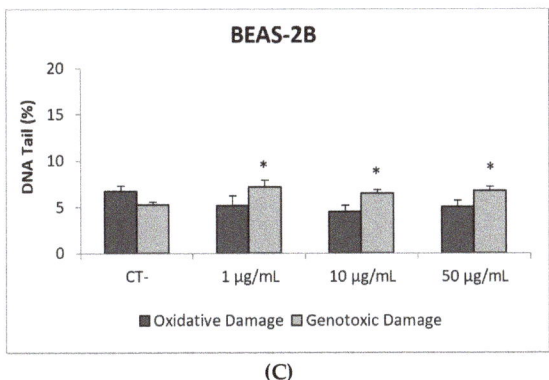

Figure 6. Results from the SiO$_2$NPs (NM203), on A549 and BEAS-2B cells. (**A**) Toxicity curves for both cell lines. (**B**) Genotoxicity results obtained in A549 cells. (**C**) Genotoxicity results obtained in BEAS-2B cells. Genotoxicity data are plotted as mean ± SEM of two independent experiments. * $p \leq 0.05$, *** $p \leq 0.001$ (one way-ANOVA). CT, control.

No studies using BEAS-2B cells have been found testing the genotoxicity of SiO$_2$NPs and using the comet assay. Nevertheless, two studies reported data using the A549 cell line. In the first study, short periods of incubation (15 min and 4 h) did not induce DNA strand breaks or FPG sensitive sites, when testing two different SiO$_2$NPs sizes (16 and 60 nm) [31]. The second study evaluated the effects of non-cytotoxic concentration of SiO$_2$NPs, with an average diameter of 39.6 nm, in treatments lasting for 24 h. Results indicated that the exposure did not increase the intracellular levels of ROS or the primary DNA damage, as measured with the comet assay [32]. Interestingly, SiO$_2$NPs exerted a synergistic action on the effects of lead, amplifying the levels of ROS and DNA damage induced by lead [32].

Regarding CeO$_2$NPs, they have widespread use in industry, cosmetic and consumer products. Its use as automobile exhaust catalysts draws special attention, due to their extensive release into the environment. At present, there is a growing interest in this compound, since it has been proposed for biomedical use, due to the potent regenerative antioxidant properties. Although in vivo exposures to CeO$_2$NPs can exert respiratory tract adverse effects, such as sensory irritation and airflow limitation [33], its analogous activity to two key antioxidant enzymes, such as superoxide dismutase and catalase, explains its role as a potent free radical scavenger. Among the proposed health effects, the potential application in neurodegenerative pathologies stands out [34].

Our results indicate that CeO$_2$NPs (NM212) does not exert any toxic effect in the used cell lines. In addition, non-genotoxic effects were observed in both A549 and BEAS-2B (Figure 7). It is interesting to note the observed reduction of oxidative DNA damage observed in treated A549 cells, which would support the antioxidant potential of CeO$_2$NPs.

Although some authors have reported the genotoxic effects of CeO$_2$NPs, there is no general agreement about this point [35]. It has been proposed that the apparent discordant reported data are the result of both the pro-oxidant and anti-oxidant role of CeO$_2$NPs. Nevertheless, in a recent study using a wide set of cell lines, from both tumoral and non-tumoral origin, only anti-oxidant effects were observed [36]. Regarding the use of BEAS-2B and A549 cells to evaluate the genotoxic effects of CeO$_2$NPs, only three studies have been found in the literature using the comet assay. In BEAS-2B cells, no induction of intracellular ROS of DNA damage was observed [37], but positive induction of DNA damage was observed in A549 cells [24]. In that study, the effects were mainly observed after short exposures (3 h), while only a slight effect at the highest tested dose (42 μg/mL) was observed. Conversely, Frieke-Kuper et al. used both cell lines and demonstrated that in both cases exposures lasting for 24 h of CeO$_2$NPs induced significant levels of DNA damage, as evaluated using the comet assay [38]. Nevertheless, the use of an in vitro 3D human bronchial epithelial model indicated that the mucociliary defense prevents CeO$_2$NPs from reaching the respiratory epithelial cells [38].

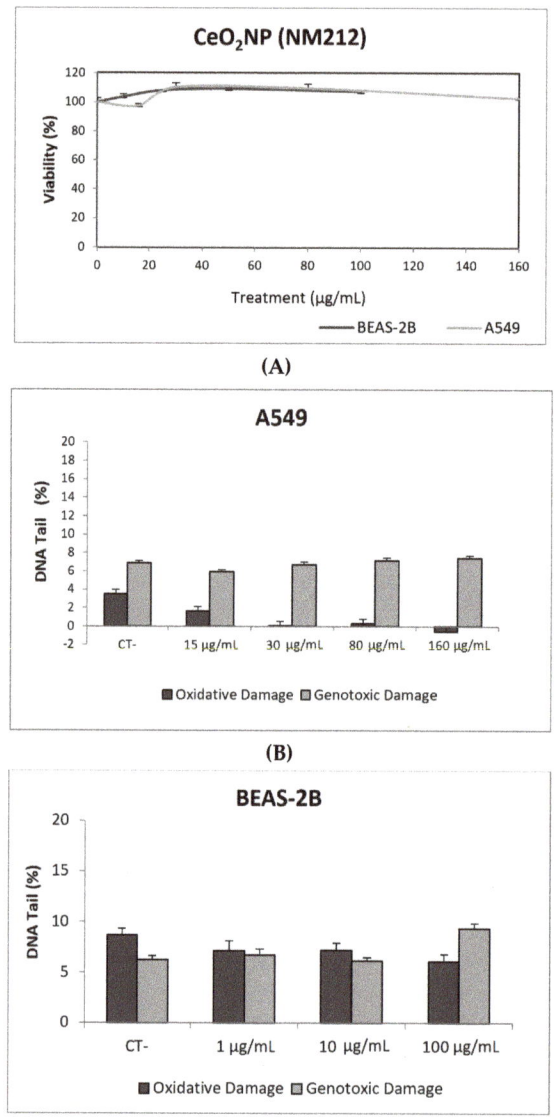

Figure 7. Results from the CeO$_2$NPs (NM212), on A549 and BEAS-2B cells. (**A**) Toxicity curves for both cell lines. (**B**) Genotoxicity results obtained in A549 cells. (**C**) Genotoxicity results obtained in BEAS-2B cells. Genotoxicity data are plotted as mean ± SEM of two independent experiments. It should be noted that there is a significant reduction in the levels of oxidative DNA damage observed in the A549 cells. CT, control.

The wide spectrum of applications of AgNPs in biomedicine, and in related fields, explain their extended use [39]. Due to their proved antimicrobial efficacy, AgNPs are incorporated into different materials such as textile fibers and wound dressings. This explains that, although the production of AgNPs is significantly lower than that of other NMs, they constitute the most popular advertised nanomaterial in the Nanotechnology Consumer Products Inventory [40]. Among the different harmful effects associated with AgNPs exposure, it has been extensively reported that may cause genotoxicity, although additional data are required to assess its carcinogenic potential [41].

In our study, AgNPs induced significant cytotoxicity in both cell lines, BEAS-2B cells showing a higher sensitivity (Figure 8). In addition, AgNPs exposure was also able to induce genotoxic damage in both cell lines. Nevertheless, when the FPG enzyme was used to detect the induction of oxidatively damaged DNA, only A549 cells showed this type of damage (Figure 8). Until now, four studies have been published testing AgNPs in BEAS-2B using the comet assay [42–45]. Interestingly, completely different genotoxicity data were reported in the indicated studies. Thus, AgNPs with a size ranging from 20–200 nm, were unable to induce DNA strand breaks in treatments lasting for 4 h [44]. Contrarily, positive DNA strand breaks were observed using different types of AgNPs as citrate coated (10, 40 and 75 nm), PVP coated (10 nm), and uncoated (50 nm). Positive induction of primary DNA damage was observed for all forms, but only after treatments lasting for 24 h. In contrast, negative results were obtained for short exposures (4 h), and no induction of intracellular ROS was detected, assuming that the observed DNA damage was not a as result of the oxidative stress status [45]. These results are opposed to those reported by Nymark et al., who indicated DNA strand breaks, together with intracellular ROS induction, when BEAS-2B cells were exposed to PVP-coated AgNPs (average diameter 42.5 ± 14.5 nm) for treatments lasting 4 and 24 h [43]. The genotoxic potential of AgNPs using A549 cells has also reported variability of data, with negative results using nanoparticles sized 20–200 nm and exposures lasting for 4 h [44], and negative results in PVK-coated AgNPs sized 20 nm, although small sizes (20 nm) induced a significant induction of DNA damage [46]. This positive induction was also observed in cells exposed for 24 h to 20–50 nm diameter nanoparticles [47]. The size of AgNPs has been considered as one of the characteristics modulating genotoxicity. High levels of DNA damage were observed for the smaller sized AgNPs (50 nm) when three different sizes (50, 80 and 200 nm) were evaluated [48]. Similar results were reported when 20 and 200 nm were compared. In that case, higher levels of DNA damage were observed when cells were exposed to 20 nm AgNPs, in exposures lasting for 2 and 24 h. The use of the FPG enzyme demonstrated that most of the damage was caused by oxidation at DNA bases [49]. Finally, it should be indicated that, using the same type of AgNPs as in our study (NM300K), El Yamani et al. reported positive induction of DNA damage, independently of the exposure time (3 or 24 h), where the observed damage was mainly due to oxidative damage, as measured combining the comet assay with the use of FPG enzyme [24].

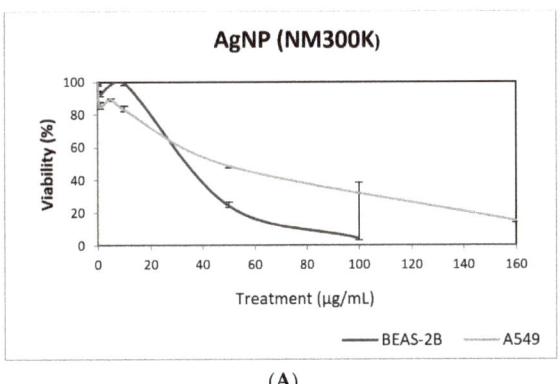

(A)

Figure 8. *Cont.*

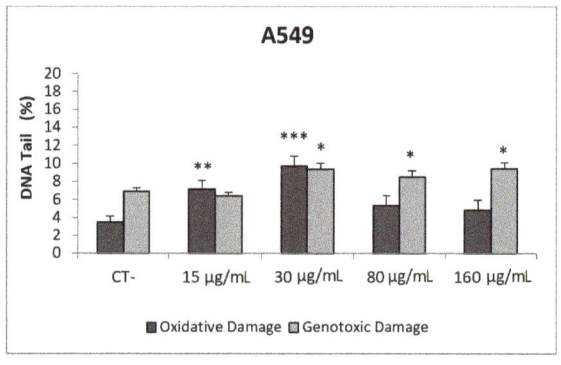

(B)

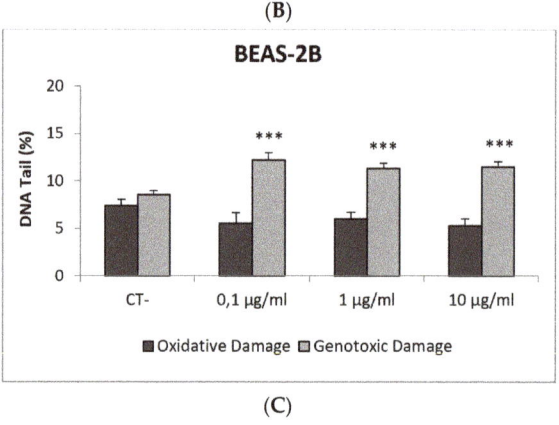

(C)

Figure 8. Results from the AgNPs (NM300K), on A549 and BEAS-2B cells. (**A**) Toxicity curves for both cell lines. (**B**) Genotoxicity results obtained in A549 cells. (**C**) Genotoxicity results obtained in BEAS-2B cells. Genotoxicity data are plotted as mean ± SEM of two independent experiments. * $p \leq 0.05$, ** $p \leq 0.01$, *** $p \leq 0.001$ (one way-ANOVA). CT, control.

MWCNTs are fibrous materials formed from honeycomb crystal lattice layers of graphite wrapped into a multiple tube shape. They are applied in multiple fields, including in their use as semiconductors, solar cell mobiles, and optical instruments. From the toxicological point of view, they are considered to have carcinogenic potential, causing lung tumors [50]. However, the underlying mechanisms are not well understood and, in particular, the reported genotoxicity data are conflicting [51].

In our study, MWCNT (NM401) did not exert toxic effects on A549 cells, but toxicities around 50% were observed in the BEAS-2B cell exposed to the whole range of tested concentrations (Figure 9A). Regarding the ability of this NM to induce DNA damage, our results indicate that direct genotoxicity was not observed at any of the tested concentrations, in any of the used cell lines. Nevertheless, oxidative DNA damage was observed in the A549 cell line, but only at the lowest concentrations (15 and 30 µg/mL) (Figure 9). Using BEAS-2B cells, the literature mainly reports negative results [52–54]. Although the comparison of straight and tangled MWCNTs demonstrated that the straight forms were positive at low concentrations, tangled MWCNTs showed to be only positive at the highest tested dose [55]. The A549 cell line has also been used in studies testing the genotoxic potential of MWCNTs in the comet assay, with contradictory results. Negative results were reported in exposures lasting for 24–72 h [54,56], although a positive response in the comet assay without FPG was also observed [57,58]. Nevertheless, both studies got negative results when the comet assay was complemented with the use of the FPG enzyme. The role of modifications in the MWCNTs structure has been evaluated, comparing the pristine versus the functionalized forms. Positive effects were reported, independently if the pristine from was compared with the OH-functionalized form [58] or with the acid-treated forms [59]. However, when A549 cells were used to test pristine versus carboxyl MWCNTs, only positive results were obtained in the comet assay. Interestingly, both MWCNTs forms gave positive induction of strand breaks when BEAS-2B cells were used [53].

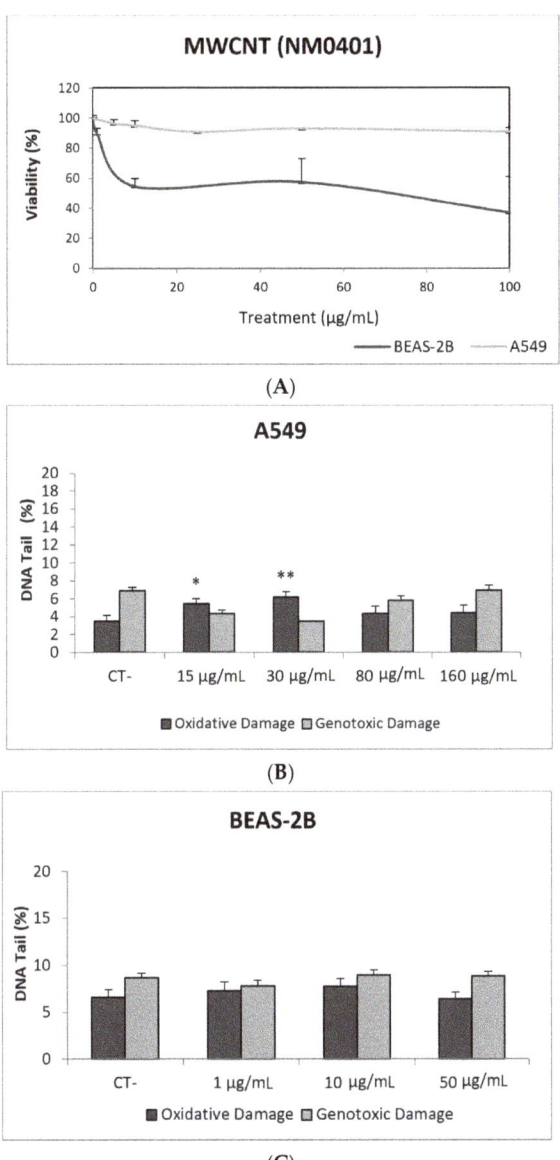

Figure 9. Results from the MWCNTs (NM401), on A549 and BEAS-2B cells. (**A**) Toxicity curves for both cell lines. (**B**) Genotoxicity results obtained in A549 cells. (**C**) Genotoxicity results obtained in BEAS-2B cells. Genotoxicity data are plotted as mean ± SEM of two independent experiments. * $p \leq 0.05$, ** $p \leq 0.01$ (one way-ANOVA). CT, control.

4. Conclusions

A summary of the results reported above is shown in Figure 10. From the reported data, we can conclude that the comet assay is a sensitive tool to determine the ability of NMs to produce DNA damage. According to the obtained results, the tested nanomaterials can be classified as weak genotoxic agents and, in such cases, most of the obtained results do not follow a clear dose–response pattern. This can result from the inherent variability associated with sampling size, an important factor when the increases in the levels of genetic damage are small. Alternatively, it is feasible that the cell uptake of nanomaterials is not always associated with their concentration in the culture media. At high concentrations, aggregation can occur, reducing the cell uptake. Furthermore, the observed differences between cell lines indicate that the selection of the cell-type is an important factor when the comet assay is used for testing NMs. In our case, we have demonstrated the highest sensitivity of the A549 cell line, regarding BEAS-2B cells. This is especially true when the induction of oxidative damage on DNA bases was evaluated. Thus, the positive induction of oxidative damage in A549 cells exposed to ZnONPs, SiO$_2$NPs, AgNPs, and MWCNT was not obtained in BEAS-2B cells. This could be due to the important antioxidant capacity of this cell line [60]. In fact, different behaviors of both cell lines have also been observed by other authors regarding different genetic endpoints. Thus, A549 cells were more sensitive when exposed to cadmium than BEAS-2B cells, the higher sensitivity of A549 cells being associated to changes in cell type-specific gene expression patterns, including the induction of genes coding for metallothioneins, the oxidative stress response, cell cycle control, mitotic signaling, apoptosis and DNA repair pathways [61]. Similarly, A549 cells were more sensitive when exposed to TiO$_2$NPs than BEAS-2B cells, and this sensitivity was associated with changes in the expression of DNA repair genes [62]. Finally, the use of hydrophobic plastic supports (HBF) permits an easy throughput approach of the comet assay and, in addition, the use of FPG enzyme has become a powerful tool to understand the mechanism of action of the tested nanomaterials, detecting those inducing oxidative DNA damage on the DNA bases.

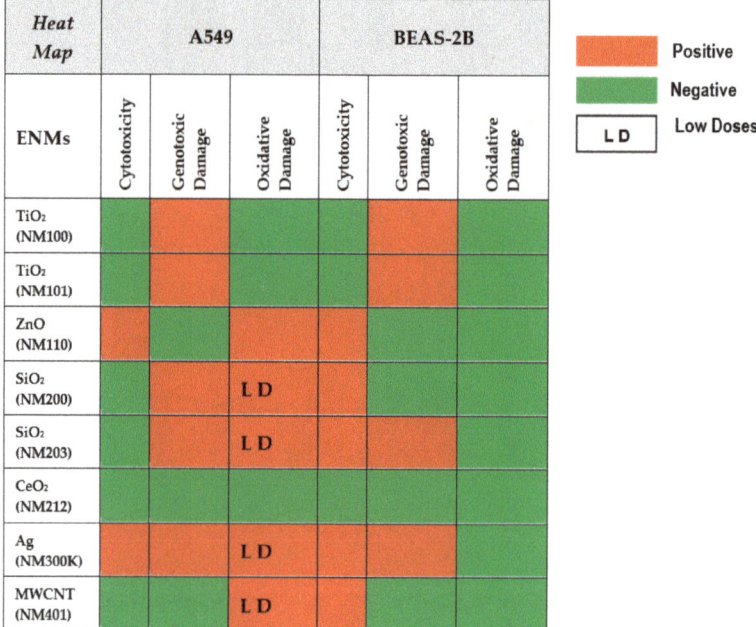

Figure 10. Heat map summarizing the overall results of testing the eight nanomaterials in the two cell lines. Toxicity, genotoxicity and oxidative damage induction are schematically represented.

Author Contributions: R.M. and A.H. planned the experiments. A.G.-R., L.R., L.V., N.X. and A.V. carried out the experimental part. A.G.-R., L.R. and L.V. analysed the data, carried out the statistical analysis, and prepared tables/figures. A.H. and R.M. wrote the final manuscript.

Funding: This investigation was supported by the EC FP7 NANoREG (Grant Agreement NMP4-LA-2013-310584). A. García-Rodríguez was funded by a postgraduate fellowship (PIF) from the Universitat Autònoma de Barcelona. L. Vila was funded by a postgraduate fellowship from the Generalitat de Catalunya.

Declaration of Interest: The authors declare that there is no conflict of interest.

References

1. Hansen, S.F.; Heggelund, L.R.; Revilla Besora, P.; Mackevica, A.; Boldrin, A.; Baun, A. Nanoproducts—What is available to European consumers? *Environ. Sci. Nano* **2016**, *3*, 169–180. [CrossRef]
2. Singh, N.; Manshian, B.; Jenkins, G.J.; Griffiths, S.M.; Williams, P.M.; Maffeis, T.G.; Wright, C.J.; Doak, S.H. NanoGenotoxicology: The DNA damaging potential of engineered nanomaterials. *Biomaterials* **2009**, *30*, 3891–3914. [CrossRef] [PubMed]
3. Gonzalez, L.; Cundari, E.; Leyns, L.; Kirsch-Volders, M. Towards a new paradigm in nano-genotoxicology: Facing complexity of nanomaterials' cellular interactions and effects. *Basic Clin. Pharmacol. Toxicol.* **2017**, *121*, 23–29. [CrossRef] [PubMed]
4. Azqueta, A.; Shaposhnikov, S.; Collins, A.R. DNA oxidation: Investigating its key role in environmental mutagenesis with the comet assay. *Mutat. Res.* **2009**, *674*, 101–108. [CrossRef] [PubMed]
5. Azqueta, A.; Collins, A.R. The essential comet assay: A comprehensive guide to measuring DNA damage and repair. *Arch. Toxicol.* **2013**, *87*, 949–968. [CrossRef] [PubMed]
6. Collins, A.; Koppen, G.; Valdiglesias, V.; Dusinska, M.; Kruszewski, M.; Møller, P.; Rojas, E.; Dhawan, A.; Benzie, I.; Coskun, E.; et al. The comet assay as a tool for human biomonitoring studies: The ComNet project. *Mutat. Res. Rev. Mutat. Res.* **2014**, *759*, 27–39. [CrossRef] [PubMed]
7. Karlsson, H.L.; Di Bucchianico, S.; Collins, A.R.; Dusinska, M. Can the comet assay be used reliably to detect nanoparticle-induced genotoxicity? *Environ. Mol. Mutagen.* **2015**, *56*, 82–96. [CrossRef]
8. Møller, P.; Hemmingsen, J.G.; Jensen, D.M.; Danielsen, P.H.; Karottki, D.G.; Jantzen, K.; Roursgaard, M.; Cao, Y.; Kermanizadeh, A.; Klingberg, H.; et al. Applications of the comet assay in particle toxicology: Air pollution and engineered nanomaterials exposure. *Mutagenesis* **2015**, *30*, 67–83. [CrossRef]
9. Elespuru, R.; Pfuhler, S.; Aardema, M.J.; Chen, T.; Doak, S.-H.; Doherty, A.; Farabaugh, C.S.; Kenny, J.; Manjanatha, M.; Mahadevan, B.; et al. Genotoxicity assessment of nanomaterials: Recommendations on best practices, assays, and methods. *Toxicol. Sci.* **2018**, *164*, 391–416. [CrossRef]
10. Vila, L.; Rubio, L.; Annangi, B.; García-Rodríguez, A.; Marcos, R.; Hernández, A. Frozen dispersions of nanomaterials are a useful operational procedure in nanotoxicology. *Nanotoxicology* **2017**, *11*, 31–40. [CrossRef]
11. Johnston, H.; Pojana, G.; Zuin, S.; Jacobsen, N.R.; Møller, P.; Loft, S.; Semmler-Behnke, M.; McGuiness, C.; Balharry, D.; Marcomini, A.; et al. Engineered nanomaterial risk. Lessons learnt from completed nanotoxicology studies: Potential solutions to current and future challenges. *Crit. Rev. Toxicol.* **2013**, *43*, 1–20. [CrossRef] [PubMed]
12. Nanogenotox. Available online: http://www.nanogenotox.eu/files/PDF/Deliverables/nanogenotox%20deliverable%203_wp4_%20dispersion%20protocol.pdf (accessed on 28 May 2019).
13. Shi, H.; Magaye, R.; Castranova, V.; Zhao, J. Titanium dioxide nanoparticles: A review of current toxicological data. *Part. Fibre Toxicol.* **2013**, *10*, 15. [CrossRef]
14. Charles, S.; Jomini, S.; Fessard, V.; Bigorgne-Vizade, E.; Rousselle, C.; Michel, C. Assessment of the in vitro genotoxicity of TiO_2 nanoparticles in a regulatory context. *Nanotoxicology* **2018**, *12*, 357–374. [CrossRef] [PubMed]
15. Bhattacharya, K.; Davoren, M.; Boertz, J.; Schins, R.P.; Hoffmann, E.; Dopp, E. Titanium dioxide nanoparticles induce oxidative stress and DNA-adduct formation but not DNA-breakage in human lung cells. *Part. Fibre Toxicol.* **2009**, *6*, 17. [CrossRef] [PubMed]

16. Ursini, C.L.; Cavallo, D.; Fresegna, A.M.; Ciervo, A.; Maiello, R.; Tassone, P.; Buresti, G.; Casciardi, S.; Iavicoli, S. Evaluation of cytotoxic, genotoxic and inflammatory response in human alveolar and bronchial epithelial cells exposed to titanium dioxide nanoparticles. *J. Appl. Toxicol.* **2014**, *34*, 1209–1219. [CrossRef] [PubMed]
17. Vales, G.; Rubio, L.; Marcos, R. Long-term exposures to low doses of titanium dioxide nanoparticles induce cell transformation, but not genotoxic damage in BEAS-2B cells. *Nanotoxicology* **2015**, *9*, 568–578. [CrossRef] [PubMed]
18. Wan, R.; Mo, Y.; Feng, L.; Chien, S.; Tollerud, D.J.; Zhang, Q. DNA damage caused by metal nanoparticles: Involvement of oxidative stress and activation of ATM. *Chem. Res. Toxicol.* **2012**, *25*, 1402–1411. [CrossRef]
19. Falck, G.C.; Lindberg, H.K.; Suhonen, S.; Vippola, M.; Vanhala, E.; Catalán, J.; Savolainen, K.; Norppa, H. Genotoxic effects of nanosized and fine TiO_2. *Hum. Exp. Toxicol.* **2009**, *28*, 339–352. [CrossRef]
20. Di Bucchianico, S.; Cappellini, F.; Le Bihanic, F.; Zhang, Y.; Dreij, K.; Karlsson, H.L. Genotoxicity of TiO_2 nanoparticles assessed by mini-gel comet assay and micronucleus scoring with flow cytometry. *Mutagenesis* **2017**, *32*, 127–137. [CrossRef]
21. Gea, M.; Bonetta, S.; Iannarelli, L.; Giovannozzi, A.M.; Maurino, V.; Bonetta, S.; Hodoroaba, V.D.; Armato, C.; Rossi, A.M.; Schilirò, T. Shape-engineered titanium dioxide nanoparticles (TiO_2-NPs): Cytotoxicity and genotoxicity in bronchial epithelial cells. *Food Chem. Toxicol.* **2019**, *127*, 89–100. [CrossRef]
22. Jugan, M.L.; Barillet, S.; Simon-Deckers, A.; Herlin-Boime, N.; Sauvaigo, S.; Douki, T.; Carriere, M. Titanium dioxide nanoparticles exhibit genotoxicity and impair DNA repair activity in A549 cells. *Nanotoxicology* **2012**, *6*, 501–513. [CrossRef] [PubMed]
23. Armand, L.; Tarantini, A.; Beal, D.; Biola-Clier, M.; Bobyk, L.; Sorieul, S.; Pernet-Gallay, K.; Marie-Desvergne, C.; Lynch, I.; Herlin-Boime, N.; et al. Long-term exposure of A549 cells to titanium dioxide nanoparticles induces DNA damage and sensitizes cells towards genotoxic agents. *Nanotoxicology* **2016**, *10*, 913–923. [CrossRef] [PubMed]
24. El Yamani, N.; Collins, A.R.; Rundén-Pran, E.; Fjellsbø, L.M.; Shaposhnikov, S.; Zienolddiny, S.; Dusinska, M. In vitro genotoxicity testing of four reference metal nanomaterials, titanium dioxide, zinc oxide, cerium oxide and silver: Towards reliable hazard assessment. *Mutagenesis* **2017**, *32*, 117–126. [CrossRef] [PubMed]
25. Singh, S. Zinc oxide nanoparticles impacts: Cytotoxicity, genotoxicity, developmental toxicity, and neurotoxicity. *Toxicol. Mech. Methods* **2019**, *29*, 300–311. [CrossRef] [PubMed]
26. Annangi, B.; Rubio, L.; Alaraby, M.; Bach, J.; Marcos, R.; Hernández, A. Acute and long-term in vitro effects of zinc oxide nanoparticles. *Arch. Toxicol.* **2016**, *90*, 2201–2213. [CrossRef] [PubMed]
27. Roszak, J.; Catalán, J.; Järventaus, H.; Lindberg, H.K.; Suhonen, S.; Vippola, M.; Stępnik, M.; Norppa, H. Effect of particle size and dispersion status on cytotoxicity and genotoxicity of zinc oxide in human bronchial epithelial cells. *Mutat. Res. Genet. Toxicol. Environ. Mutagen.* **2016**, *805*, 7–18. [CrossRef] [PubMed]
28. Karlsson, H.L.; Cronholm, P.; Gustafsson, J.; Möller, L. Copper oxide nanoparticles are highly toxic: A comparison between metal oxide nanoparticles and carbon nanotubes. *Chem. Res. Toxicol.* **2008**, *21*, 726–732. [CrossRef] [PubMed]
29. Murugadoss, S.; Lison, D.; Godderis, L.; Van Den Brule, S.; Mast, J.; Brassinne, F.; Sebaihi, N.; Hoet, P.H. Toxicology of silica nanoparticles: An update. *Arch. Toxicol.* **2017**, *91*, 2967–3010. [CrossRef] [PubMed]
30. Yazdimamaghani, M.; Moos, P.J.; Dobrovolskaia, M.A.; Ghandehari, H. Genotoxicity of amorphous silica nanoparticles: Status and prospects. *Nanomedicine* **2019**, *16*, 106–125. [CrossRef]
31. Gonzalez, L.; Thomassen, L.C.; Plas, G.; Rabolli, V.; Napierska, D.; Decordier, I.; Roelants, M.; Hoet, P.H.; Kirschhock, C.E.; Martens, J.A.; et al. Exploring the aneugenic and clastogenic potential in the nanosize range: A549 human lung carcinoma cells and amorphous monodisperse silica nanoparticles as models. *Nanotoxicology* **2010**, *4*, 382–395. [CrossRef]
32. Lu, C.F.; Yuan, X.Y.; Li, L.Z.; Zhou, W.; Zhao, J.; Wang, Y.M.; Peng, S.Q. Combined exposure to nano-silica and lead induced potentiation of oxidative stress and DNA damage in human lung epithelial cells. *Ecotoxicol. Environ. Saf.* **2015**, *122*, 537–544. [CrossRef] [PubMed]
33. Li, Y.; Li, P.; Yu, H.; Bian, Y. Recent advances (2010–2015) in studies of cerium oxide nanoparticles' health effects. *Environ. Toxicol. Pharmacol.* **2016**, *44*, 25–29. [CrossRef] [PubMed]
34. Rzigalinski, B.A.; Carfagna, C.S.; Ehrich, M. Cerium oxide nanoparticles in neuroprotection and considerations for efficacy and safety. *Wiley Interdiscip. Rev. Nanomed. Nanobiotechnol.* **2017**, *9*, 4. [CrossRef] [PubMed]

35. de Souza, T.A.J.; Rocha, T.L.; Franchi, L.P. Detection of DNA damage induced by cerium dioxide nanoparticles: From models to molecular mechanism activated. *Adv. Exp. Med. Biol.* **2018**, *1048*, 215–226. [PubMed]
36. Rubio, L.; Annangi, B.; Vila, L.; Hernández, A.; Marcos, R. Antioxidant and anti-genotoxic properties of cerium oxide nanoparticles in a pulmonary-like cell system. *Arch. Toxicol.* **2016**, *90*, 269–278. [CrossRef] [PubMed]
37. Rubio, L.; Marcos, R.; Hernández, A. Nanoceria acts as antioxidant in tumoral and transformed cells. *Chem. Biol. Interact.* **2018**, *291*, 7–15. [CrossRef] [PubMed]
38. Frieke Kuper, C.; Gröllers-Mulderij, M.; Maarschalkerweerd, T.; Meulendijks, N.M.; Reus, A.; van Acker, F.; Zondervan-van den Beuken, E.K.; Wouters, M.E.; Bijlsma, S.; Kooter, I.M. Toxicity assessment of aggregated/agglomerated cerium oxide nanoparticles in an in vitro 3D airway model: The influence of mucociliary clearance. *Toxicol. In Vitro* **2015**, *29*, 389–397. [CrossRef]
39. Marin, S.; Vlasceanu, G.M.; Tiplea, R.E.; Bucur, I.R.; Lemnaru, M.; Marin, M.M.; Grumezescu, A.M. Applications and toxicity of silver nanoparticles: A recent review. *Curr. Top. Med. Chem.* **2015**, *15*, 1596–1604. [CrossRef]
40. Vance, M.E.; Kuiken, T.; Vejerano, E.P.; McGinnis, S.P.; Hochella, M.F., Jr.; Rejeski, D.; Hull, M.S. Nanotechnology in the real world: Redeveloping the nanomaterial consumer products inventory. *Beilstein J. Nanotechnol.* **2015**, *6*, 1769–1780. [CrossRef]
41. Hadrup, N.; Sharma, A.K.; Loeschner, K. Toxicity of silver ions, metallic silver, and silver nanoparticle materials after in vivo dermal and mucosal surface exposure: A review. *Regul. Toxicol. Pharmacol.* **2018**, *98*, 257–267. [CrossRef]
42. Kim, H.R.; Kim, M.J.; Lee, S.Y.; Oh, S.M.; Chung, K.H. Genotoxic effects of silver nanoparticles stimulated by oxidative stress in human normal bronchial epithelial (BEAS-2B) cells. *Mutat. Res.* **2011**, *726*, 129–135. [CrossRef] [PubMed]
43. Nymark, P.; Catalán, J.; Suhonen, S.; Järventaus, H.; Birkedal, R.; Clausen, P.A.; Jensen, K.A.; Vippola, M.; Savolainen, K.; Norppa, H. Genotoxicity of polyvinylpyrrolidone-coated silver nanoparticles in BEAS 2B cells. *Toxicology* **2013**, *313*, 38–48. [CrossRef] [PubMed]
44. Cronholm, P.; Karlsson, H.L.; Hedberg, J.; Lowe, T.A.; Winnberg, L.; Elihn, K.; Wallinder, I.O.; Möller, L. Intracellular uptake and toxicity of Ag and CuO nanoparticles: A comparison between nanoparticles and their corresponding metal ions. *Small* **2013**, *9*, 970–982. [CrossRef] [PubMed]
45. Gliga, A.R.; Skoglund, S.; Wallinder, I.O.; Fadeel, B.; Karlsson, H.L. Size-dependent cytotoxicity of silver nanoparticles in human lung cells: The role of cellular uptake, agglomeration and Ag release. *Part. Fibre Toxicol.* **2014**, *11*, 11. [CrossRef] [PubMed]
46. Rosário, F.; Hoet, P.; Nogueira, A.J.A.; Santos, C.; Oliveira, H. Differential pulmonary in vitro toxicity of two small-sized polyvinylpyrrolidone-coated silver nanoparticles. *J. Toxicol. Environ. Health A* **2018**, *81*, 675–690. [CrossRef]
47. Wang, J.; Che, B.; Zhang, L.W.; Dong, G.; Luo, Q.; Xin, L. Comparative genotoxicity of silver nanoparticles in human liver HepG2 and lung epithelial A549 cells. *J. Appl. Toxicol.* **2017**, *37*, 495–501. [CrossRef] [PubMed]
48. Huk, A.; Izak-Nau, E.; Reidy, B.; Boyles, M.; Duschl, A.; Lynch, I.; Dušinska, M. Is the toxic potential of nanosilver dependent on its size? *Part. Fibre Toxicol.* **2014**, *11*, 65. [CrossRef]
49. Kruszewski, M.; Grądzka, I.; Bartłomiejczyk, T.; Chwastowska, J.; Sommer, S.; Grzelak, A.; Zuberek, M.; Lankoff, A.; Dusinska, M.; Wojewódzka, M. Oxidative DNA damage corresponds to the long term survival of human cells treated with silver nanoparticles. *Toxicol. Lett.* **2013**, *219*, 151–159. [CrossRef]
50. Kobayashi, N.; Izumi, H.; Morimoto, Y. Review of toxicity studies of carbon nanotubes. *J. Occup. Health* **2017**, *59*, 394–407. [CrossRef]
51. Møller, P.; Jacobsen, N.R. Weight of evidence analysis for assessing the genotoxic potential of carbon nanotubes. *Crit. Rev. Toxicol.* **2017**, *47*, 867–884. [CrossRef]
52. Lindberg, H.K.; Falck, G.C.; Singh, R.; Suhonen, S.; Järventaus, H.; Vanhala, E.; Catalán, J.; Farmer, P.B.; Savolainen, K.M.; Norppa, H. Genotoxicity of short single-wall and multi-wall carbon nanotubes in human bronchial epithelial and mesothelial cells in vitro. *Toxicology* **2013**, *313*, 24–37. [CrossRef] [PubMed]
53. Ursini, C.L.; Cavallo, D.; Fresegna, A.M.; Ciervo, A.; Maiello, R.; Buresti, G.; Casciardi, S.; Bellucci, S.; Iavicoli, S. Differences in cytotoxic, genotoxic, and inflammatory response of bronchial and alveolar human lung epithelial cells to pristine and COOH-functionalized multiwalled carbon nanotubes. *BioMed Res. Int.* **2014**, *2014*, 359506. [CrossRef]

54. Louro, H.; Pinhão, M.; Santos, J.; Tavares, A.; Vital, N.; Silva, M.J. Evaluation of the cytotoxic and genotoxic effects of benchmark multi-walled carbon nanotubes in relation to their physicochemical properties. *Toxicol. Lett.* **2016**, *262*, 123–134. [CrossRef] [PubMed]
55. Catalán, J.; Siivola, K.M.; Nymark, P.; Lindberg, H.; Suhonen, S.; Järventaus, H.; Koivisto, A.J.; Moreno, C.; Vanhala, E.; Wolff, H.; et al. In vitro and in vivo genotoxic effects of straight versus tangled multi-walled carbon nanotubes. *Nanotoxicology* **2016**, *10*, 794–806. [CrossRef] [PubMed]
56. Thurnherr, T.; Brandenberger, C.; Fischer, K.; Diener, L.; Manser, P.; Maeder-Althaus, X.; Kaiser, J.P.; Krug, H.F.; Rothen-Rutishauser, B.; Wick, P. A comparison of acute and long-term effects of industrial multiwalled carbon nanotubes on human lung and immune cells in vitro. *Toxicol. Lett.* **2011**, *200*, 176–186. [CrossRef] [PubMed]
57. Cavallo, D.; Fanizza, C.; Ursini, C.L.; Casciardi, S.; Paba, E.; Ciervo, A.; Fresegna, A.M.; Maiello, R.; Marcelloni, A.M.; Buresti, G.; et al. Multi-walled carbon nanotubes induce cytotoxicity and genotoxicity in human lung epithelial cells. *J. Appl. Toxicol.* **2012**, *32*, 454–464. [CrossRef] [PubMed]
58. Ursini, C.L.; Cavallo, D.; Fresegna, A.M.; Ciervo, A.; Maiello, R.; Buresti, G.; Casciardi, S.; Tombolini, F.; Bellucci, S.; Iavicoli, S. Comparative cyto-genotoxicity assessment of functionalized and pristine multiwalled carbon nanotubes on human lung epithelial cells. *Toxicol. In Vitro* **2012**, *26*, 831–840. [CrossRef] [PubMed]
59. Visalli, G.; Bertuccio, M.P.; Iannazzo, D.; Piperno, A.; Pistone, A.; Di Pietro, A. Toxicological assessment of multi-walled carbon nanotubes on A549 human lung epithelial cells. *Toxicol. In Vitro* **2015**, *29*, 352–362. [CrossRef]
60. Kinnula, V.L.; Yankaskas, J.R.; Chang, L.; Virtanen, I.; Linnala, A.; Kang, B.H.; Crapo, J.D. Primary and immortalized (BEAS 2B) human bronchial epithelial cells have significant antioxidative capacity in vitro. *Am. J. Respir. Cell. Mol. Biol.* **1994**, *11*, 568–576. [CrossRef]
61. Fischer, B.M.; Neumann, D.; Piberger, A.L.; Risnes, S.F.; Köberle, B.; Hartwig, A. Use of high-throughput RT-qPCR to assess modulations of gene expression profiles related to genomic stability and interactions by cadmium. *Arch. Toxicol.* **2016**, *90*, 2745–2761. [CrossRef]
62. Biola-Clier, M.; Beal, D.; Caillat, S.; Libert, S.; Armand, L.; Herlin-Boime, N.; Sauvaigo, S.; Douki, T.; Carriere, M. Comparison of the DNA damage response in BEAS-2B and A549 cells exposed to titanium dioxide nanoparticles. *Mutagenesis* **2017**, *32*, 161–172. [CrossRef] [PubMed]

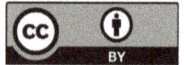

© 2019 by the authors. Licensee MDPI, Basel, Switzerland. This article is an open access article distributed under the terms and conditions of the Creative Commons Attribution (CC BY) license (http://creativecommons.org/licenses/by/4.0/).

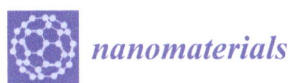

Article

Hepato(Geno)Toxicity Assessment of Nanoparticles in a HepG2 Liver Spheroid Model

Elisabeth Elje [1,2], Espen Mariussen [1], Oscar H. Moriones [3,4], Neus G. Bastús [3], Victor Puntes [3,5,6], Yvonne Kohl [7], Maria Dusinska [1] and Elise Rundén-Pran [1,*]

[1] Health Effects Laboratory, Department for Environmental Chemistry, NILU—Norwegian Institute for Air Research, Instituttveien 18, 2007 Kjeller, Norway; eel@nilu.no (E.E.); ema@nilu.no (E.M.); mdu@nilu.no (M.D.)
[2] Department of Molecular Medicine, Institute of Basic Medical Sciences, Faculty of Medicine, University of Oslo, Sognsvannsveien 9, 0372 Oslo, Norway
[3] Institut Català de Nanociència y Nanotecnologia (ICN2-UAB-CSIC-BIST), Campus UAB, Bellaterra, 08193 Barcelona, Spain; oscarhernando.moriones@icn2.cat (O.H.M.); neus.bastus@icn2.cat (N.G.B.); victor.puntes@icn2.cat (V.P.)
[4] Universitat Autònoma de Barcelona (UAB), Campus UAB, Bellaterra, 08193 Barcelona, Spain
[5] Vall d'Hebron Institut de Recerca (VHIR), 08035 Barcelona, Spain
[6] Institució Catalana de Recerca i Estudis Avançats (ICREA), 08010 Barcelona, Spain
[7] Fraunhofer Institute for Biomedical Engineering IBMT, Joseph-von-Fraunhofer-Weg 1, 66280 Sulzbach, Germany; yvonne.kohl@ibmt.fraunhofer.de
* Correspondence: erp@nilu.no

Received: 31 January 2020; Accepted: 11 March 2020; Published: 18 March 2020

Abstract: (1) In compliance with the 3Rs policy to reduce, refine and replace animal experiments, the development of advanced in vitro models is needed for nanotoxicity assessment. Cells cultivated in 3D resemble organ structures better than 2D cultures. This study aims to compare cytotoxic and genotoxic responses induced by titanium dioxide (TiO_2), silver (Ag) and zinc oxide (ZnO) nanoparticles (NPs) in 2D monolayer and 3D spheroid cultures of HepG2 human liver cells. (2) NPs were characterized by electron microscopy, dynamic light scattering, laser Doppler anemometry, UV-vis spectroscopy and mass spectrometry. Cytotoxicity was investigated by the alamarBlue assay and confocal microscopy in HepG2 monolayer and spheroid cultures after 24 h of NP exposure. DNA damage (strand breaks and oxidized base lesions) was measured by the comet assay. (3) Ag-NPs were aggregated at 24 h, and a substantial part of the ZnO-NPs was dissolved in culture medium. Ag-NPs induced stronger cytotoxicity in 2D cultures (EC_{50} 3.8 µg/cm^2) than in 3D cultures ($EC_{50} > 30$ µg/cm^2), and ZnO-NPs induced cytotoxicity to a similar extent in both models (EC_{50} 10.1–16.2 µg/cm^2). Ag- and ZnO-NPs showed a concentration-dependent genotoxic effect, but the effect was not statistically significant. TiO_2-NPs showed no toxicity ($EC_{50} > 75$ µg/cm^2). (4) This study shows that the HepG2 spheroid model is a promising advanced in vitro model for toxicity assessment of NPs.

Keywords: advanced in vitro model; comet assay; genotoxicity; hepatotoxicity; liver spheroids; nanoparticles; 3D culture; HepG2

1. Introduction

During the last decades, concerns have been raised about the potential human health risk of nanoparticles (NPs) due to the increased development and production of NPs with novel properties [1,2]. NPs are produced in a huge variety of forms and in large volumes, and they are used in a broad range of applications in everyday life. For example, NPs of titanium dioxide (TiO_2) are used as a pigment in paint, food and cosmetics [3]; zinc oxide (ZnO) is used in cosmetics due to its UV-blocking properties [4]; and silver (Ag) is used as a disinfection agent in medical equipment and consumer products, on account of its antimicrobial activity [5]. Thus, humans are likely to be exposed to NPs, either intentionally or accidentally, during production and usage [6]. Transport of NPs across biological barriers has been observed by elemental analysis in both rodents and humans [7–11]. As an example, gold NPs have been reported to reach the systemic circulation in humans, after inhalation, and translocate to other organs [8,9].

Several *in vivo* studies show that NPs accumulate in the liver, which is an important target organ for NPs and other xenobiotics due to its metabolic activity [12–18]. Induction of hepatotoxicity is one of the most common reasons for a medicine to be rejected or removed from the market [19,20]. Therefore, there is a need for sensitive hepatotoxicity screening methods for drug development and hazard assessment of chemicals or new materials, such as NPs. When considering the 3Rs—replacement, reduction and refinement—to minimize the use of animal experiments, hepatotoxicity should be assessed by reliable in vitro models. A great advantage of in vitro hepatocellular models for studying hepatotoxicity is the possibility of using human cells, either as primary cells or cell lines. The use of human hepatocyte cell lines, such as HepG2, C3A, Huh7 and HepaRG, has many advantages compared to primary cells. They are relatively easy to culture and have an unlimited life span, a relatively stable phenotype, high availability and low costs; moreover, inter-donor variations are avoided [21]. However, when comparing in vitro cell culture models in standard two-dimensional (2D) monolayers with complex organs, the cell lines in 2D culture display a limited hepatocytic functionality [21].

The liver-like functionality of the human hepatocellular carcinoma cell line HepG2 is enhanced when the cells are cultured in a three-dimensional (3D) arrangement. This increases the cell-to-cell contacts and intercellular communication [22] and changes the protein expression and metabolic status of the cells [21–23]. HepG2 cells in 3D cultures show upregulation of genes involved in liver-specific xenobiotic and lipid metabolism, whereas genes related to the extracellular matrix, cytoskeleton and cell adhesion have higher expression in 2D cultures [22,24].

The use of spheroids as 3D cultures in hepatotoxicity assessment is an increasing field of interest, and HepG2 spheroids, prepared with and without using scaffolds, have been applied for toxicity experiments with both NPs [6,25,26] and chemicals [27,28]. However, the differences in toxic responses between cells cultured in 2D and 3D are not yet clear. The scaffold-free HepG2 spheroid model was characterized in [27], where we demonstrated its applicability for testing genotoxicity of standard chemicals by the modified enzyme-linked comet assay, which measures DNA strand breaks (SBs) and oxidized DNA lesions. Interestingly, we found differences in sensitivity between the 2D and 3D models [27]. The comet assay has also been performed with Ag-, ZnO- and TiO_2-NPs and carbon nanotubes on a commercialized spheroid model with primary liver cells [6], and it has been shown to work well with different 3D models [6,27,29,30]. However, the comet assay has—to our knowledge—not yet been applied in HepG2 spheroids for genotoxicity testing of NPs. By using the miniaturized version of the comet assay, the throughput is increased. High-throughput methods are needed to reduce and replace animal experiments and to align with the increasing amounts of NPs being produced [31]. HepG2 spheroids have also been applied in the micronucleus test for chromosomal aberration testing, showing higher sensitivity than a standard 2D model to exposure to benzo(a)pyrene and 2-amino-1-methyl-6-phenylimidazo(4,5-b)pyridine [28]. In contrast, Dubiak-Szepietowska et al. (2016) found that liver 3D cultures are more resistant than 2D to cytotoxicity induced by NPs of Ag, SiO_2 and ZnO [25].

This study aimed to evaluate cytotoxicity and genotoxicity in HepG2 2D and 3D cultures after 24 h exposure to TiO_2-, Ag- and ZnO-NPs and to identify any differences in responses in 2D and 3D cultures. The tested NPs were selected on the basis of high production volumes and applications in consumer and medical products.

2. Materials and Methods

2.1. Cultivation of HepG2 Cells and Preparation of Spheroidal Cultures

HepG2 cells, provided from the ECACC (European Collection of Authenticated Cell Cultures) (cell line no. 85011430, Salisbury, United Kingdom) were cultured in 2D and 3D arrangements, as previously explained in detail [27]. In brief, HepG2 cells were cultured in Dulbecco's modified Eagle's medium (DMEM D6046 with low glucose and 4 mM L-glutamine, Sigma-Aldrich, Oslo, Norway) supplemented with 10% v/v fetal bovine serum (FBS, 26140-079, Thermo Fisher Scientific, Oslo, Norway), 100 U/mL penicillin and 100 µg/mL streptomycin (5070-63, Thermo Fisher Scientific, Oslo, Norway). Spheroid generation was performed, using the hanging drop technique, with 2500 cells per 20 µL drop. After four days of incubation of the cells at 37 °C with 5% CO_2 as hanging drop, the spheroids were transferred to a low adhesion plate. After one week, the spheroids had a diameter of approximately 800 µm [27] and were exposed to NPs as explained below. In parallel, 2D cultures were seeded in a 96-well plate with 20000 cells/well the day before exposure.

2.2. Nanoparticle Dispersions and Preparation for Toxicity Studies

TiO_2-NPs were provided by Catalan Institute of Nanoscience and Nanotechnology (ICN2, Spain) in colloidal dispersion and stored at 4 °C. TiO_2-NPs, of a mean size of approximately 4 nm in diameter, were prepared by a precipitation method following and adapting the method of Pottier et al. [32]. The stock solution of Ti^{4+} (0.7 M) was prepared by dissolving the Titanium (IV) isopropoxide (TTIP, Fluka Chemika) precursor in an HCl (3 mol/L) solution. For the production of TiO_2 anatase NPs, an aqueous Ti^{4+} stock solution (50 mL) was diluted in Milli-Q water (350 mL), at room temperature. The pH of the mixture was fixed at 11 by the addition of NaOH (3 M). Suspensions were aged at 70 °C for 24 h, and the solid was collected by centrifugation. Samples were further purified by 3 centrifuging cycles and re-suspended in an aqueous solution of tetramethylammonium hydroxide (TMAOH, Sigma-Aldrich) (100 M). Samples were characterized by transmission electron microscopy, dynamic light scattering and UV-Vis spectroscopy. The former was used to determine the particle size and size distribution. On the day of exposure, the TiO_2-NPs were diluted in FBS (1:1), and thereafter diluted 1:9 in cell culture medium, without FBS, to a concentration of 455 µg/mL (stock dispersion).

Ag-NPs (NM300K) were provided by Fraunhofer Institute for Molecular Biology and Applied Ecology (IME, Schmallenberg, Germany) and ZnO-NPs (NM110, JRCNM01100a) by the Joint Research Centre (Ispra, Italy). Stock dispersions of Ag- and ZnO-NPs were prepared according to the NANOGENOTOX protocol [33]. Briefly, the Ag- or ZnO-NPs were mixed with a bovine serum albumin (BSA) water solution (0.05% m/v, product nr A9418, Sigma-Aldrich), in a 20 mL scintillation vial (Wheaton Industries, Millville, NJ, USA), to a final concentration of 2.56 mg/mL (stock dispersion). To the ZnO-powder, 30 µL 100% ethanol (product nr 600068, Antibac AS, Asker, Norway) per 15.4 mg NP powder was added before BSA-water, to facilitate dispersion. The NP/BSA–water mixtures were sonicated on ice with a sonicator probe Labsonic®P Probe 3 mm (853 5124, Sartorius Stedim Biotech, Göttingen, Germany) and Labsonic®P (Sartorius Stedim Biotech), at 50% amplitude for 15 min (100% cycle, 100 watts), or with an ultrasound homogenizer Sonopuls (Bandelin, Germany), at 50% amplitude for 15 min (100% cycle). The dispersion solution of NM300K (NM300K DISP) was not included in the study, based on negative results from other studies on cytotoxicity and DNA damage [34–36].

Working concentrations of all the NPs were prepared by serial dilution of the stock dispersion in the culture medium. HepG2 cells in 2D and 3D culture were exposed for 24 h to TiO_2-NPs, Ag-NPs or ZnO-NPs (1–75 µg/cm^2 in 2D system, corresponding to 3–212 µg/mL in both systems; see Supplementary Tables S1 and S2 for details). As a negative control, complete NP-free culture medium was used. The same volumes (100 µL per well) and concentrations of NPs were used for both 2D and 3D cultures. NP dispersions were prepared, at most, two hours before cell exposure and NP characterization.

For characterization purposes (next sections), the NP stock solutions were also prepared in water dispersions, without proteins present, as described above, but in water instead of FBS/medium and BSA-water.

2.3. Size and Morphology Measurements of the NPs by Electron Microscopy

TiO_2-NP diameters were obtained from the analysis of transmission electron microscopy (TEM) images acquired with a FEI Tecnai G2 F20 S-TWIN HR(S) TEM equipped with an energy-dispersive X-ray spectroscopy (EDX) detector, operated at an accelerated voltage of 200 kV. Microliters of the samples were prepared by drop-casting 10 µL of the sample on a carbon-coated copper TEM grid and leaving to dry at room temperature. In addition, scanning electron microscopy was done with a FEI Magellan 400L XHR SEM, in scanning mode, operated at 1 kV, and in transmission mode, operated at 20 kV/STEM, for bigger sizes. The average size and size distribution of the samples were measured by using ImageJ software, by counting at least 300 particles from different regions of the grid. TEM images of Ag- and ZnO-NPs were acquired, but the size distribution was not measured.

2.4. Hydrodynamic Diameter and Zeta Potential Measurements of the NPs

The hydrodynamic size and surface charge of the NPs were determined by Dynamic Light Scattering and Laser Doppler Anemometry, respectively, using a Zetasizer Nano ZS (Malvern Instruments, Malvern, UK) instrument equipped with a light source wavelength of 532 nm and a fixed scattering angle of 173°. Aliquots of one milliliter of the colloidal NP dispersions at a concentration of 10% (v/v) were placed into specific plastic cuvettes, and the software was arranged with the parameters of refractive index and absorption coefficient, and the solvent viscosity at 25 °C. Each value was the average of at least 3 independent measurements. All measurements used the Smoluchowski model.

2.5. UV-Vis Measurements of the NP Dispersions

UV-visible spectra were acquired with an Agilent Cary 60 UV-Vis spectrophotometer. A 10% (v/v) colloidal NP dispersion was placed in a cell, and the spectral analysis was performed in the 200–800 nm wavelength range, at room temperature.

2.6. Analysis of Silver and Zinc Ions in NP Dispersions

Samples for analysis of dissolved silver and zinc and potential dissolution of the NPs were taken from cell-free exposure medium parallel to the start of exposure. The concentrations 1, 10, 30 and 100 µg/cm^2 were selected, corresponding to 2.8–283 µg/mL. Medium without NPs was used as control. The samples were transferred to Amicon Ultra centrifugal filter unit tubes (Millipore, product no UFC900324) containing a 3 KDa filter unit [37]. The tubes were preconditioned before use with ultrapure water at 3900 g for 10 min. The samples were centrifuged at 3900 g for 30 min, to let the particles remain in the filter and the dissolved Ag and Zn to go through with the filtrate.

An aliquot of the filtrate containing released ions from the NPs was added to supra pure nitric acid, at a final concentration of 1% (v/v). The concentrations of dissolved zinc and silver (defined as <3 kDa fraction) were determined by the use of an inductively coupled plasma mass spectrometer (ICP-MS) type Agilent 7700× (Agilent, Santa Clara, CA, USA), using the method accredited according to requirements of NS-EN/IEC 17025 (NILU-U-110). Then, ^{115}In was added to all standards, blanks and samples, as internal standard, and detection limits were 0.006 ng/mL Ag and 0.6 ng/mL Zn. Certified reference material (1640a Trace Elements in Natural Water, NIST) were analyzed in every run. One sample per concentration was used in three independent experiments ($n = 3$).

2.7. Fluorescence Imaging of the Spheroids

After NP exposure, the spheroids were washed with PBS before live and dead cells were stained by fluorescein diacetate (FDA, Invitrogen, Thermo Fisher Scientific, Oslo, Norway) and propidium iodide (PI, Invitrogen, Thermo Fisher Scientific), respectively. After incubation with 30 μg/mL FDA and 40 μg/mL PI for 10 min in the dark, at room temperature, the spheroids were washed with PBS and transferred to a glass-bottomed culture slide (μ-slide 8-well glass bottom, Ibidi) for imaging with confocal microscope Zeiss LSM 700, using the software ZEN2010 (Zeiss). Excitation and emissions peaks were 535 and 617 nm for PI and 498 and 517 nm for FDA. At least three spheroids were imaged from each sample in two independent experiments ($n = 2$). Z-stack images were captured from the spheroid surface and approximately 150 μm inside, toward the center of the spheroid, as described in [27]. The images were merged by using maximum intensity in ImageJ [38].

2.8. Viability Measurements by AlamarBlue Assay

The alamarBlue assay measures the ability of the cells to metabolize resazurin by reducing it to the fluorescent molecule resorufin. The metabolic capacity represents the viability of the cell culture relative to the control sample. The assay was performed to evaluate the cell viability in the 3D and 2D cultures after NP exposure, as described in [27]. In brief, 2D and 3D cultures were washed with PBS and incubated with alamarBlue solution (10% w/v) for 3 h, before fluorescence was measured quantitatively on a plate reader (excitation = 530 nm; emission = 590 nm). Chlorpromazine hydrochloride (Sigma-Aldrich, Oslo, Norway), 100 μM, was included as positive control for the assay, based on results from [27], giving cell viability below 30% for both 2D and 3D cultures after 24 h exposure. At least two and three parallel culture wells were used per concentration for 2D and 3D cultures, respectively, and at least two wells per culture well were used for determining average fluorescence. To control for potential interference between the NPs and the alamarBlue solution, cell-free control samples, with and without NPs, were included.

To compare potential cytotoxic effects of NPs with their corresponding salts, HepG2 cells in 2D configuration were exposed to solutions of silver nitrate ($AgNO_3$) and zinc chloride ($ZnCl_2$). Both $AgNO_3$ (product nr 319430, Fluka) and $ZnCl_2$ (product nr 793523, Sigma-Aldrich, Oslo, Norway) were dissolved in complete cell culture medium (5 mM) before being further diluted upon cell exposure (1–5000 μM). Cells (2D) were exposed in 96-well plates, with at least 3 parallel exposure wells, for 24 h.

2.9. DNA Damage Measured by the Comet Assay

The enzyme-linked alkaline comet assay with inclusion of formamidopyrimidine DNA glycosylase (Fpg, gift from NorGenoTec AS Professor Andrew Collins and Dr. Sergey Shaposhnikov, Norway) was used to measure the level of DNA SBs and oxidized bases in 2D and 3D cultures. Fpg measures oxidized and ring open purines and DNA alkylated bases [39,40] and converts these lesions to SBs. The detailed procedure of the modified comet assay in 2D and 3D models is described in [27]. In brief, disaggregated cultures were embedded in low-melting-point agarose on precoated slides, before being submerged in lysis solution (2.5 M NaCl, 0.1 M EDTA, 10 mM Tris, 10% v/v Triton X-100, pH 10, 4 °C) for at least 1 h. The miniaturized version of the comet assay was used, with 12 mini-gels on each slide, similarly to [36]. Slides with samples for Fpg incubation were washed twice for 8 min in buffer F (40 mM HEPES, 0.1 M KCl, 0.5 mM EDTA, 0.2 mg/mL BSA, pH 8, 4 °C), Fpg diluted in buffer F was added, covered with a polyethylene foil and incubated at 37 °C for 30 min, in a humid box. All slides with cells embedded in gels were placed in the electrophoresis tank with electrophoresis solution (0.3 M NaOH, 1 mM EDTA, pH > 13, 4 °C), to let the DNA unwind for 20 min before running electrophoresis for 20 min (25 V, 1.25 V/cm, Consort EV202). Slides were neutralized in PBS and H_2O and dried horizontally, before staining with SYBR®gold (Sigma-Aldrich, Oslo, Norway). Comets were imaged using a Leica DMI 6000 B microscope (Leica Microsystems), equipped with a SYBR®photographic filter (Thermo Fischer Scientific, Oslo, Norway), and scored using the software Comet Assay IV 4.3.1

(Perceptive Instruments, Bury St Edmunds, UK). Median % DNA in tail from around 50 comets per gel was used as a measure of DNA SBs. Oxidized DNA lesions were calculated as net Fpg-sensitive sites, i.e., as the difference in % DNA in tail between samples with Fpg incubation and samples without incubation. Hydrogen peroxide, H_2O_2 (50 µM, Sigma-Aldrich, Oslo, Norway), and the photosensitizer Ro 19-8022 (2 µM, kindly provided by Hoffmann La Roche) with light irradiation were included as positive controls for DNA SBs and Fpg activity, respectively. The photosensitizer with light induces oxidized purines, mainly 8-oxoGuanine, which is detected by the Fpg [39,41]. At least 2 and 3 gels were prepared for each concentration, for 2D and 3D cultures, respectively, in each experiment.

2.10. Statistical Analysis

Results are presented as mean with standard error of the mean (SEM) of 3 independent experiments ($n = 3$), unless otherwise mentioned. Effects were compared to nontreated cells, and statistical analysis by one-way ANOVA, multiple comparisons and post-test Dunnett were performed in GraphPad Prism 7. Comparison of 2D and 3D cultures were performed by two-way ANOVA, multiple comparisons and post-test Sidak. The *p*-values are marked by * as $p < 0.05$, ** as $p < 0.01$, *** as $p < 0.001$ and **** as $p < 0.0001$. EC_{50} values were calculated in Prism, using nonlinear regression analysis (Hill function).

3. Results

3.1. Characterization of the NPs

Characterization of the NPs was performed in water (TiO_2-NPs 455 µg/mL, Ag- and ZnO-NPs 2.56 mg/mL), stock dispersions (TiO_2-NPs 455 µg/mL in TMAOH and culture medium with FBS, Ag- and ZnO-NPs 2.56 mg/mL in BSA-water) and working dispersions (212 µg/mL in medium), at 0 and 24 h after preparation. A summary of the physical and chemical characteristics of the pristine NPs used is shown in Table 1.

3.1.1. Electron Microscopy Analysis for Size and Shape of the NPs

The primary size and shape of the NPs in water were determined by electron microscopy imaging (Figure 1). The TiO_2-NPs were quasi-spherical, with a mean diameter of 5.54 ± 0.98 nm (Figure 1A), the Ag-NPs were spherical (Figure 1B) and the ZnO-NPs were aggregated with irregular shapes (Figure 1C).

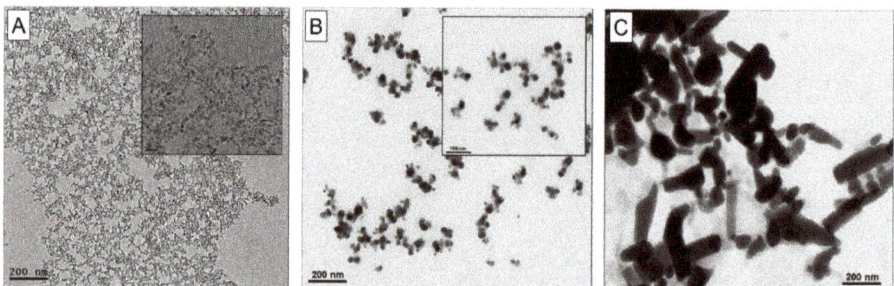

Figure 1. Representative transmission electron microscopy (TEM) images of (**A**) quasi-spherical TiO_2-NPs, and representative scanning transmission electron microscopy (STEM) images of (**B**) spherical Ag-NPs and (**C**) irregular ZnO-NPs in pure water. Scale bar = 200 nm. Scale bar in inserts: (**A**) 20 nm and (**B**) 100 nm.

Table 1. Characterization of pristine nanoparticles (NPs). TiO_2-NPs were provided by ICN2, Ag-NPs by Fraunhofer IME and ZnO-NPs by JRC. TMAOH: tetramethylammonium hydroxide. PGT: polyoxyethylene glycerol trioleate. PEG: polyethylene glycol, TEM: transmission electron microscopy. NA: not available.

NP	Code	Product Type	Solvent	Polymorph	Morphology	Surface Functionali-zation	TEM Diameter (nm)	Surface Area (m²/g)	Ref.
TiO_2	-	Dispersion	TMAOH	Anatase	Quasi-sphere	TMAOH	5.54 ± 0.98	NA	[42]
Ag	NM300K	Dispersion	PGT (4%), Tween 20 (4%)	Metallic	Sphere	PEG	<20 nm	NA	[43]
ZnO	NM110/JRCNM01100a	Powder	-	Zincite	Variable	Uncoated	147 ± 149	12.4 ± 0.2	

3.1.2. UV-Vis Spectroscopy for Analysis of Particle Stability

UV−vis spectra of the NP dispersions prepared in pure water (t = 0 h), as stock dispersions (t = 0 and 24 h) and as working dispersions (t = 0 and 24 h) are shown in Figure 2. When comparing Ag-NPs diluted in pure water and in water with BSA (stock), no red-shift is observed (Figure 2A,B). The red-shift is indicative of the formation of a dense dielectric layer onto the NP surface consistent with the absorption of proteins on their surface, and no stable protein corona formation was thus measured for Ag-NPs, which can be ascribed to the presence of polyethylene glycol at their surface. The UV-vis spectra of Ag-NPs working dispersions have an increased absorbance signal at high wavelengths and a decrease in the peak intensity, indicative of aggregation. The UV-vis spectra of TiO$_2$- and ZnO-NPs (Figure 2C–F) lack absorption peaks in the visible region, and no changes in time were observed. The small peak that appears in the visible region around 500 nm, as shown in Figure 2B,D,F, is due to the presence of phenol red in the culture medium.

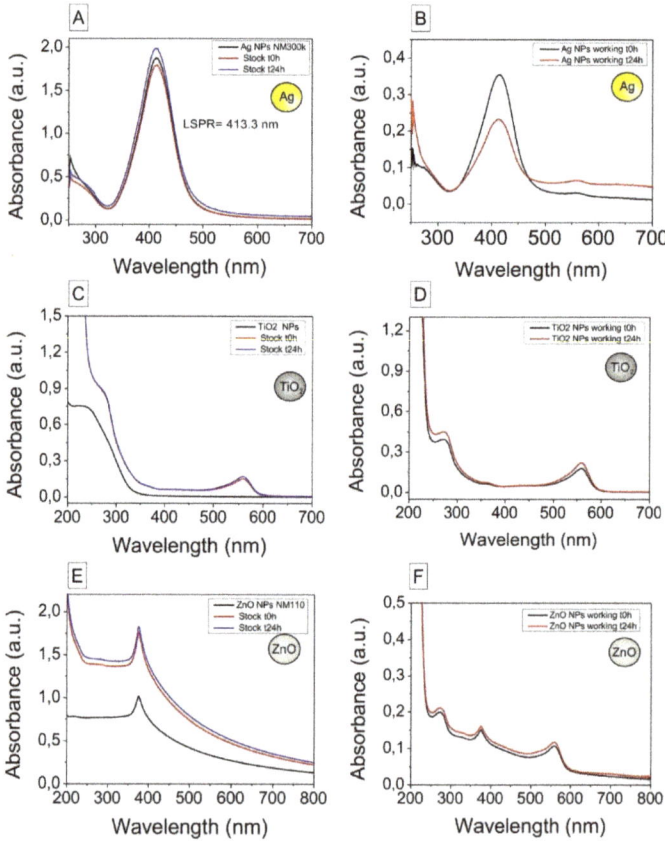

Figure 2. UV−vis spectra of the nanoparticle dispersions diluted in pure water (t = 0 h), as stock dispersions (t = 0 and 24 h) and as working dispersions (t = 0 and 24 h). Samples were diluted 1:200 (Ag), 1:10 (TiO$_2$) and 1:20 (ZnO) in pure water for analysis. (**A**) Ag-NPs in pure water and stock dispersion (2.56 mg/mL). (**B**) Ag-NPs working dispersion (212 µg/mL, t = 0 and 24 h). (**C**) TiO$_2$-NPs in water and stock dispersion (455 µg/mL, t = 0 and 24 h). (**D**) TiO$_2$-NPs working dispersion (212 µg/mL, t = 0 and 24 h). (**E**) ZnO-NPs in pure water and stock dispersion (2.56 mg/mL, t = 0 and 24 h). (**F**) ZnO-NPs working dispersion (212 µg/mL, t = 0 and 24 h). The peak at 560 nm can be ascribed to the presence of phenol red in the culture medium.

3.1.3. Hydrodynamic Diameter and Zeta Potential

The hydrodynamic diameter and zeta potential of the Ag-, ZnO- and TiO$_2$-NPs in pure water (t = 0 h only) are summarized in Supplementary Table S3; NP stock dispersions are in Table 2, and NP working dispersions are in Table 3. Representative size distribution curves are shown in Supplementary Figures S1 and S2.

Table 2. Hydrodynamic diameter and zeta potential (ZP) of nanoparticle (NP) stock dispersions (concentrations: TiO$_2$ 455 µg/mL; Ag and ZnO 2.56 mg/mL). For analysis, samples were diluted 1:10 in pure water. Numbers are given as mean ± standard deviation (SD) (n = 3). PDI: polydispersity index, a.u.: arbitrary unit.

NP	Time (h)	Hydrodynamic Diameter (nm), by Intensity	PDI (a.u.)	ZP (mV)
TiO$_2$-NPs	0	193.6 ± 6.2	0.262 ± 0.013	−16.1 ± 1.80
	24	207.4 ± 43.1	0.242 ± 0.008	−14.3 ± 0.61
Ag-NPs (NM300K)	0	54.2 ± 3.48	0.364 ± 0.023	−9.84 ± 3.94
	24	57.5 ± 1.50	0.459 ± 0.026	−8.79 ± 2.41
ZnO-NPs (NM110)	0	373.8 ± 21.5	0.199 ± 0.046	−15.8 ± 0.70
	24	400.1 ± 11.9	0.166 ± 0.032	−14.8 ± 0.30

Table 3. Hydrodynamic diameter and zeta potential (ZP) of nanoparticle (NP) working dispersions (concentration 212 µg/mL, corresponding to 75 µg/cm^2). For analysis, samples were diluted 1:10 in pure water. Numbers are given as mean ± standard deviation (SD) (n = 3). PDI: polydispersity index; a.u.: arbitrary unit.

NP	Time (h)	Hydrodynamic Diameter (nm), by Intensity	PDI (a.u.)	ZP (mV)
TiO$_2$-NPs	0	217.3 ± 27.3	0.285 ± 0.013	−5.73 ± 1.62
	24	189.8 ± 16.2	0.235 ± 0.022	−7.49 ± 2.63
Ag-NPs (NM300K)	0	37.3 ± 0.04	0.283 ± 0.065	−14.4 ± 1.99
	24	508.8 ± 29.5	0.452 ± 0.095	−20.1 ± 1.45
ZnO-NPs (NM110)	0	346.1 ± 9.6	0.258 ± 0.020	−23.8 ± 0.30
	24	338.0 ± 21.7	0.281 ± 0.032	−24.9 ± 0.25

The hydrodynamic diameter (by intensity) was for all NPs higher than the pristine NP size. At the start of the experiment, the mean hydrodynamic diameter (by intensity) was 54.2 nm for Ag-NPs, 373.8 nm for ZnO-NPs and 193.6 nm for TiO$_2$-NPs. The hydrodynamic diameter of the TiO$_2$- and ZnO-NPs increased slightly between 0 and 24 h, for both the stock and working dispersions. In contrast, the increase in hydrodynamic diameter of the Ag-NPs was strong between 0 and 24 h, and the polydispersity index (PDI) was relatively high at 24 h, indicating a broader size distribution. The mean hydrodynamic diameter of samples without NPs showed the presence of proteins in the dispersions, measured with high variations (BSA-water 152.7 nm ± 43.0 nm with PDI 0.406 ± 0.003; medium 120.2 nm ± 59.9 nm with PDI 0.299 ± 0.128).

The zeta potential measurements also showed an evolution of the NPs' surface charge. A drop in the surface charge, toward the average value of proteins, was observed when comparing the dispersions without proteins (Supplementary Table S3) with stock (Table 2) and working dispersions (Table 3). Zeta potential curves are shown in Supplementary Figure S3. The zeta potential of NP free BSA-water was −2.15 ± 1.01 mV, and the corresponding value of medium was −5.77 ± 2.49 mV.

3.1.4. ICP-MS Analysis of Dissolved Ag and Zn in NP Dispersions

The concentrations of dissolved Ag and Zn in the <3 kDa filtrates were analyzed by ICP-MS. Medium without NPs had a Zn concentration of 25.7 µg/L (25.4–150.9 µg/L) or 0.4 µM (0.2–2.3 µM) whereas the Ag concentration was below the detection limit (<0.006 µg/L). A substantial amount of Zn was measured in the filtrate of the medium with added ZnO-NPs, ranging from 8 to 87 µM. In the filtrates from medium with added Zn-NPs (10–100 µg/cm^2), the Zn concentration was nearly the same (79 to 87 µM) (Table 4). The concentrations of dissolved Ag in the filtrate of the medium with added Ag-NPs ranged from 0.00008 to 0.014 µM (Table 4).

Table 4. Concentrations of dissolved Ag and Zn in dispersions of Ag- and ZnO-nanoparticles (NPs) in cell culture medium. Zn concentrations in medium without NPs was 25.7 µg/L (25.4–150.9 µg/L) or 0.4 µM (0.2–2.3 µM). Ag content was below the limit of detection (<0.006 µg/L). Numbers are given as median (interquartile range) (n = 3). * Theoretical concentration of total Ag or Zn in the dispersion (not ZnO).

NP	Nominal Concentration			Measured Dissolved Ag/Zn Concentration (<3 kDa)		
	µg/cm^2	µg/L *	µM *	µg/L	µM	% of Nominal
Ag-NPs (NM300K)	1	2827.4	26.2	0.0090 (0.0089–0.0399)	0.00008 (0.00008–0.00037)	0.0003
	10	28274.3	262.1	0.0920 (0.0804–1.2723)	0.001 (0.001–0.012)	0.0003
	30	84823.0	786.3	1.49 (0.88–4.08)	0.014 (0.008–0.038)	0.0018
	100	282743.3	2621.1	0.20 (0.12–6.98)	0.002 (0.001–0.065)	0.00007
ZnO-NPs (NM110)	1	2271.5	34.7	519.7 (428.0–611.3)	7.9 (6.5–9.4)	22.9
	10	22715.0	347.5	5166.9 (4998.8–5693.0)	79.0 (76.5–87.1)	22.7
	30	68144.9	1042.4	5177.1 (4898.0–5436.3)	79.2 (74.9–83.2)	7.6
	100	227149.6	3474.8	5700.5 (5627.4–6057.8)	87.2 (86.1–92.7)	2.5

3.2. Cytotoxicity of Ag-NPs, ZnO-NPs and TiO$_2$-NPs in 2D and 3D Cultures

Effects of Ag-NPs, ZnO-NPs and TiO$_2$-NPs on the viability of HepG2 cells in 2D and 3D cultures were measured after 24 h exposure, using alamarBlue assay and confocal imaging. No interference of NPs with the alamarBlue assay was found (results not shown). The relative cell viability decreased in a concentration-dependent manner after exposure to ZnO- and Ag-NPs, but not for TiO$_2$-NPs, in both 2D and 3D cultures (Figure 3). For ZnO-NPs, calculated EC$_{50}$ values were in the same range for 2D and 3D cultures: 10.1 and 16.2 µg/cm^2, respectively (Table 5). The induced cytotoxicity of Ag-NP was higher in 2D cultures compared to 3D cultures, with EC$_{50}$ values of 3.8 and >30 µg/cm^2, respectively (Table 5).

Table 5. EC$_{50}$ values from alamarBlue assay in HepG2 2D and 3D cultures after 24 h exposure to TiO$_2$-NPs, Ag-NPs or ZnO-NPs. EC$_{50}$ values of metal compartments are given in parentheses.

Substance	2D			3D		
	EC$_{50}$ (µg/cm^2)	EC$_{50}$ (µg/mL)	EC$_{50}$ (µM)	EC$_{50}$ (µg/cm^2)	EC$_{50}$ (µg/mL)	EC$_{50}$ (µM)
TiO$_2$-NP	>75.0 (>45.0)	>212.1 (>127.1)	>2655.2	>75.0 (>45.0)	>212.1 (>127.1)	>2655.2
Ag-NP	3.8	10.7	99.2	>30.0	>84.8	>786.4
ZnO-NP	10.1 (8.1)	28.5 (22.9)	350.4	16.2 (13.0)	45.7 (36.7)	561.4
AgNO$_3$	1.2 (0.8)	3.4 (2.2)	20.1	-	-	-
ZnCl$_2$	17.5 (8.4)	49.4 (23.7)	362.7	-	-	-

To investigate the distribution of viable and dead cells in the spheroid culture after exposure to Ag- and ZnO-NPs, confocal microscopy and imaging was performed on exposed spheroids with live and dead cell staining by FDA and PI, respectively. Increased numbers of dead cells on the spheroid surface were seen after exposure to Ag- and ZnO-NPs at the highest concentration, and correspondingly, fewer viable cells were detected. Limited fluorescence could be detected from the spheroid core, and the viability of cells in this region could therefore not be determined. Representative images show a projection of z-stack images from the spheroid surface to approximately 150 µm into the spheroid

(Figure 4). The confocal microscopy analysis showed a clear induction of cell death on the spheroid surface after exposure of Ag- and ZnO-NPs.

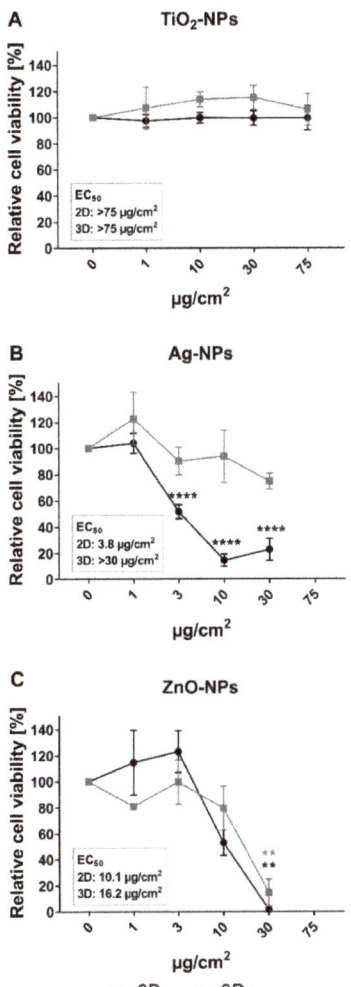

Figure 3. Cytotoxicity of TiO$_2$-, Ag- and ZnO-NPs measured by alamarBlue assay in 2D and 3D HepG2 cultures. Cell viability was measured as metabolic capacity and calculated relative to negative control cultures (set to 100%). (**A**) No significant effects were seen on the viability of 2D (black curve) and 3D (gray curve) cultures after 24 h exposure to TiO$_2$-NPs. The cell viability was reduced after 24 h incubation with (**B**) Ag-NP and (**C**) ZnO-NP for both 2D and 3D cultures. The effect of the exposure was significantly different in 2D and 3D cultures after exposure to Ag-NP at concentrations 10 and 30 µg/cm^2, evaluated by two-way ANOVA with post-test Sidak. Values are presented as mean ± SEM of 2–6 independent experiments: (**A**) n = 2, 3, (**B**) n = 4–6 and (**C**) n = 3. The concentration 75 µg/cm^2 was excluded for testing of Ag-NP and ZnO-NP (b and c) because of high cytotoxicity in previously published experiments [36]. ** $p < 0.01$; **** $p < 0.0001$.

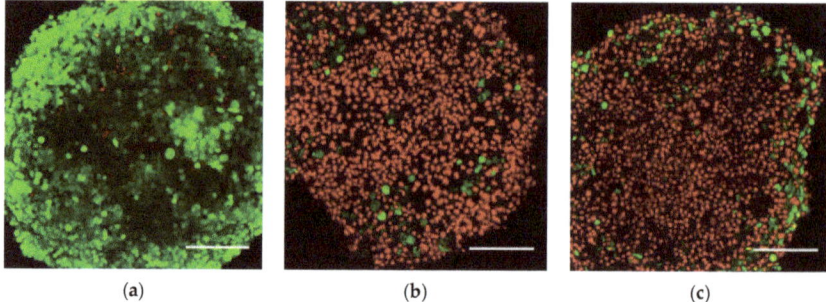

Figure 4. Representative confocal images of HepG2 spheroids exposed for 24 h to (**a**) culture medium, (**b**) Ag-NPs and (**c**) ZnO-NPs. Spheroids were exposed to 30 µg/cm^2 (85 µg/mL) of Ag- and ZnO-NPs for 24 h, before staining. Dead cells were stained with propidium iodide (PI) (**red**) and viable cells with fluorescein diacetate (FDA) (**green**). The images are z-stack projections from the spheroid surface and approximately 150 µm down toward the core. An increase in number of dead cells on the surface of the spheroids was seen after exposure to Ag-NPs and ZnO-NPs. Scale bar = 200 µm. Representative images from two independent experiments (n = 2), each with at least three parallel spheroids.

3.3. Cytotoxicity of Zn^{2+} and Ag^+ Ion Solutions in 2D and 3D Cultures

To compare the cytotoxicity of Ag- and ZnO-NPs with corresponding salts, the alamarBlue assay was performed after exposure of HepG2 cells in the 2D model to AgNO$_3$ and ZnCl$_2$ solutions. Some precipitation was seen upon mixing the AgNO$_3$ solution into the cell culture medium, most likely due to precipitation of AgCl due to a high presence of Cl$^-$ in the medium. The relative cell viability of the HepG2 cells after AgNO$_3$ and ZnCl$_2$ exposure decreased in a concentration-related manner (Supplementary Figure S4). The EC$_{50}$ values were 20.1 µM for AgNO$_3$ and 362.7 µM for ZnCl$_2$ (Table 5), which are higher than the amounts of dissolved Ag and Zn measured in the NP dispersions (Section 3.1.4). If we used the same concentration units as the NPs, the EC$_{50}$ values of AgNO$_3$ and ZnCl$_2$ would correspond to 0.8 µg/cm^2 (2.2 µg/mL) Ag$^+$ ions, and 8.4 µg/cm^2 (23.7 µg/mL) Zn^{2+} ions, assuming the compounds were freely dissolved in the solution. The EC$_{50}$ values after exposure to ZnO-NPs and ZnCl$_2$ were similar. The EC$_{50}$ value for Ag-NPs exposure was higher than for AgNO$_3$, showing higher cytotoxicity of the salt solution than the NPs in this test system.

3.4. Genotoxicity in 2D and 3D Cultures Measured by the Comet Assay

The levels of DNA SBs and oxidized base lesions were measured by the enzyme-linked comet assay after 24 h exposure with NPs. In both 2D and 3D cultures, a trend with a concentration-dependent increasing level of DNA SBs was seen after exposure to Ag-NPs and ZnO-NPs; however, a statistically significant increase was found only at cytotoxic concentrations in the 2D cultures (from exposure of 3 µg/cm^2 Ag-NPs and at 10 µg/cm^2 ZnO-NPs in 2D cultures). No effect on the level of DNA damage was observed after exposure to TiO$_2$-NPs in either 2D or 3D cultures (Figure 5). The background level of DNA damage was measured in unexposed HepG2 cells from 2D and 3D cultures and found to be similar for DNA SBs, with 5.0 ± 0.8 (2D, n = 9) and 6.2 ± 1.0 (3D, n = 7) % DNA in tail as average in all experiments (Supplementary Figure S5). For oxidized DNA base lesions, the background level was higher in 3D cultures compared to 2D, with levels of net Fpg sites at 3.7 ± 0.7 (2D, n = 9) and 7.6 ± 2.1 (3D, n = 7) % DNA in tail (Supplementary Figure S5). As a positive control for DNA SBs, cells were treated for 5 min with 50 µM H$_2$O$_2$; this induced a high level of DNA damage in both 2D and 3D cultures (Supplementary Figure S5). The control sample for Fpg enzyme activity, cells treated with Ro 19-8022 plus light, showed DNA damage within the expected range; the % DNA in tail was increased by at least 20 percentage points compared to without Fpg incubation (results not shown).

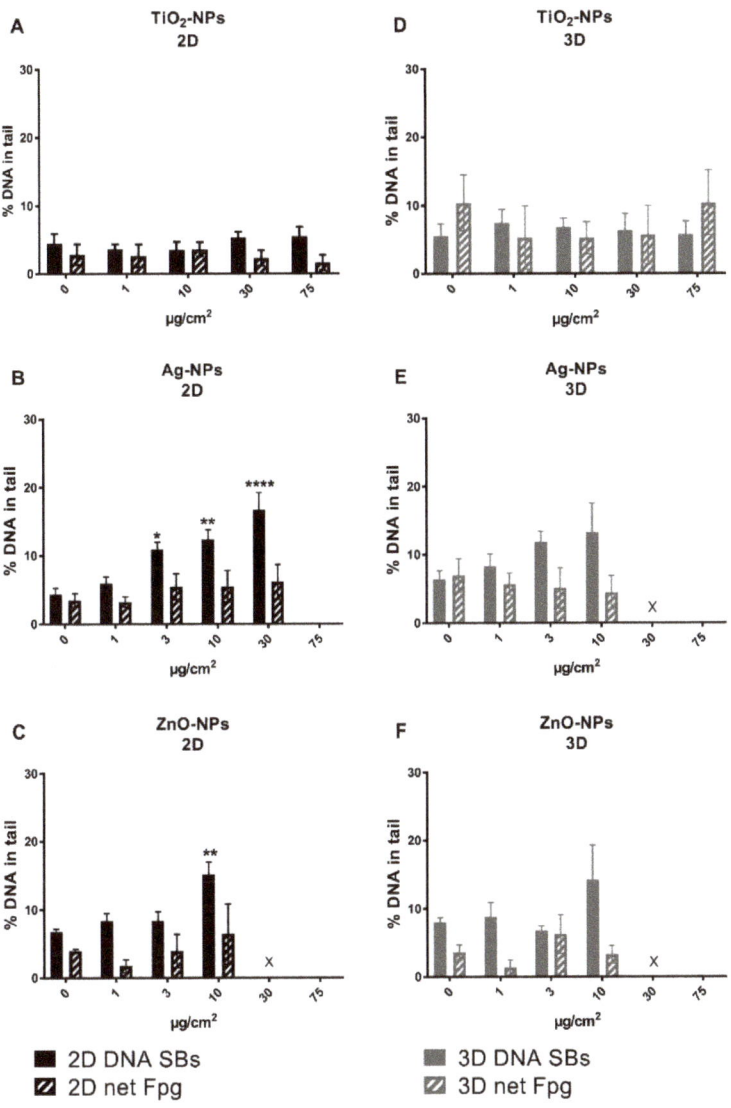

Figure 5. DNA damage in 2D and 3D cultures after exposure to TiO_2-, Ag- and ZnO-NPs measured by the comet assay. The 2D (**A–C**) and 3D (**D–F**) cultures were exposed to TiO_2-, Ag- and ZnO-NPs for 24 h. No increase in DNA damage was seen after exposure to TiO_2-NPs. Ag- and ZnO-NPs induced an increase in DNA SBs; however, this was statistically significant only at cytotoxic concentrations. Moreover, $n = 3$ for TiO_2- and ZnO-NPs, and $n = 6$ for Ag-NPs except at 3 µg/cm², where $n = 4$. X: not measured due to cytotoxicity and too low cell number. The concentration 75 µg/cm² was excluded in the experiments with Ag-NPs and ZnO-NPs (**B,C** and **E,F**) because of high cytotoxicity in previously published experiments [36]. * $p < 0.05$, ** $p < 0.01$, *** $p < 0.001$ and **** $p < 0.0001$.

4. Discussion

There is a huge demand to develop in vitro models that more closely resemble the *in vivo* situation, for toxicity assessment of NPs and chemicals. These models should be standardized in regard to critical toxicity endpoints. Here, we have focused on the liver spheroid model and evaluated it for reliability in detecting cytotoxicity and genotoxicity of NPs.

This study investigated potential differences in induction of cell death and DNA damage, depending on whether the liver cells were cultured in 2D or 3D arrangements, by applying the enzyme-linked comet assay, accompanied with cytotoxicity tests, on HepG2 spheroids and monolayers exposed to TiO_2-, Ag- and ZnO-NPs. HepG2 spheroids were prepared with a reproducible scaffold-free technique described in detail in Elje et al. (2019). Levels of DNA SBs in unexposed cells were found to be similar to the previous study [27]. However, 3D cultures had a higher background level of oxidized DNA lesions than 2D cultures, which can indicate a higher basal level of oxidative stress in the 3D model. This should be investigated further.

As toxicity of NPs is highly dependent upon physicochemical properties, it is important to characterize NP behavior under the given experimental conditions. The strong increase in the hydrodynamic size and the high PDI value for Ag-NPs indicate that the working dispersion of Ag-NPs had aggregated after 24 h of exposure. These results are in accordance with the UV-vis spectra, in which a decrease in intensity of the silver plasmon band, along with the increased absorbance at higher wavelengths, is shown. Ag-NP absorption is highly sensitive to the aggregation state of the NPs, due to strong surface plasmon resonance interactions between close NPs (at distances about their diameter) [44]. The UV-vis results, combined with the changes in size distribution and zeta potential, suggest that the amount of BSA protein per Ag-NP was too low to form a homogenous and dense coating, and that the stabilization of the NPs was likely to be electrostatic. Consequently, the ionic strength of the culture medium may contribute to the aggregation of the NPs. The increase in hydrodynamic diameter of TiO_2- and ZnO-NPs after 24 h can be explained by the formation of a loosely bound soft protein corona. In terms of NP stabilization by proteins, no significant information can be drawn from the UV-vis spectra of TiO_2- and ZnO-NPs. The wide band gap nature of these materials and their inability to absorb energy in the visible range explain the absence of absorption peaks in the visible region. Thus, the attenuation of transmitted light comes from the combination of absorption and Rayleigh scattering. Other studies using the same Ag-NPs (NM300K) and ZnO-NPs (NM110) have reported smaller hydrodynamic sizes and higher stability [6,36,43,45]. As NPs' behavior depends on their surroundings [46], this highlights the importance of performing NP characterization with the same conditions as used in the experiments.

Exposure of HepG2 cells to TiO_2-NPs did not induce any cytotoxicity or genotoxicity in 2D and 3D cultures. TiO_2-NPs have also been reported in other studies to be less toxic than other nano-metal oxides [47], and their toxicity is dependent on their physicochemical properties [48–50]. Toxic effects have been seen in both in vitro and *in vivo* studies [36,51,52] and are not related to dissolution of metal ions [47].

ZnO-NPs exposure induced cytotoxicity to a similar extent in both 2D and 3D HepG2 cultures. Elevated DNA damage was observed in 2D and 3D cultures at the highest concentrations; however, significant induction of DNA damage was found only in 2D cultures and at cytotoxic concentrations. Similarly, exposure to Ag-NPs induced cell death and a concentration-dependent increase in DNA damage, though statistically significant only at cytotoxic concentrations. The reduced viability seen with the alamarBlue assay was strongest in 2D cultures and did not reach statistical significance in the 3D cultures. However, when the spheroids were examined with confocal microscopy, many dead cells were seen at the surface of the exposed 3D cultures. As expected for a relatively complex model that closely resembles organ structure, higher variability was found in 3D cultures compared to 2D cultures. This can explain why statistically significant results were more difficult to achieve.

Significant induction of DNA SBs after ZnO- and Ag-NPs exposure was seen only at cytotoxic concentrations, in contrast to previously reported results for A549 and TK6 cells with the same NPs and nearly identical comet assay protocols [36]. This can be explained by the cell lines used, as the HepG2 cells seem to be less sensitive to genotoxic compounds than A549 and TK6 cells. Cowie et al. studied genotoxic response to metal and polymeric NPs in human and mammalian cells of different origin and found large differences in sensitivity of cells, with TK6 cells giving one of the best concentration-dependent response [53]. The discrepancy can also be related to the differences in cell cycle and exposure times. As demonstrated in a study applying the comet assay with Fpg to spheroids of primary liver cells (InSphero model), the genotoxic effect of NPs increased after repeated or longer exposures [6]. This was shown using the same Ag- and ZnO-NPs as in the present study, in addition to TiO$_2$-NPs and carbon nanotubes. Ag- and ZnO-NPs were the most potent NPs for inducing DNA SBs in the spheroidal culture, showing similar effects as in 2D cultured C3A HepG2 derivative cells [6,54]. Ag-NPs also induce an increase in DNA oxidation [6]. The presence of non-parenchymal cells can possibly explain the higher response to the NPs in the InSphero model compared to the HepG2 spheroids. The HepG2 spheroids show relatively high metabolic capacity and appear to be a good advanced in vitro model for the liver [21–24]. The commercial primary cell InSphero co-culture model is more complex than the HepG2 spheroids. However, the HepG2 spheroids used in this study are easy to prepare, have low costs and high interlaboratory reproducibility [27], and are thus a convenient and reliable alternative to commercial models.

Underlying mechanisms of NP toxicity include oxidative stress and dissolution of the NPs. In the case of metal or metal oxide NPs, toxicity can be caused by dissolution of ions, direct action of the NPs or interaction between NPs and the cellular environment [1,47,55–57]. Both ZnO- and Ag-NPs are generally found to induce toxicity in 2D cultures, as well as liver damage *in vivo* [17,18,55,56]. For metal NPs, there is always a question of whether toxicity is due to direct effect of the NPs or to dissolved ions. We found that a substantial number of ions was released at the start of the exposure (Table 4), with dissolved Zn concentrations of 10–100 µg/cm^2. Increased intracellular Zn^{2+} levels resulting from dissolution of ZnO-NPs have been reported to be correlated with high levels of reactive oxygen species (ROS) and apoptosis [56]. However, Sharma et al. (2012) found that the released zinc ions were less important for the toxic effects of ZnO-NPs in HepG2 cells [58]. Other critical factors for cytotoxicity and genotoxicity of ZnO-NPs are size, shape, surface composition and semiconductor characteristics [55,56,58]. Other studies have showed that ZnO-NPs dissolve rapidly in cell culture medium DMEM, with a subsequent slow increase over time [59], and that the dissolution is dependent upon factors such as pH, ionic strength and HCO$_3^-$ and HPO$_4^{2-}$ concentrations, and less on the initial NP concentration [60]. That the level of dissolved Zn reached a plateau is most likely explained by a saturation of dissolved zinc in the medium. In the 2D model, ZnCl$_2$ and ZnO-NPs had similar EC$_{50}$ values for cytotoxicity by alamarBlue assay. The level of dissolved Zn from the ZnO-NPs corresponded to a nontoxic concentration of ZnCl$_2$. These results indicate that the cytotoxic effect of ZnO-NP was caused by either by ZnO-NPs or the combination of ZnO-NPs and Zn^{2+} ions, and not only by released Zn^{2+} ions.

Dissolution and release of ions has been linked also with toxicity induced by Ag-NPs [47,55]. Oxidation of Ag(0) on the surface of the NPs, as well as other forms of interactions, will lead to particle corrosion and release of Ag$^+$ [61–64], which, after cellular uptake, can cause mitochondrial dysfunction [64,65]. In the present study, low levels of dissolved Ag were found in the Ag-NPs exposure dispersions shortly after exposure, and the amounts were lower than the measured EC$_{50}$ for cytotoxicity of AgNO$_3$. Higher amounts of dissolved Ag have been found in other studies using the same Ag-NPs [6,37,54], and the differences may be related to distinct exposure media, different incubation times and sample preparation. However, most Ag$^+$ released from the NPs will not remain freely dissolved in the cell culture medium, due to the high ionic strength of cell culture media and presence of halides (0.12 M total dissolved Cl [66]), amino acids and proteins. Unbound Ag$^+$ will precipitate as AgCl and Ag$_2$S [62,65] or bind to proteins due to high affinity to thiol groups (SH-groups) [67]. Precipitation was observed when preparing AgNO$_3$, and a substantial part of the AgNO$_3$ solution was most likely precipitated AgCl (K$_{SP}$ 1.77 × 10^{-10} M^2 [68]) and not freely dissolved

Ag$^+$ ions [69,70]. For the Ag-NPs dispersion, precipitated nano- and microcrystals may have been trapped in the filter during sample preparation for ion analysis and thus not detected as dissolved Ag. Consequently, the low level of freely dissolved Ag cannot be correlated with the persistence of the Ag-NPs in the presence of halides. Thus, it is unclear to what extent the Ag-NPs dissolve under the given experimental conditions. Oxidative stress is a likely underlying mechanism of Ag-NP-induced toxicity [64], as the corrosion of Ag-NPs is REDOX active and produces ROS [49,50]. A mechanism for induction of ROS production of Ag-NPs consists of interactions with proteins, subsequent altered protein function [71] and activation of signaling pathways involved in ROS production [64]. An increased intracellular level of ROS can activate cell-death-regulating pathways, such as p53, AKT and MAP kinase [72]. Thus, it is not clear if the toxicity of Ag-NPs in 2D and 3D cultures was caused by the ions released from the Ag-NPs, the Ag-NPs or both.

The differences in sensitivity to NP-induced toxicity on 2D and 3D cultures could possibly be related to the exposure scenarios. While the cells in the 2D cultures were growing on the bottom of flat wells, the spheroids were cultured slightly above the bottom of U-shaped wells. The cultures are most likely exposed to the same NP concentration (µg/mL) only if the exposure medium is a stable colloidal dispersion during the experimental time, which would be the case for TiO_2- and ZnO-NPs. The Ag-NPs were aggregated at the end of the exposure time, and sedimentation of the aggregates would increase the concentration of NPs reaching the cells in the 2D cultures, while decreasing it for the 3D cultures. Possibly this can explain the stronger effect on viability of the 2D cultures compared with 3D cultures. As spheroidal cultures are exposed directly only on the spheroid surface, the exposure of cells in the interior is dependent on penetration of the compound inside the spheroid. Toxicity to cells in the interior of the spheroid could also occur via cell signaling pathways activated in the cells on the surface of the spheroid. As shown in Elje et al., short exposure to H_2O_2 was not sufficient to induce the same levels of DNA SBs in HepG2 2D and 3D cultures. The induced damage was around ten times higher in the 2D cultures, possibly explained by too short a time for the compound to reach the cells in the interior of the spheroid [27]. Fleddermann et al. found that SiO_2-NPs were distributed through the whole HepG2 spheroid when the NPs were mixed with cells before spheroid formation. However, when exposing the already formed spheroids for 24 h, NPs were seen only to a depth of 20 µm [26]. Cell types, cell densities, physicochemical characteristics of the NPs (including size distribution) and ion release may influence the penetration inside the spheroid [73–77].

Several studies have shown differences in sensitivity to induced toxicity in 3D and 2D cultures [25,27–29,73,78]. We have previously found similar cytotoxicity in 2D and 3D HepG2 cultures, but higher sensitivity in the 3D culture for induced DNA damage by MMS [27]. Increased sensitivity in genotoxicity was also seen after exposure to 11 chemicals in a HepaRG spheroid model [29]. In agreement with this, benzo(a)pyrene and 2-amino-1-methyl-6-phenylimidazo(4,5-b)pyridine, which both require metabolic activation for induction of genotoxicity, induced a higher micronucleus frequency in HepG2 spheroids compared to monolayer cultures [28]. Other studies showed a greater resistance of the 3D cultures to toxicity of various drugs and chemicals [73,78]. Thus, the development of advanced 3D models for toxicity testing in vitro can give a more realistic model for human hazard and risk assessment. Slight modifications of experimental protocols may be needed for 3D cultures when comparing them to 2D cultures, to be able to control the concentration of the tested NPs or chemical that reaches the cells. Introduction of non-parenchymal cells, such as endothelial cells, stellate cells or macrophages, in co-cultures with hepatocytes, will make the model more complex and can further increase the relevance to the human liver.

5. Conclusions

With the increasing production of NPs and, thus, the risk of exposure to humans, the development of advanced in vitro models is especially important with respect to time, costs and the 3Rs. This study has shown that the HepG2 spheroid model can be applied successfully for the testing of NP-induced cytotoxic and genotoxic effects. The toxic responses in 2D and 3D cultures can be different, as seen after exposure to Ag-NPs where the 3D cultures were more resistant, but also similar, as TiO$_2$-NPs induced no effect, and ZnO-NPs induced a strong cytotoxic effect in both models. The 2D cultures reflected concentration-dependent responses better; higher variability was seen in 3D cultures, and thus statistically significant results were more difficult to achieve. Ultimately, 3D cultures may be a more realistic model when compared to the human liver, as the spheroid model involves more complex cell arrangements and exposure scenario. The HepG2 spheroid model is thus a promising 3D model for use in nanotoxicology.

Supplementary Materials: The following are available online at http://www.mdpi.com/2079-4991/10/3/545/s1. Figure S1: DLS size distribution (by intensity) of nanoparticle dispersions. Figure S2: DLS size distribution (by number) of nanoparticle dispersions. Figure S3: Zeta potential of nanoparticle dispersions. Figure S4: Cytotoxicity results from alamarBlue assay on HepG2 2D model after AgNO$_3$ and ZnCl$_2$ exposure. Figure S5: Untreated and H$_2$O$_2$-exposed controls in the comet assay. Table S1: Theoretical nanoparticle concentrations applied to the 2D and 3D cultures during 24 h exposure. Table S2: Theoretical Ag and Zn content in the applied nanoparticle dispersions of Ag (NM300k) and ZnO (NM110). Table S3: Characterization of NPs in pure water.

Author Contributions: Conceptualization, E.E., M.D., E.M., E.R.-P. and Y.K.; methodology, E.E., M.D., E.M., E.R.-P., Y.K. and V.P.; software, M.D., E.M., E.E. and E.R.-P.; validation, M.D., E.M. and E.R.-P.; formal analysis, E.E., M.D., E.M., E.R.-P., V.P., O.H.M. and N.G.B.; investigation, E.E., E.M. and O.H.M.; resources, M.D., E.M., E.R.-P. and V.P.; data curation, E.E. and O.H.M.; writing—original draft preparation, E.E.; writing—review and editing, E.E., E.M., O.H.M., N.G.B., V.P., Y.K., M.D. and E.R.-P.; visualization, E.E. and O.H.M.; supervision, E.R.-P., E.M., M.D., Y.K. and V.P.; project administration, E.R.-P., E.M. and M.D.; funding acquisition, M.D., E.R.-P. and E.M. All authors have read and agreed to the published version of the manuscript.

Funding: This research was funded by the European Commission under the Horizon2020 program (grant agreement No. 685817, HISENTS, and grant agreement No. 814425, RiskGONE), the hCOMET project (COST Action, CA 15132) and the Norwegian Research Council (272412/F40).

Acknowledgments: The authors would like to thank Michelle Hesler (IBMT) and Iren E. Sturtzel (NILU) for technical assistance, Marit Vadset (NILU) for performing ICP-MS analysis, Hoffmann La Roche for providing the Ro 19-8022, Fraunhofer IME for providing the Ag-NPs, and JRC for providing the ZnO-NPs. Further, the authors thank Andrew Collins and Sergey Shaposhnikov at NorGenoTec AS, Norway, for providing the Fpg. Andrew Collins also kindly edited the manuscript with English corrections.

Conflicts of Interest: The authors declare no conflict of interest.

References

1. Nel, A.; Xia, T.; Mädler, L.; Li, N. Toxic potential of materials at the nanolevel. *Science* **2006**, *311*, 622–627. [CrossRef]
2. Donaldson, K.; Stone, V.; Kreyling, W.; Borm, P.J.A. Nanotoxicology. *Occup. Environ. Med.* **2004**, *61*, 727–728. [CrossRef]
3. Weir, A.; Westerhoff, P.; Fabricius, L.; Hristovski, K.; von Goetz, N. Titanium dioxide nanoparticles in food and personal care products. *Environ. Sci. Technol.* **2012**, *46*, 2242–2250. [CrossRef]
4. Vaseem, M.; Umar, A.; Hahn, Y. Chapter 4: ZnO Nanoparticles: Growth, Properties, and Application. In *Metal Oxide Nanostructures and Their Applications*; Umar, A., Hahn, Y., Eds.; American Scientific Publishers: Valencia, CA, USA, 2010; pp. 1–36.
5. Tran, Q.H.; Nguyen, V.Q.; Le, A.-T. Silver nanoparticles: Synthesis, properties, toxicology, applications and perspectives. *Adv. Nat. Sci. Nanosci. Nanotechnol.* **2013**, *4*. [CrossRef]
6. Kermanizadeh, A.; Løhr, M.; Roursgaard, M.; Messner, S.; Gunness, P.; Kelm, J.M.; Møller, P.; Stone, V.; Loft, S. Hepatic toxicology following single and multiple exposure of engineered nanomaterials utilising a novel primary human 3D liver microtissue model. *Part. Fibre Toxicol.* **2014**, *11*, 56. [CrossRef]
7. Choi, H.S.; Ashitate, Y.; Lee, J.H.; Kim, S.H.; Matsui, A.; Insin, N.; Bawendi, M.G.; Semmler-Behnke, M.; Frangioni, J.V.; Tsuda, A. Rapid translocation of nanoparticles from the lung airspaces to the body. *Nat. Biotechnol.* **2010**, *28*, 1300–1303. [CrossRef]
8. Miller, M.R.; Raftis, J.B.; Langrish, J.P.; McLean, S.G.; Samutrtai, P.; Connell, S.P.; Wilson, S.; Vesey, A.T.; Fokkens, P.H.B.; Boere, A.J.F.; et al. Correction to "Inhaled Nanoparticles Accumulate at Sites of Vascular Disease". *ACS Nano* **2017**, *11*, 10623–10624. [CrossRef]

9. Miller, M.R.; Raftis, J.B.; Langrish, J.P.; McLean, S.G.; Samutrtai, P.; Connell, S.P.; Wilson, S.; Vesey, A.T.; Fokkens, P.H.B.; Boere, A.J.F.; et al. Inhaled Nanoparticles Accumulate at Sites of Vascular Disease. *ACS Nano* **2017**, *11*, 4542–4552. [CrossRef]
10. Kafa, H.; Wang, J.T.; Rubio, N.; Klippstein, R.; Costa, P.M.; Hassan, H.A.; Sosabowski, J.K.; Bansal, S.S.; Preston, J.E.; Abbott, N.J.; et al. Translocation of LRP1 targeted carbon nanotubes of different diameters across the blood-brain barrier in vitro and in vivo. *J. Control. Release* **2016**, *225*, 217–229. [CrossRef]
11. Braakhuis, H.M.; Kloet, S.K.; Kezic, S.; Kuper, F.; Park, M.V.; Bellmann, S.; van der Zande, M.; Le Gac, S.; Krystek, O.; Peters, R.J.; et al. Progress and future of in vitro models to study translocation of nanoparticles. *Arch. Toxicol.* **2015**, *89*, 1469–1495. [CrossRef]
12. Sykes, E.A.; Dai, Q.; Tsoi, K.M.; Hwang, D.M.; Chan, W.C.W. Nanoparticle exposure in animals can be visualized in the skin and analysed via skin biopsy. *Nat. Commun.* **2014**, *5*, 3796. [CrossRef] [PubMed]
13. Choi, C.H.J.; Alabi, C.A.; Webster, P.; Davis, M.E. Mechanism of active targeting in solid tumors with transferrin-containing gold nanoparticles. *PNAS* **2010**, *107*, 1235–1240. [CrossRef] [PubMed]
14. Arami, H.; Khandhar, A.; Liggitt, D.; Krishnan, K.M. In vivo delivery, pharmacokinetics, biodistribution and toxicity of iron oxide nanoparticles. *Chem. Soc. Rev.* **2015**, *44*, 8576–8607. [CrossRef] [PubMed]
15. Wang, B.; He, X.; Zhang, Z.; Zhao, Y.; Feng, W. Metabolism of nanomaterials in vivo: Blood circulation and organ clearance. *Acc. Chem. Res.* **2013**, *46*, 761–769. [CrossRef]
16. Roy, R.; Kumar, S.; Tripathi, A.; Dwivedi, P.D. Interactive threats of nanoparticles to the biological system. *Immunol. Lett.* **2014**, *158*, 79–87. [CrossRef]
17. Wu, T.; Tang, M. Review of the effects of manufactured nanoparticles on mammalian target organs. *J. Appl. Toxicol.* **2018**, *38*, 25–40. [CrossRef]
18. Cao, Y.; Gong, Y.; Liao, W.; Luo, Y.; Wu, C.; Wang, M.; Yang, Q. A review of cardiovascular toxicity of TiO_2, ZnO and Ag nanoparticles (NPs). *Biometals* **2018**, *31*, 457–476. [CrossRef]
19. Fung, M.; Thornton, A.; Mybeck, K.; Wu, J.S.; Hornbuckle, K.; Muniz, E. Evaluation of the Characteristics of Safety Withdrawal of Prescription Drugs from Worldwide Pharmaceutical Markets-1960 to 1999 Therapeutic Innovation & Regulatory. *Science* **2001**, *35*, 293–317. [CrossRef]
20. Devarbhavi, H. An Update on Drug-induced Liver Injury. *J. Clin. Exp. Hepatol.* **2012**, *2*, 247–259. [CrossRef]
21. Godoy, P.; Hewitt, N.J.; Albrecht, U.; Andersen, M.E.; Ansari, N.; Bhattacharya, S.; Bode, J.G.; Bolleyn, J.; Borner, C.; Böttger, J.; et al. Recent advances in 2D and 3D in vitro systems using primary hepatocytes, alternative hepatocyte sources and non-parenchymal liver cells and their use in investigating mechanisms of hepatotoxicity, cell signaling and ADME. *Arch. Toxicol.* **2013**, *87*, 1315–1530. [CrossRef]
22. Kyffin, J.A.; Sharma, P.; Leedale, J.; Colley, H.E.; Murdoch, C.; Mistry, P.; Webb, S.D. Impact of cell types and culture methods on the functionality of in vitro liver systems—A review of cell systems for hepatotoxicity assessment. *Toxicology* **2018**, *48*, 262–275. [CrossRef] [PubMed]
23. Hurrell, T.; Ellero, A.A.; Masso, Z.F.; Cromarty, A.D. Characterization and reproducibility of HepG2 hanging drop spheroids toxicology in vitro. *Toxicology* **2018**, *50*, 86–94. [CrossRef] [PubMed]
24. Chang, T.T.; Hughes-Fulford, M. Monolayer and spheroid culture of human liver hepatocellular carcinoma cell line cells demonstrate distinct global gene expression patterns and functional phenotypes. *Tissue Eng. Part A* **2009**, *15*, 559–567. [CrossRef] [PubMed]
25. Dubiak-Szepietowska, M.; Karczmarczyk, A.; Jönsson-Niedziolka, M.; Winckler, T.; Feller, K.H. Development of complex-shaped liver multicellular spheroids as a human-based model for nanoparticle toxicity assessment in vitro. *Toxicol. Appl. Pharmacol.* **2016**, *294*, 78–85. [CrossRef] [PubMed]
26. Fleddermann, J.; Susewind, J.; Peuschel, H.; Koch, M.; Tavernaro, I.; Kraegeloh, A. Distribution of SiO_2 nanoparticles in 3D liver microtissues. *Int. J. Nanomed.* **2019**, *14*, 1411–1431. [CrossRef] [PubMed]
27. Elje, E.; Hesler, M.; Rundén-Pran, E.; Mann, P.; Mariussen, E.; Wagner, S.; Dusinska, M.; Kohl, Y. The comet assay applied to HepG2 liver spheroids. *Mutat. Res. Genet. Toxicol. Environ.* **2019**, *845*, 403033. [CrossRef]
28. Shah, U.K.; Mallia, J.O.; Singh, N.; Chapman, K.E.; Doak, S.H.; Jenkins, G.J.S. A three-dimensional in vitro HepG2 cells liver spheroid model for genotoxicity studies. *Mutat. Res.* **2018**, *825*, 51–58. [CrossRef]
29. Mandon, M.; Huet, S.; Dubreil, E.; Fessard, V.; Le Hegarat, L. Three-dimensional HepaRG spheroids as a liver model to study human genotoxicity in vitro with the single cell gel electrophoresis assay. *Sci. Rep.* **2019**, *9*, 10548. [CrossRef]

30. Reisinger, K.; Blatz, V.; Brinkmann, J.; Downs, T.R.; Fischer, A.; Henkler, F.; Hoffmann, S.; Krul, C.; Liebsch, M.; Luch, A. Validation of the 3D Skin Comet assay using full thickness skin models: Transferability and reproducibility. *Mutat. Res. Genet. Toxicol. Environ.* **2018**, *827*, 27–41. [CrossRef]
31. Collins, A.R.; Annangi, B.; Rubio, L.; Marcos, R.; Dorn, M.; Merker, C.; Estrela-Lopis, I.; Cimpan, M.R.; Ibrahim, M.; Cimpan, E. High throughput toxicity screening and intracellular detection of nanomaterials. *Wiley Interdiscip. Rev. Nanomed. Nanobiotechnol.* **2017**, *9*. [CrossRef]
32. Pottier, A.; Cassaignon, S.; Chaneac, C.; Villain, F.; Tronc, E.; Jolivet, J.-P. Size tailoring of TiO$_2$ anatase nanoparticles in aqueous medium and synthesis of nanocomposites. Characterization by Raman spectroscopy. *J. Mater. Chem.* **2003**, *13*, 877–882. [CrossRef]
33. The Generic NANOGENOTOX dispersion protocol—Standard Operation Procedure (SOP) and Background Documentation. Available online: https://www.anses.fr/en/system/files/nanogenotox_deliverable_5.pdf (accessed on 20 January 2020).
34. Kleiven, M.; Macken, A.; Oughton, D.H. Growth inhibition in Raphidocelis subcapita—Evidence of nanospecific toxicity of silver nanoparticles. *Chemosphere* **2019**, *221*, 785–792. [CrossRef] [PubMed]
35. Maria, V.L.; Ribeiro, M.J.; Guilherme, S.; Soares, A.M.V.M.; Scott-Fordsmand, J.J.; Amorim, M.J.B. Silver (nano)materials cause genotoxicity in Enchytraeus crypticus, as determined by the comet assay. *Environ. Toxicol. Chem.* **2018**, *37*, 184–191. [CrossRef] [PubMed]
36. El Yamani, N.; Collins, A.R.; Rundén-Pran, E.; Fjellsbø, L.M.; Shaposhnikov, S.; Zienolddiny, S.; Dusinska, M. In vitro genotoxicity testing of four reference metal nanomaterials, titanium dioxide, zinc oxide, cerium oxide and silver: Towards reliable hazard assessment. *Mutagenesis* **2017**, *32*, 117–126. [CrossRef]
37. Kleiven, M.; Rossbach, L.M.; Gallego-Urrea, J.A.; Brede, D.A.; Oughton, D.H.; Coutris, C. Characterizing the behavior, uptake, and toxicity of NM300K silver nanoparticles in Caenorhabditis elegans. *Environ. Toxicol. Chem.* **2018**, *37*, 1799–1810. [CrossRef]
38. Schindelin, J.; Arganda-Carreras, I.; Frise, E.; Kaynig, V.; Longair, M.; Pietzsch, T.; Preibisch, S.; Rueden, C.; Saalfeld, S.; Schmid, B. Fiji: An open-source platform for biological-image analysis. *Nat. Methods* **2012**, *9*, 676–682. [CrossRef]
39. Dusinska, M.; Collins, A. Detection of oxidised purines and UV-induced photoproducts in DNA, by inclusion of lesion-specific enzymes in the comet assay (single cell gel electrophoresis). *ALTA-Altern. Lab. Anim.* **1996**, *24*, 405–411.
40. Speit, G.; Schütz, P.; Bonzheim, I.; Trenz, K.; Hoffmann, H. Sensitivity of the FPG protein towards alkylation damage in the comet assay. *Toxicol. Lett.* **2004**, *146*, 151–158. [CrossRef]
41. Azqueta, A.; Slyskova, J.; Langie, S.A.S.; Gaivao, I.O.; Collins, A. Comet assay to measure DNA repair: Approach and applications. *Front. Genet.* **2014**, *5*, 288. [CrossRef]
42. Klein, C.L.; Comero, S.; Stahlmecke, B.; Romazanov, J.; Kuhlbusch, T.A.J.; Van Doren, E.; De Temmerman, P.-J.; Mast, J.; Wick, P.; Krug, H.; et al. *NM-Series of Representative Manufactured Nanomaterials, NM-300 Silver*; Publications Office of the European Union: Luxembourg, 2011.
43. Singh, C.; Friedrichs, S.; Levin, M.; Birkedal, R.; Jensen, K.A.; Pojana, G.; Wohlleben, W.; Schulte, S.; Wiench, K.; Turney, T.; et al. *NM-Series of Representative Manufactured Nanomaterials—Zinc Oxide NM-110, NM-111, NM-112, NM-113: Characterisation and Test Item Preparation*; Publications Office of the European Union: Luxembourg, 2011.
44. Piella, J.; Bastus, N.G.; Puntes, V. Size-Dependent Protein-Nanoparticle Interactions in Citrate-Stabilized Gold Nanoparticles: The Emergence of the Protein Corona. *Bioconj. Chem.* **2017**, *28*, 88–97. [CrossRef]
45. Safar, R.; Doumandji, Z.; Saidou, T.; Ferrari, L.; Nahle, S.; Rihn, B.H.; Joubert, O. Cytotoxicity and global transcriptional responses induced by zinc oxide nanoparticles NM 110 in PMA-differentiated THP-1 cells. *Toxicol. Lett.* **2019**, *308*, 65–73. [CrossRef] [PubMed]
46. Nel, A.E.; Mädler, L.; Velegol, D.; Xia, T.; Hoek, E.M.V.; Somasundaran, P.; Klaessig, F.; Castranova, V.; Thompson, M. Understanding biophysicochemical interactions at the nano–bio interface. *Nat. Mater.* **2009**, *8*, 543. [CrossRef]
47. Vimbela, G.V.; Ngo, S.M.; Fraze, C.; Yang, L.; Stout, D.A. Antibacterial properties and toxicity from metallic nanomaterials. *Int. J. Nanomed.* **2017**, *12*, 3941–3965. [CrossRef] [PubMed]
48. Wang, J.; Fan, Y. Lung injury induced by TiO$_2$ nanoparticles depends on their structural features: Size, shape, crystal phases, and surface coating. *Int. J. Mol. Sci.* **2014**, *15*, 22258–22278. [CrossRef] [PubMed]

49. Bastús, N.G.; Casals, E.; Vàzquez-Campos, S.; Puntes, S. Reactivity of engineered inorganic nanoparticles and carbon nanostructures in biological media. *Nanotoxicology* **2008**, *2*, 99–112. [CrossRef]
50. Casals, E.; Gonzalez, E.; Puntes, V.F. Reactivity of inorganic nanoparticles in biological environments: Insights into nanotoxicity mechanisms. *J. Phys. D Appl. Phys.* **2012**, *45*, 443001. [CrossRef]
51. Zhang, X.; Li, W.; Yang, Z. Toxicology of nanosized titanium dioxide: An update. *Arch. Toxicol.* **2015**, *89*, 2207–2217. [CrossRef]
52. Shi, H.; Magaye, R.; Castranova, V.; Zhao, J. Titanium dioxide nanoparticles: A review of current toxicological data. *Part. Fibre Toxicol.* **2013**, *10*, 15. [CrossRef]
53. Cowie, H.; Magdolenova, Z.; Saunders, M.; Drlickova, M.; Correia, S.C.; Halamoda, B.K.; Gombau, L.; Gaudagnini, R.; Lorenzo, Y.; Walker, L.; et al. Suitability of human and mammalian cells of different origin for the assessment of genotoxicity of metal and polymeric engineered nanoparticles. *Nanotoxicology* **2015**, *9* (Suppl. 1), 57–65. [CrossRef]
54. Kermanizadeh, A.; Pojana, G.; Gaiser, B.K.; Birkedal, R.; Bilanicova, D.; Wallin, H.; Jensen, K.A.; Sellergren, B.; Hutchison, G.R.; Marcomini, A.; et al. In vitro assessment of engineered nanomaterials using a hepatocyte cell line: Cytotoxicity, pro-inflammatory cytokines and functional markers. *Nanotoxicology* **2013**, *7*, 301–313. [CrossRef]
55. Ivask, A.; Juganson, K.; Bondarenko, O.; Mortimer, M.; Aruoja, V.; Kasemets, K.; Blinova, I.; Heinlaan, M.; Slaveykova, V.; Kahru, A. Mechanisms of toxic action of Ag, ZnO and CuO nanoparticles to selected ecotoxicological test organisms and mammalian cells in vitro: A comparative review. *Nanotoxicology* **2014**, *8* (Suppl. 1), 57–71. [CrossRef]
56. Krol, A.; Pomastowski, P.; Rafinska, K.; Railean-Plugaru, V.; Buszewski, B. Zinc oxide nanoparticles: Synthesis, antiseptic activity and toxicity mechanism. *Adv. Colloid Interface Sci.* **2017**, *249*, 37–52. [CrossRef]
57. Sirelkhatim, A.; Mahmud, S.; Seeni, A.; Kaus, N.H.M.; Ann, L.C.; Bakhori, S.K.M.; Hasan, H.; Mohamad, D. Review on Zinc Oxide Nanoparticles: Antibacterial Activity and Toxicity Mechanism. *Nano-Micro Lett.* **2015**, *7*, 219–242. [CrossRef]
58. Sharma, V.; Singh, P.; Pandey, A.K.; Dhawan, A. Induction of oxidative stress, DNA damage and apoptosis in mouse liver after sub-acute oral exposure to zinc oxide nanoparticles. *Mutat. Res.* **2012**, *745*, 84–91. [CrossRef]
59. Reed, R.B.; Ladner, D.A.; Higgins, C.P.; Westerhoff, P.; Ranville, J.F. Solubility of nano-zinc oxide in environmentally and biologically important matrices. *Environ. Toxicol. Chem.* **2012**, *31*, 93–99. [CrossRef]
60. Li, M.; Lin, D.; Zhu, L. Effects of water chemistry on the dissolution of ZnO nanoparticles and their toxicity to Escherichia coli. *Environ. Pollut.* **2013**, *173*, 97–102. [CrossRef]
61. McShan, D.; Ray, P.C.; Yu, H. Molecular toxicity mechanism of nanosilver. *J. Food Drug Anal.* **2014**, *22*, 116–127. [CrossRef]
62. Behra, R.; Sigg, L.; Clift, M.J.D.; Herzog, F.; Minghetti, M.; Johnston, B.; Petri-Fink, A.; Rothen-Ruthishauser, B. Bioavailability of silver nanoparticles and ions: From a chemical and biochemical perspective. *J. R. Soc. Interface* **2013**, *10*, 20130396. [CrossRef]
63. Adamczyk, Z.; Ocwieja, M.; Mrowiec, H.; Walas, S.; Lupa, D. Oxidative dissolution of silver nanoparticles: A new theoretical approach. *J. Colloid Interface Sci.* **2016**, *469*, 355–364. [CrossRef]
64. Akter, M.; Sikder, M.T.; Rahman, M.M.; Ullah, A.K.M.A.; Hossain, K.F.B.; Banik, S.; Hosokawa, T.; Saito, S.; Kurasaki, M. A systematic review on silver nanoparticles-induced cytotoxicity: Physicochemical properties and perspectives. *J. Adv. Res.* **2018**, *9*, 1–16. [CrossRef]
65. Reidy, B.; Haase, A.; Luch, A.; Dawson, K.A.; Lynch, I. Mechanisms of Silver Nanoparticle Release, Transformation and Toxicity: A Critical Review of Current Knowledge and Recommendations for Future Studies and Applications. *Materials* **2013**, *6*, 2295–2350. [CrossRef]
66. Product Information, Dulbecco's Modified Eagle's Medium (DME). Available online: https://www.sigmaaldrich.com/content/dam/sigma-aldrich/docs/Sigma/Formulation/d6046for.pdf (accessed on 20 January 2020).
67. Kędziora, A.; Speruda, M.; Krzyżewska, E.; Rybka, J.; Łukowiak, A.; Bugla-Płoskońska, G. Similarities and Differences between Silver Ions and Silver in Nanoforms as Antibacterial Agents. *J. Mol. Sci.* **2018**, *19*, 444. [CrossRef]
68. Solubility Product Constants. Available online: https://www.periodni.com/solubility_product_constants.htmL (accessed on 20 January 2020).

69. Kaiser, J.P.; Roesslein, M.; Diener, L.; Wichser, A.; Nowack, B.; Wick, P. Cytotoxic effects of nanosilver are highly dependent on the chloride concentration and the presence of organic compounds in the cell culture media. *J. Nanobiotechnol.* **2017**, *15*, 5. [CrossRef]
70. Loza, K.; Sengstock, C.; Chernousova, S.; Köller, M.; Epple, M. The predominant species of ionic silver in biological media is colloidally dispersed nanoparticulate silver chloride. *RSC Adv.* **2014**, *4*, 35290–35297. [CrossRef]
71. Saptarshi, S.R.; Duschl, A.; Lopata, A.L. Interaction of nanoparticles with proteins: Relation to bio-reactivity of the nanoparticle. *J. Nanobiotechnol.* **2013**, *11*, 26. [CrossRef]
72. Li, Y.; Guo, M.; Lin, Z.; Zhao, M.; Xiao, M.; Wang, C.; Xu, T.; Chen, T.; Zhu, B. Polyethylenimine-functionalized silver nanoparticle-based co-delivery of paclitaxel to induce HepG2 cell apoptosis. *Int. J. Nanomed.* **2016**, *11*, 6693–6702. [CrossRef]
73. Evans, S.J.; Clift, M.J.D.; Singh, N.; Mallia, J.O.; Burgum, M.; Wills, J.W.; Wilkinson, T.S.; Jenkins, G.J.S.; Doak, S.H. Critical review of the current and future challenges associated with advanced in vitro systems towards the study of nanoparticle (secondary) genotoxicity. *Mutagenesis* **2017**, *32*, 233–241. [CrossRef]
74. Konstantinova, V.; Ibrahim, M.; Lie, S.A.; Birkeland, E.S.; Neppelberg, E.; Marthinussen, M.C.; Costea, D.E.; Cimpan, M.R. Nano-TiO$_2$ penetration of oral mucosa: In vitro analysis using 3D organotypic human buccal mucosa models. *J. Oral Pathol. Med.* **2017**, *46*, 214–222. [CrossRef]
75. Hao, F.; Jin, X.; Liu, Q.S.; Zhou, Q.; Jiang, G. Epidermal Penetration of Gold Nanoparticles and Its Underlying Mechanism Based on Human Reconstructed 3D Episkin Model. *ACS Appl. Mater. Interfaces* **2017**, *9*, 42577–42588. [CrossRef]
76. England, C.G.; Priest, T.; Zhang, G.; Sun, X.; Patel, D.N.; McNally, N.R.; van Berkel, V.; Gobin, A.M.; Frieboes, H.B. Enhanced penetration into 3D cell culture using two and three layered gold nanoparticles. *Int. J. Nanomed.* **2013**, *8*, 3603–3617. [CrossRef]
77. Conte, C.; Mastrotto, F.; Taresco, V.; Tchoryk, A.; Quaglia, F.; Stolnik, S.; Alexander, C. Enhanced uptake in 2D- and 3D- lung cancer cell models of redox responsive PEGylated nanoparticles with sensitivity to reducing extra- and intracellular environments. *J. Control. Release* **2018**, *277*, 126–141. [CrossRef]
78. Ham, S.L.; Joshi, R.; Thakuri, P.S.; Tavana, H. Liquid-based three-dimensional tumor models for cancer research and drug discovery. *Exp. Biol. Med.* **2016**, *241*, 939–954. [CrossRef]

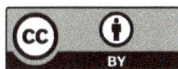

© 2020 by the authors. Licensee MDPI, Basel, Switzerland. This article is an open access article distributed under the terms and conditions of the Creative Commons Attribution (CC BY) license (http://creativecommons.org/licenses/by/4.0/).

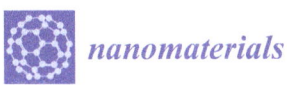

Article

In Vitro Genotoxicity of Polystyrene Nanoparticles on the Human Fibroblast Hs27 Cell Line

Anna Poma [1],*, Giulia Vecchiotti [1], Sabrina Colafarina [1], Osvaldo Zarivi [1], Massimo Aloisi [1], Lorenzo Arrizza [2], Giuseppe Chichiriccò [1] and Piero Di Carlo [3,4]

1. Department of Life, Health and Environmental Sciences, University of L'Aquila, I-67100 L'Aquila, Italy
2. Center for Microscopy, University of L'Aquila, I-67100 L'Aquila, Italy
3. Department of Psychological, Health & Territorial Sciences, University "G. d'Annunzio" of Chieti-Pescara, I-66100 Chieti, Italy
4. Center of Excellence on Aging and Translational Medicine—Ce.S.I.-Me.T. University "G. d'Annunzio" of Chieti-Pescara, I-66100 Chieti, Italy
* Correspondence: annamariagiuseppina.poma@univaq.it

Received: 2 August 2019; Accepted: 5 September 2019; Published: 11 September 2019

Abstract: Several studies have provided information on environmental nanoplastic particles/debris, but the in vitro cyto-genotoxicity is still insufficiently characterized. The aim of this study is to analyze the effects of polystyrene nanoparticles (PNPs) in the Hs27 cell line. The viability of Hs27 cells was determined following exposure at different time windows and PNP concentrations. The genotoxic effects of the PNPs were evaluated by the cytokinesis-block micronucleus (CBMN) assay after exposure to PNPs. We performed ROS analysis on HS27 cells to detect reactive oxygen species at different times and treatments in the presence of PNPs alone and PNPs added to the *Crocus sativus* L. extract. The different parameters of the CBMN test showed DNA damage, resulting in the increased formation of micronuclei and nuclear buds. We noted a greater increase in ROS production in the short treatment times, in contrast, PNPs added to *Crocus sativus* extract showed the ability to reduce ROS production. Finally, the SEM-EDX analysis showed a three-dimensional structure of the PNPs with an elemental composition given by C and O. This work defines PNP toxicity resulting in DNA damage and underlines the emerging problem of polystyrene nanoparticles, which extends transversely from the environment to humans; further studies are needed to clarify the internalization process.

Keywords: polystyrene nanoparticles; nanoplastics; genotoxicity; Hs27 human fibroblasts

1. Introduction

Global plastic production to date is highly related to the environmental pollution by plastic materials [1]. Microplastics (MPs), as fragments <5 mm, but also as fragments with lower dimensions (below 1 mm), are released into the environment [2–4].

Once released, MP particles will degrade gradually into nanosized plastics, but at the same time, nanoplastics (NPs, <1000 nm) may be emitted directly into the environment [5]. In recent years, the different aspects of toxicity regarding microplastics have been found in different environmental organisms [5–12]. According to the literature, the upper dimensional limit of nanoplastics goes from a minimum of 100 nm to a maximum of 1000 nm [13–15].

Plastics are synthetic or semi-synthetic polymeric materials obtained from natural components such as cellulose, oil, and coal that are used in the most disparate products for their manageability and their rapid production. They are excellent insulators, resistant to corrosion and degradation, which are not optimal for the fate of the environment. Normally produced at a high temperature and by cooling, the individual monomers bind together and form long carbon chains. The most important and used material is polystyrene: an aromatic polymer formed by styrene and petrochemical derivatives including packaging, electronic, and household products.

Plastics as microplastics have also been reported for a long time in the marine environment [2].

The way in which NPs are formed is still largely unknown. The process is sequential: from a macroplastic, one passes through the micro- to then arrive at the nanoplastic. It can be assumed that there is dependence on the plastic material. Polystyrene is the most abundant and reaches concentrations of the order of 10^8 particles per milliliter [16].

NPs are a subject of study that is still very undervalued and not widespread. The NPs, having reduced dimensions, suffer the impacts of water molecules and suspended ones avoid sedimentation [17]. Being hydrophobic, they can also aggregate with each other based on the pH and the composition of the liquid, for example, polystyrene nanoparticles in the sea aggregate stably by altering their dispersion capacities, mainly in relation to the dimensions. Aggregation, through weak ties, depends on the number and strength of collisions [17]. NPs can also form hetero-aggregation with other materials, which favors their spread [18].

The toxicity, as demonstrated, is not due to the macro components as well as the degradation products of the same, which become more reactive and dimensionally favored to overcome the biological barriers of animals and plants. This damage not only afflicts the ecosystems they live in, but also humans indirectly. First, there is a variation in the trophic chains; second, there is the phenomenon of bioaccumulation: when an animal food reaches the "human table", it is very likely that it contains not only the plastic directly ingested, but also all that the organisms had consumed, of which the same was fed (biomagnification). The effects of NPs on humans are still mostly unknown, although paradoxically more serious given their small size; thanks to these, they can overcome many biological barriers and enter into circulation, something not possible with the larger dimensions of microplastics. It is important to clarify how these NPs interact with humans and the food chain [18]; two fundamental characteristics of NPs must be taken into consideration: the size/shape and loads, which are the most effective in terms of internalization by cells. NPs of spherical shape are much better absorbed than those of elongated shape and both bind receptor proteins that vary their expression. It is fundamental to investigate such interactions to be able to elaborate a predictive toxicity system. Moreover, the interactions between the surface charges of nanoparticles and the biological membranes are fundamental. Using polystyrene NPs, it was found that these were phagocytosed by macrophages and not internalized by "tissue" cells [18]. Regarding the charge of nanoparticles, the positive NPs are internalized more quickly than the negatively charged ones. [19]. NPs may enter the animal and human food chain [20]. Mussels (*Mytilus edulis*) take NPs and PNPs (polystyrene nanoparticles) in the intestine [21,22] and unicellular green algae adsorb PNPs (<100 nm) [23]. The scallop (*Placopecten magellanicus*) internalizes protein coated polystyrene microparticles [24]. PNPs < 100 nm is present in the marine food chain from algae to fish [25]. PNPs < 500 nm may reach the circulation due to gut absorption in sea urchin embryos [7].

The effects of PNPs (<500 nm) have been tested in vivo in rat [26,27] and in vitro in oral and intestinal models [28]. Very little information is available on the toxicity of PNPs toward human cells and organisms and on the potential risks of adsorbed PNPs [29,30]. Considering the nanosize and the surface exposed of NPs and PNPs, it is urgent to pay more attention to the toxic effects of NPs in environment and human health.

In this work, we focused our attention on polystyrene nanoparticle genotoxicity by considering that NPs induce DNA damage [31,32]. We evaluated the cyto- and genotoxic effects of PNPs on the human fibroblast foreskin Hs27 cell line. The use of human skin fibroblasts as the cell system to test PNP genotoxicity is related to dermo-cosmetics product components enriched by polystyrene microbeads (i.e., scrubs, shampoos, soap, toothpaste and personal care products) [33], which may be fragmented in toxic and genotoxic PNPs and microplastics [34,35].

It will take time for the scientific community to build up the body of hazard and environmental exposure data for a full risk assessment of microplastics and NPs of the types applied in cosmetics and personal care product formulations.

In this context, we investigated the cyto-genotoxic potential of the PNPs after exposing the Hs27 human foreskin fibroblast cell line to different concentrations in the culture medium; following the treatment, we evaluated the viability and metabolic activity of the cells by the MTS assay test of cell proliferation associated with a preliminary screening improved by growth curve. Moreover, we detected reactive oxygen species (ROS) production with PNPs alone and PNPs added with an antioxidant extract of *Crocus sativus* L. stigmas. To estimate the PNP genotoxic potential, we used the cytokinesis-block micronucleus (CBMN) assay. Finally, we carried out PNP morphological analysis through scanning electron microscopy (SEM) equipped with an x-ray microanalysis system to obtain a chemical and semiquantitative characterization of the single elements of the PNPs.

2. Materials and Methods

2.1. Cell Culture

The in vitro toxicological study was conducted in a cell line, the fibroblast Hs27 (human foreskin, cultures from Public Health England, supplied by Sigma-Aldrich Srl, Milan, Italy).

Cell culture media, trypsin, and all reagents used, unless otherwise indicated, were purchased from Euroclone SpA. The cells were cultured in Dulbecco's Modified Eagle Medium (DMEM) containing 10% fetal bovine serum, 100 UI/mL Penicillin/Streptomycin, 2 mM L-glutamine, in a HERAEUS incubator (Hera cell 150, Thermo Electron Corporation, Langenselbold, Germany) set with the following parameters: 5% CO_2 atmosphere, 37 °C temperature. The culture maintenance was carried out under sterile conditions under a biological laminar flow hood. The cells were detached with 0.05% trypsin-0.02% EDTA.

2.2. Polystyrene Nanoparticles

The polystyrene nanoparticles (PNPs) were purchased to Sigma Aldrich (catalogue No. 43,302). The particle size was 100 nm, the diameter was 0.100 mm, and the density 1.05 gr/cm^3. The particles are in aqueous suspension (10% WT).

2.3. Saffron: Crocus sativus L. Stigmas Extract

Plant material (*Crocus sativus* L.) was kindly furnished by local farmers in the area of the "Zafferano dell'Aquila PDO" consortium, Navelli, AQ (Italy). Plant extraction (stigmas) was performed according to [36], in our case, however, the extraction was carried out in aqueous solution [37].

2.4. Cell–Growth Curve

The cells were seeded at a density of 10,000 cells/cm^2 in a six multi-well (35 mm in diameter) and when 90% of confluence was achieved, they were counted in a Bürker camera with the dye exclusion Trypan Blue, diluted 1:10. The determination was carried out for 4, 24, and 48 h at different concentrations of 5, 25, and 75 μg/mL of PNPs. In particular, the cells were treated with the different concentrations of PNPs, then readings were taken for each concentration at different times of exposure (4, 24, and 48 h).

Each experimental condition represents a technical triplicate, data refer to the mean and standard error of three independent experiments.

2.5. MTS [3-(4,5-dimethylthiazol-2-yl)-5-(3-carboxymethoxyphenyl)-2-(4-sulfophenyl)-2H-tetrazolium] Test

The viability of Hs27 cell line was determined by the MTS assay using a CellTiter Cell Proliferation Test Kit (Promega, Madison, MI, USA). The analysis was performed according to the manufacturer's protocol. The effect of PNPs (size 100 nm) on cell proliferation was assessed following exposure for

4, 24, and 48 h at different concentrations (5 µg/mL, 25 µg/mL, and 75 µg/mL). Cells were seeded at 5000 cells/cm^2 and treated after 24 h with different concentrations of PNPs (5 µg/mL, 25 µg/mL, and 75 µg/mL) at the established times in a humidified incubator in a controlled atmosphere (5% CO_2, 80% humidity, 37 °C). Each experimental condition represents a technical triplicate and data refer to the mean and standard error of three independent experiments. The positive controls (cells treated with 0.1% Triton X-100) were performed with each series of experiments (4, 24, and 48 h). Cell culture absorbance was measured at 490 nm, and cell proliferation was evaluated [38].

2.6. ROS (Reactive Oxygen Species) Detection

Cellular ROS concentration was determined according to the "Total ROS Assay Kit 520 nm". Briefly, 10,000 cells/cm^2 were seeded in 96-well plates, after 24 h, cells were incubated at 37 °C for 60 min with ROS stain 1X (Thermo Fisher Scientific Inc., Waltham, MA, USA ref. 88-5930) resuspended in dimethyl sulfoxide (DMSO). After incubation, the medium was removed, DMEM was added in the control cells and DMEM containing 5, 25, and 75 µg/mL of PNPs in treated cells. The H_2O_2 (150 µM) was added as the positive control. Another plate was performed with the same conditions (5, 25, and 75 µg/mL of PNPs), in which an antioxidant extract of *Crocus sativus* stigmas was added at 25 µg/mL final concentration [37].

Both plates were read at different times in a microplate reader (Perkin-Elmer Victor 3) (λexc 490, λemi535) at T0, T15, T30, T45, T60 min, and T24 h. The fluorescence data T0–T24 h were evaluated for statistical analysis. Each experimental condition represents a technical triplicate, data refer to the mean and standard error.

2.7. Cytokinesis-Block Micronucleus (CBMN) Assay

CBMN was carried out with slight modifications according to the protocol of Fenech [39] and OECD guidelines [40]. The Hs27 cell line was seeded in each flask with 2.5×10^5 cells/flask, and after 24 h of culture, the cells were exposed to different concentrations (5 µg/mL, 25 µg/mL, and 75 µg/mL) of PNPs for 48 h. Colchicine was used as a positive control at 5 µg/mL. Cytochalasin B (3 µg/mL) no longer than 24 h after stimulation by PNPs was added to the cell cultures.

Cells were harvested after an additional 24 h and centrifuged for 8 min at 1100 rpm; next, the supernatant was removed, and cells treated for 1 min with 0.075 M KCl hypotonic solution.

Following, the cells were processed and analyzed according to the criteria of Fenech guidelines [39].

Three biological replicates for each sample were used for CBMN analysis with three technical replicates (slides) each.

For each experimental condition, we calculated the cytokinesis block proliferation index (CBPI) to determine the frequency of mononuclear cells, bi- and multinucleated, using the following formula: ((N° mononucleated cells) + (2 × N° binucleated cells) + (3 × N° multinucleated cells))/(total number of cells). Furthermore, for each experimental condition we evaluated the total cells and nuclear buds (NBUDs) as a biomarker of genotoxicity.

2.8. Analysis of Polystyrene Particles (PNPs) by Scanning Electron Microscopy SEM

The study of the morphology and the elemental analysis of PNPs were carried out by scanning electron microscopy (Gemini Field Emission SEM 500, ZEISS, Milan, Italy) equipped with an x-ray microanalysis system (EDS Oxford Inca 250 x-act) at the Center of Microscopies, University of L'Aquila.

For PNP characterization, the sample (1 µL) was deposited on a dedicated sample carrier (stub) and then dehydrated in air. Finally, a thin film (5 nm) of chromium was deposited onto the sample using Sputter Quorum 150T ES to make it conductive for measurement purposes.

The SEM observations were carried out at different magnifications, and morphological analysis of the particles was performed simultaneously to obtain the EDS microanalysis of the selected particles.

2.9. Statistical Analysis

For the data statistical analysis, we used the Student's *t* test (unpaired) with post-hoc correction, comparing the value of the treated cells with the respective untreated control, through independent tests. For statistically significant values, * = $p < 0.05$; ** = $p < 0.005$; *** = $p < 0.0005$.

The data were analyzed using the GraphPad Prism software, version 6.0 (© 1995–2015 GraphPad Software, Inc. San Diego, CA 92108). Three independent experiments were performed for all assays applied.

3. Results

3.1. Cell Growth Curve and MTS

Preliminary results are reported in the growth curve for the Hs27 cell line with PNP treatment at different concentrations (Figure 1). In Figure 1, it can be seen that with respect to the control in every experimental condition up to 4 h, there was no significant proliferation decrease, regardless of the concentration. Differences appeared after 24 h, but control and the highest concentration still showed almost identical results. The exposure of the cells to 75 µg/mL of PNPs at 48 h showed a sudden decrease. The trend of the growth curve was due to the possible tendency of the nanoparticles to aggregate (PNPs in this work as in general the nanoparticles do [30]), this explains why at the lower concentrations there were no statistically significant results; on the contrary, at the concentration of 75 µg/mL and at a longer time of incubation (48 h), we can assume that PNP particles aggregates tend to enhance and interact with cell proliferation.

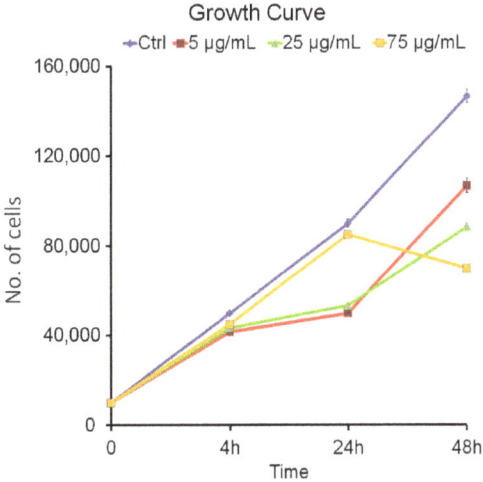

Figure 1. Growth curve in the Hs27 cells was determined by Trypan Blue (counting dye method). The effects of polystyrene nanoparticles (PNPs) exposure were evaluated following exposure at 4, 24, and 48 h at 5, 25, and 75 µg/mL concentrations and compared to the control cells. Error bars represent the standard error of the mean.

The cytotoxicity of the PNPs was measured by the MTS cell viability test, which evaluates the metabolic activation of Hs27 cells after treatment at different concentrations.

The test determines whether cells increase their metabolic activity, measuring the reduction of MTS by a formazan soluble in the culture medium, as MTS reduction only occurs in viable and metabolically active cells. Compared to the control cells, the data at 4 h showed a significant viability increase at 75 µg/mL (about 33%). After 24 h, again, the treatment at 75 µg/mL of PNPs was statistically significant; finally at 48 h, the results showed an increase only at 5 µg/mL PNPs, which was about 20%.

Triton-X-100 0.1% was used as a positive control and induced a significant decrease in viability after 4, 24, and 48 h treatment in PNPs (Figure 2). We speculate that the observed viability trend is not dose dependent and that there is no significant variation in cell viability.

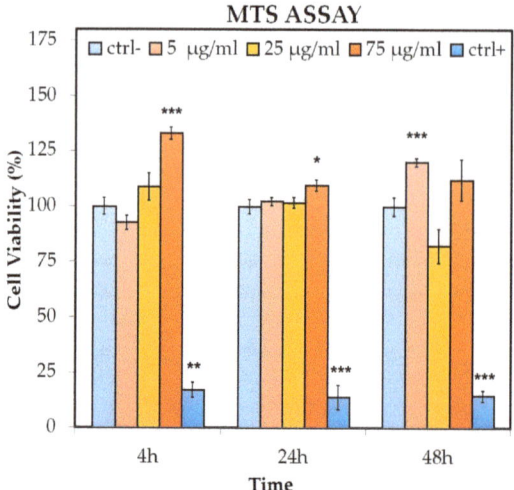

Figure 2. MTS [3-(4,5-dimethylthiazol-2-yl)-5-(3-carboxymethoxyphenyl)-2-(4-sulfophenyl)-2H-tetrazolium] test in Hs27 cells: the effects of polystyrene nanoparticles (PNPs) on cell proliferation were evaluated following exposures at 4, 24, and 48 h at 5, 25, and 75 µg/mL concentrations and compared to the control cells. Triton-X-100 0.1% was used as a positive control. Significance values * = $p < 0.05$; ** = $p < 0.005$; *** = $p < 0.0005$; error bars represent the standard error of the mean.

3.2. Tests of Micronuclei with Block of Cytokinesis with Cytochalasin B "CBMN Assay"

From the data obtained from the micronucleus test, we calculated the CBPI index "Cytokinesis Block Proliferation Index" to evaluate the cellular proliferation progression and therefore the cytostatic and cytotoxic effects, followed by the different concentrations of PNPs (5, 25, and 75 µg/mL).

Compared to the control condition, the CBPI obtained from the cells incubated with the PNPs was, in every condition data, not statistically significant (Figure 3a). Regarding the induction of micronuclei (BNMN), we observed a significant increase dose-dependent at 25 µg/mL and 75 µg/mL where we observed an increase of about 38% and 52%, respectively (Figure 3b). Furthermore, we analyzed the presence of NBUDs (Figure 3c), which originate from the nucleus as extroflections of nucleoplasmic material or as micronuclei connected to the nucleus by a bridge [40]. Our result shows a significant decrease at 5 µg/mL (about 30%) with respect to the control, and on the contrary, an increase at 75 µg/mL of about 50%. In Figure 4, we can see DNA damage as micronuclei and NBUDs in Hs27 cells after PNP treatment.

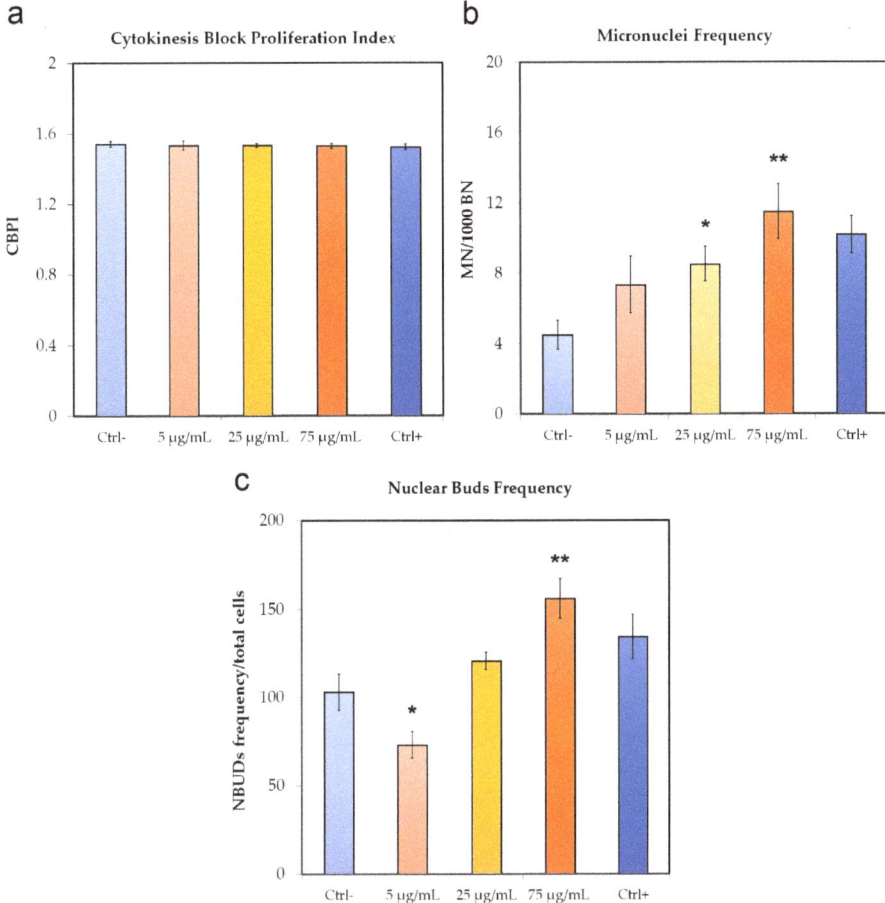

Figure 3. Micronuclei (BNMN), CBPI, and Nuclear Bud (NBUDs) expression in the Hs27 cells treated with polystyrene nanoparticles (PNPs): CBPI, "Cytokinesis Block Proliferation Index" (**a**), Micronuclei (**b**) and Nuclear Buds (**c**) were evaluated at 5, 25, and 75 µg/mL concentrations after exposure to PNPs. CBPI = ((N° mononucleated cells) + (2 × N° binucleated cells) + (3 × N° multinucleated cells))/(total cell number). The number of micronuclei refers to 1000 binucleated cells. The number of Nuclear Buds refers to a total of 1000 binucleated cells. Colchicine (5 µg/mL) was used as a positive control. Significance values * = $p < 0.05$; ** = $p < 0.005$; *** = $p < 0.0005$; error bars represent the standard error of the mean.

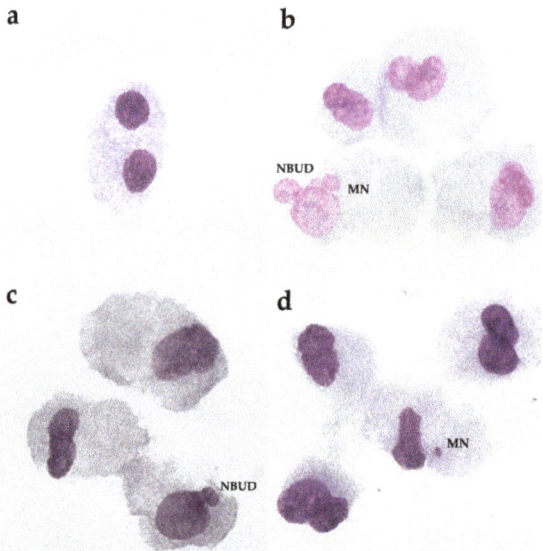

Figure 4. CBMN assay in the Hs27 cells: DNA damage after PNP treatment. (**a**) Binucleated cell, (**b**) cell with micronuclei and nuclear bud, (**c**) cell with nuclear bud, (**d**) cell with micronuclei. Magnification 100×.

3.3. ROS Detection

Time course experiments were performed to comparatively evaluate the possible ROS production in Hs27 cells at different concentrations of PNPs (5, 25, and 75 µg/mL) and PNPs added with an antioxidant extract of *Crocus sativus* stigmas (25 µg/mL). Figure 5a shows that treatment with 5 µg/mL NPs induces highly significant stimulation of ROS production in the cell line, starting from T15 min/T0 of treatment. At T30 min/T0, we statistically increased in ROS production at 5 µg/mL ($p < 0.0005$) and 25 µg/mL ($p < 0.05$) concentrations. The increase ROS level at T1 h/T0 was still statistically significant with respect to the control at 5 µg/mL ($p < 0.005$) and 25 µg/mL ($p < 0.05$) concentrations, but we also noticed that the same concentrations with respect to T30 min/T0 had a strong decrease in ROS production. At T24 h/T0, there are no significant variations in ROS production with respect to the control cells. In Figure 5b, we reported the level of ROS production with PNPs added together with saffron extract: we observed that in the presence of the extract, the ROS production was lower. Significant data obtained by comparing the PNP treatment and PNPs added with saffron are reported in Table 1, and it is noticeable that there was a significant decrease in reactive oxygen species at 5 µg/mL and T15 min/T0, T30 min/T0, and T1 h/T0. In particular at T30 min/T0, we had a ROS decrease by about 30%. Regarding the 25 µg/mL concentration, the results were statistically significant at T30 min/T0 and T1 h/T0 and a ROS reduction of about 18% and 22%, respectively.

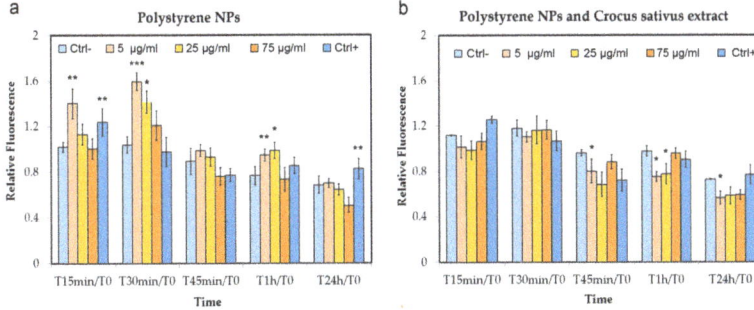

Figure 5. ROS detection in Hs27 cells: the effects of polystyrene nanoparticles (PNPs) on ROS production were evaluated following exposure at 0, 15, 30, 45, 60 min, and after 24 h at 5, 25, and 75 µg/mL concentrations. Each time refers to T0. Hs27 ROS production with PNPs (**a**) and Hs27 ROS production added with antioxidant stigmas extract of *Crocus sativus* (25 µg/mL) (**b**). H_2O_2 (150 µM) was used as a positive control. Significance values * = $p < 0.05$; ** = $p < 0.005$; *** = $p < 0.0005$; error bars represent the standard error of the mean.

Table 1. ROS detection comparison in Hs27 cells treated with polystyrene nanoparticles (PNPs) and PNPs added with the *Crocus sativus* stigmas extract. Values are means ± SD.

Time Ratio	5 µg/mL		P Value	25 µg/mL		P Value
	PNPs	PNPs with *Crocus s.*		PNPs	PNPs with *Crocus s.*	
T15 min/T0	1.4 ± 0.004	1.01 ± 0.004	<0.05	1.13 ± 0.005	0.99 ± 0.002	
T30 min/T0	1.60 ± 1.2 × 10^{-5}	1.10 ± 0.001	<0.0005	1.41 ± 0.007	1.16 ± 0.001	<0.05
T1 h/T0	0.95 ± 0.0013	0.75 ± 0.001	<0.005	0.99 ± 0.007	0.78 ± 0.002	<0.05

3.4. Analysis of PNPs by SEM Scanning Electron Microscopy

PNPs information were obtained by evaluating their morphology and elemental composition. With electron microscopy, we undertook a morphological analysis through different images to test the particle size (Figure 6). Regarding the composition, an investigation was made with EDS microanalysis to assess whether there were impurities such as heavy metals that could affect the experiment. During the analysis of the sample, properly treated, we noticed that polystyrene nanospheres tended to form a reticular structure thanks to their homogeneous shape. Furthermore, it could be seen that the average particle size was around 100 nm, according to the manufacturer's specifications (Figure 6).

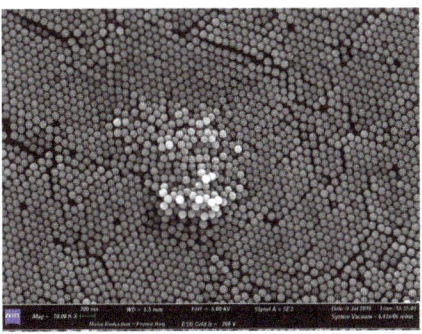

Figure 6. Scanning electron microscopy (SEM): morphological analysis of polystyrene nanoparticles (PNPs) with scanning electron microscopy.

Taking advantage of EDX spectroscopy (energy dispersive x-ray analysis), we evaluated the elemental composition of the sample (Figure 7). The technique provides information on the elemental composition, hence the spectrum only shows the presence of the carbon elements, reinforcing the idea that the only component was polystyrene and oxygen due to the presence of the water residue.

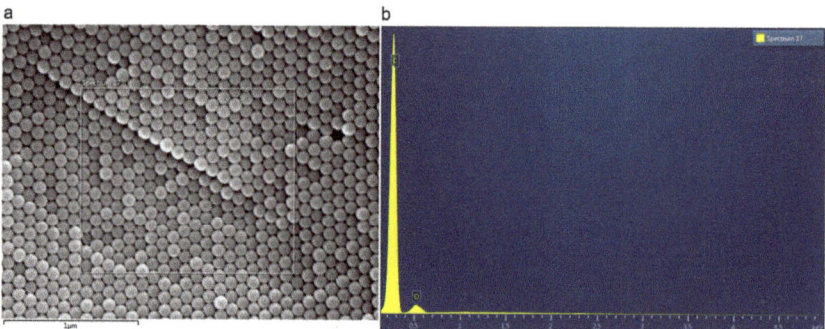

Figure 7. Energy dispersive x-ray analysis (EDX spectroscopy) analysis of polystyrene nanoparticles (PNPs) to characterize elemental composition, area of sample (**a**) and relative elemental spectrum (**b**).

4. Discussion

Global plastic production increases annually [41], with an estimated 4.8 to 12.7 million metric tons of plastic entering the oceans each year [42], posing a threat to seabirds [43], fish [44], turtles [45], and marine mammals [46]. Dispersed plastic is a new emergency for environmental health, and the greatest danger is derived from the products of their degradation. NPs are dispersed in the soil, air, and water; in particular PNPs are the most subjected to degradation. Some new evidence of the toxic potential of PNPs has emerged from the present study, particularly with regard to the genotoxicity.

Tests of the viability of MTS cells by evaluating the metabolic activity of Hs 27 cells exclude an inhibitory action of PNPs on metabolic activity; this activity increased after PNP treatment most likely as a response to cellular stress. This hypothesis is supported by the results of the CBMN tests regarding the treatments with the lowest concentrations of NPs. Genotoxic damage was observed at concentrations above 5 μg/mL, which produced results comparable to MTS tests. Thus, high concentrations of PNPs seem to be necessary to produce appreciable cell damage in relation to exposure times. These in vitro data are quite indicative of the genotoxicity of PNPs and provide indirect evidence of the ability of PNPs to penetrate cells, as widely reported for other particles of similar size to NPs [30] and PNPs [47].

From our results, it is clear that by analyzing the metabolic activity in relation to the production of ROS, treatment with PNPs is able to determine oxidative stress inside the cells. In agreement with the literature [30], the result obtained by us show a high production of ROS within the first 30 min and a decrease afterward, due to the detoxification systems that the cell puts in place. Moreover, we observed that the ROS production decreased when PNPs were added together with the saffron extract. Hence, the free radical scavenging ability of saffron [48] is also expressed in human fibroblasts in which oxidative stress is produced by PNPs. This ability is related to the phenolic/flavonoid contents of saffron *Crocus sativus* L. stigmas known to play a role in preventing oxidative damage caused by free radicals and inhibiting hydrolytic and oxidative enzymes [49]. Thus, the Hs27 human fibroblasts exposed to PNPs suffer damage both in terms of genotoxicity and oxidative stress and the antioxidant power of saffron extract may be able to contrast the ROS formation.

According to the SEM-EDX analysis, PNPs are composed exclusively of C and O, and therefore the physical–chemical properties, and consequently the toxic effects are attributable to the size, shape, surface properties, reactivity, and solubility, all characteristics that influence the ability to induce damage within the cells [50]. The more that particles reach a nanosize, the more their surface area exposed with reactive chemical groups extends.

Our current approach to study the toxicological potential of PNPs raises some important points such as to determine how the particles are internalized by the cells; particles with dimensions of about 100–200 nm are internalized through endocytosis mechanisms, in contrast, larger ones are absorbed through phagocytosis [30,51]. The available information on the toxicity of PNPs in vivo is poor [30,52,53]. In this regard, considering environmental pollution, adverse factors could be invoked for NPs and PNPs such as the risk that they can adsorb, concentrate, and release environmental pollutants into the organisms, thus acting as transporters [54–56].

Author Contributions: Conceptualization, A.P. and G.V.; Methodology, A.P., G.V., M.A., P.D.C., L.A., G.C., and S.C.; Software, G.V., O.Z., P.D.C., S.C., and L.A.; Validation, G.V., S.C., and A.P.; Formal analysis, G.V., O.Z., and P.D.C.; Investigation, G.V., A.P., L.A., M.A., and S.C.; Resources, G.V., G.C., and A.P.; Data curation, G.V., P.D.C., and S.C.; Writing—original draft preparation, A.P., G.V., and S.C.; Writing—review and editing, A.P., P.D.C., and G.V.; Visualization, G.V.; Supervision, A.P. and G.V.; Project administration, A.P. and P.D.C.; Funding acquisition, A.P., G.C., and P.D.C.

Funding: This research received no external funding.

Acknowledgments: We acknowledge Carlo Marinosci for his technical support during the experiments.

Conflicts of Interest: The authors declare no conflicts of interest.

References

1. United Nations Environment Programme. Division of Early Warning, and Assessment. In *UNEP Year Book 2011: Emerging Issues in Our Global Environment*; UNEP/Earthprint: Genève, Switzerland, 2011.
2. Andrady, A.L. Microplastics in the marine environment. *Mar. Pollut. Bull.* **2011**, *62*, 1596–1605. [CrossRef] [PubMed]
3. Cózar, A.; Echevarría, F.; González-Gordillo, J.I.; Irigoien, X.; Úbeda, B.; Hernández-León, S.; Fernández-de-Puelles, M.L. Plastic debris in the open ocean. *Proc. Natl. Acad. Sci. USA* **2014**, *111*, 10239–10244. [CrossRef] [PubMed]
4. Ter Halle, A.; Jeanneau, L.; Martignac, M.; Jardé, E.; Pedrono, B.; Brach, L.; Gigault, J. Nanoplastic in the North Atlantic subtropical gyre. *Environ. Sci. Technol.* **2017**, *51*, 13689–13697. [CrossRef] [PubMed]
5. Mattsson, K.; Jocic, S.; Doverbratt, I.; Hansson, L.A. Nanoplastics in the aquatic environment. In *Microplastic Contamination in Aquatic Environments*; Elsevier: Amsterdam, The Netherlands, 2018; pp. 379–399. [CrossRef]
6. Browne, M.A.; Niven, S.J.; Galloway, T.S.; Rowland, S.J.; Thompson, R.C. Microplastic moves pollutants and additives to worms, reducing functions linked to health and biodiversity. *Curr. Biol.* **2013**, *23*, 2388–2392. [CrossRef] [PubMed]
7. Della Torre, C.; Bergami, E.; Salvati, A.; Faleri, C.; Cirino, P.; Dawson, K.A.; Corsi, I. Accumulation and embryotoxicity of polystyrene nanoparticles at early stage of development of sea urchin embryos Paracentrotus lividus. *Environ. Sci. Technol.* **2014**, *48*, 12302–12311. [CrossRef] [PubMed]
8. Phuong, N.N.; Zalouk-Vergnoux, A.; Poirier, L.; Kamari, A.; Châtel, A.; Mouneyrac, C.; Lagarde, F. Is there any consistency between the microplastics found in the field and those used in laboratory experiments? *Environ. Pollut.* **2016**, *211*, 111–123. [CrossRef] [PubMed]
9. Ma, Y.; Huang, A.; Cao, S.; Sun, F.; Wang, L.; Guo, H.; Ji, R. Effects of nanoplastics and microplastics on toxicity, bioaccumulation, and environmental fate of phenanthrene in fresh water. *Environ. Pollut.* **2016**, *219*, 166–173. [CrossRef] [PubMed]
10. Sussarellu, R.; Suquet, M.; Thomas, Y.; Lambert, C.; Fabioux, C.; Pernet, M.E.J.; Corporeau, C. Oyster reproduction is affected by exposure to polystyrene microplastics. *Proc. Natl. Acad. Sci. USA* **2016**, *113*, 2430–2435. [CrossRef]
11. Li, J.; Qu, X.; Su, L.; Zhang, W.; Yang, D.; Kolandhasamy, P.; Shi, H. Microplastics in mussels along the coastal waters of China. *Environ. Pollut.* **2016**, *214*, 177–184. [CrossRef]
12. Horton, A.A.; Walton, A.; Spurgeon, D.J.; Lahive, E.; Svendsen, C. Microplastics in freshwater and terrestrial environments: Evaluating the current understanding to identify the knowledge gaps and future research priorities. *Sci. Total Environ.* **2017**, *586*, 127–141. [CrossRef]

13. Cole, M.; Galloway, T.S. Ingestion of nanoplastics and microplastics by Pacific oyster larvae. *Environ. Sci. Technol.* **2015**, *49*, 14625–14632. [CrossRef] [PubMed]
14. Cole, M.; Lindeque, P.; Fileman, E.; Halsband, C.; Galloway, T.S. The impact of polystyrene microplastics on feeding, function and fecundity in the marine copepod Calanus helgolandicus. *Environ. Sci. Technol.* **2015**, *49*, 1130–1137. [CrossRef] [PubMed]
15. Gigault, J.; Ter Halle, A.; Baudrimont, M.; Pascal, P.Y.; Gauffre, F.; Phi, T.L.; Reynaud, S. Current opinion: What is a nanoplastic? *Environ. Pollut.* **2018**, *235*, 1030–1034. [CrossRef] [PubMed]
16. Lambert, S.; Wagner, M. Formation of microscopic particles during the degradation of different polymers. *Chemosphere* **2016**, *161*, 510–517. [CrossRef] [PubMed]
17. Alimi, O.S.; Farner Budarz, J.; Hernandez, L.M.; Tufenkji, N. Microplastics and nanoplastics in aquatic environments: Aggregation, deposition, and enhanced contaminant transport. *Environ. Sci. Technol.* **2018**, *52*, 1704–1724. [CrossRef] [PubMed]
18. Bouwmeester, H.; Hollman, P.C.; Peters, R.J. Potential health impact of environmentally released micro-and nanoplastics in the human food production chain: Experiences from nanotoxicology. *Environ. Sci. Technol.* **2015**, *49*, 8932–8947. [CrossRef]
19. Verma, A.; Stellacci, F. Effect of surface properties on nanoparticle–cell interactions. *Small* **2010**, *6*, 12–21. [CrossRef]
20. Wright, S.L.; Kelly, F.J. Plastic and human health: A micro issue? *Environ. Sci. Technol.* **2017**, *51*, 6634–6647. [CrossRef]
21. Ward, J.E.; Kach, D.J. Marine aggregates facilitate ingestion of nanoparticles by suspension-feeding bivalves. *Mar. Environ. Res.* **2009**, *68*, 137–142. [CrossRef]
22. Wegner, A.; Besseling, E.; Foekema, E.M.; Kamermans, P.; Koelmans, A.A. Effects of nanopolystyrene on the feeding behavior of the blue mussel (Mytilus edulis L.). *Environ. Toxic. Chem.* **2012**, *31*, 2490–2497. [CrossRef]
23. Bhattacharya, P.; Lin, S.J.; Turner, J.P.; Ke, P.C. Physical adsorption of charged plastic nanoparticles affects algal photosynthesis. *J. Phys. Chem. C* **2010**, *114*, 16556–16561. [CrossRef]
24. Brillant, M.; MacDonald, B. Postingestive selection in the sea scallop (Placopectenmagellanicus) on the basis of chemical properties of particles. *Mar. Biol.* **2002**, *141*, 457–465. [CrossRef]
25. Cedervall, T.; Hansson, L.A.; Lard, M.; Frohm, B.; Linse, S. Food chain transport of nanoparticles affects behaviour and fat metabolism in fish. *PLoS ONE* **2012**, *7*, e32254. [CrossRef] [PubMed]
26. Hussain, N.; Jani, P.U.; Florence, A.T. Enhanced oral uptake of tomato lectin-conjugated nanoparticles in the rat. *Pharm. Res.* **1997**, *14*, 613–618. [CrossRef] [PubMed]
27. Kulkarni, S.A.; Feng, S.S. Effects of particle size and surface modification on cellular uptake and biodistribution of polymeric nanoparticles for drug delivery. *Pharm. Res.* **2013**, *30*, 2512–2522. [CrossRef] [PubMed]
28. Walczak, A.P.; Kramer, E.; Hendriksen, P.J.; Helsdingen, R.; van der Zande, M.; Rietjens, I.M.; Bouwmeester, H. In vitro gastrointestinal digestion increases the translocation of polystyrene nanoparticles in an in vitro intestinal co-culture model. *Nanotoxicology* **2015**, *9*, 886–894. [CrossRef] [PubMed]
29. EFSA Scientific Committee. Guidance on the risk assessment of the application of nanoscience and nanotechnologies in the food and feed chain. *EFSA J.* **2011**, *9*, 2140. [CrossRef]
30. Saquib, Q.; Faisal, M.; Al-Khedhairy, A.A.; Alatar, A.A. (Eds.) *Cellular and Molecular Toxicology of Nanoparticles*; Springer: New York, NY, USA, 2018; Volume 1048. [CrossRef]
31. Karlsson, H.L. The comet assay in nanotoxicology research. *Anal. Bioanal. Chem.* **2010**, *398*, 651–666. [CrossRef]
32. Xie, H.; Mason, M.M.; Wise, J.P. Genotoxicity of metal nanoparticles. *Rev. Environ. Health* **2011**, *26*, 251–268. [CrossRef]
33. Hernandez, L.M.; Yousefi, N.; Tufenkji, N. Are there nanoplastics in your personal care products? *Environ. Sci. Technol. Lett.* **2017**, *4*, 280–285. [CrossRef]
34. Singh, N.; Manshian, B.; Jenkins, G.J.; Griffiths, S.M.; Williams, P.M.; Maffeis, T.G.; Doak, S.H. NanoGenotoxicology: The DNA damaging potential of engineered nanomaterials. *Biomaterials* **2009**, *30*, 3891–3914. [CrossRef] [PubMed]
35. Anderson, A.G.; Grose, J.; Pahl, S.; Thompson, R.C.; Wyles, K.J. Microplastics in personal care products: Exploring perceptions of environmentalists, beauticians and students. *Marine Pollut. Bullet.* **2016**, *113*, 454–460. [CrossRef] [PubMed]
36. Menghini, L.; Leporini, L.; Vecchiotti, G.; Locatelli, M.; Carradori, S.; Ferrante, C.; Brunetti, L. Crocus sativus L. stigmas and byproducts: Qualitative fingerprint, antioxidant potentials and enzyme inhibitory activities. *Food Res. Int.* **2018**, *109*, 91–98. [CrossRef] [PubMed]

37. Lahmass, I.; Lamkami, T.; Delporte, C.; Sikdar, S.; Van Antwerpen, P.; Saalaoui, E.; Megalizzi, V. The waste of saffron crop, a cheap source of bioactive compounds. *J. Funct. Foods* **2017**, *35*, 341–351. [CrossRef]
38. Cory, A.H.; Owen, T.C.; Barltrop, J.A.; Cory, J.G. Use of an aqueous soluble tetrazolium/formazan assay for cell growth assays in culture. *Cancer Commun.* **1991**, *3*, 207–212. [CrossRef] [PubMed]
39. Fenech, M. Cytokinesis-block micronucleus cytome assay. *Nat. Protoc.* **2007**, *2*, 1084–1104. [CrossRef] [PubMed]
40. OECD Guidelines for the Testing of Chemicals, Section 4: Health Effects. Test No. 487. Vitro Mammalian Cell Micronucleus Test. Available online: www.oecd-ilibrary.org (accessed on 4 September 2019).
41. Andrady, A.L.; Neal, M.A. Applications and Societal Benefits of Plastics. *Philos. Trans. R. Soc. Lond. Ser. B* **2009**, *364*, 1977–1984. [CrossRef] [PubMed]
42. Jambeck, J.R.; Geyer, R.; Wilcox, C.; Siegler, T.R.; Perryman, M.; Andrady, A.; Narayan, R.; Law, K.L. Marine pollution. Plastic waste inputs from land into the ocean. *Science* **2015**, *347*, 768–771. [CrossRef] [PubMed]
43. Wilcox, C.; Van Sebille, E.; Hardesty, B.D. Threat of plastic pollution to seabirds is global, pervasive, and increasing. *Proc. Natl. Acad. Sci. USA* **2015**, *112*, 11899–11904. [CrossRef] [PubMed]
44. Gregory, M.R. Environmental implications of plastic debris in marine settings—Entanglement, ingestion, smothering, hangers-on, hitch-hiking and alien invasions. *Philos. Trans. R. Soc. Lond. Ser. B Biol. Sci.* **2009**, *364*, 2013–2025. [CrossRef] [PubMed]
45. Mrosovsky, N.; Ryan, G.D.; James, M.C. Leatherback turtles: The menace of plastic. *Mar. Pollut. Bull.* **2009**, *58*, 287–289. [CrossRef] [PubMed]
46. Laist, D.W. Impacts of marine debris: Entanglement of marine life in marine debris including a comprehensive list of species with entanglement and ingestion records. In *Marine Debris*; Springer: New York, NY, USA, 1997; pp. 99–139. [CrossRef]
47. Mishra, P.; Vinayagam, S.; Duraisamy, K.; Patil, S.R.; Godbole, J.; Mohan, A.; Chandrasekaran, N. Distinctive impact of polystyrene nano-spherules as an emergent pollutant toward the environment. *Environ. Sci. Poll. Res.* **2019**, *26*, 1537–1547. [CrossRef] [PubMed]
48. Bukhari, S.I.; Manzoor, M.; Dhar, M.K. A comprehensive review of the pharmacological potential of *Crocus sativus* and its bioactive apocarotenoids. *Biomed. Pharmacother.* **2018**, *98*, 733–745. [CrossRef] [PubMed]
49. Frankel, E.N. Nutritional benefits of flavonoids. In *Food Factors for Cancer Prevention*; Springer: Tokyo, Japan, 1997; pp. 613–616. [CrossRef]
50. Xia, T.; Kovochich, M.; Brant, J.; Hotze, M.; Sempf, J.; Oberley, T.; Nel, A.E. Comparison of the abilities of ambient and manufactured nanoparticles to induce cellular toxicity according to an oxidative stress paradigm. *Nano Lett.* **2006**, *6*, 1794–1807. [CrossRef] [PubMed]
51. Rabinovitch, M. Professional and non-professional phagocytes: An introduction. *Trends Cell Biol.* **1995**, *5*, 85–87. [CrossRef]
52. Rodriguez-Seijo, A.; Lourenço, J.; Rocha-Santos, T.A.P.; Da Costa, J.; Duarte, A.C.; Vala, H.; Pereira, R. Histopathological and molecular effects of microplastics in *Eisenia andrei* Bouché. *Environ. Pollut.* **2017**, *220*, 495–503. [CrossRef] [PubMed]
53. Pedà, C.; Caccamo, L.; Fossi, M.C.; Gai, F.; Andaloro, F.; Genovese, L.; Maricchiolo, G. Intestinal alterations in European sea bass *Dicentrarchus labrax* (Linnaeus, 1758) exposed to microplastics: Preliminary results. *Environ. Pollut.* **2016**, *212*, 251–256. [CrossRef]
54. Chua, E.M.; Shimeta, J.; Nugegoda, D.; Morrison, P.D.; Clarke, B.O. Assimilation of polybrominated diphenyl ethers from microplastics by the marine amphipod, *Allorchestes compressa*. *Environ. Sci. Technol.* **2014**, *48*, 8127–8134. [CrossRef]
55. Koelmans, A.A.; Besseling, E.; Foekema, E.M. Leaching of plastic additives to marine organisms. *Environ. Pollut.* **2014**, *187*, 49–54. [CrossRef]
56. Nowack, B.; Ranville, J.F.; Diamond, S.; Gallego-Urrea, J.A.; Metcalfe, C.; Rose, J.; Horne, N.; Koelmans, A.A.; Klaine, S.J. Potential scenarios for nanomaterial release and subsequent alteration in the environment. *Environ. Toxicol. Chem.* **2012**, *31*, 50–59. [CrossRef]

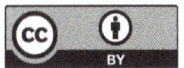

© 2019 by the authors. Licensee MDPI, Basel, Switzerland. This article is an open access article distributed under the terms and conditions of the Creative Commons Attribution (CC BY) license (http://creativecommons.org/licenses/by/4.0/).

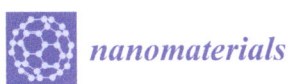

Article

Effects of Titanium Dioxide Nanoparticles on the *Hprt* Gene Mutations in V79 Hamster Cells

Alena Kazimirova [1,*], Naouale El Yamani [2], Laura Rubio [3], Alba García-Rodríguez [4], Magdalena Barancokova [1], Ricard Marcos [4,5] and Maria Dusinska [2,*]

1. Department of Biology, Faculty of Medicine, Slovak Medical University, 833 03 Bratislava, Slovakia; magdalena.barancokova@szu.sk
2. Health Effects Laboratory, Department of Environmental Chemistry, NILU-Norwegian Institute for Air Research, N-2027 Kjeller, Norway; ney@nilu.no
3. Nanobiology Laboratory, Department of Natural and Exact Sciences, Pontificia Universidad Católica Madre y Maestra, PUCMM, 80677 Santiago de los Caballeros, Dominican Republic; l.rubio@ce.pucmm.edu.do
4. Department of Genetics and Microbiology, Faculty of Biosciences, Universitat Autònoma de Barcelona, 08193 Cerdanyola del Vallès (Barcelona), Spain; albagr.garcia@gmail.com (A.G.-R.); ricard.marcos@uab.es (R.M.)
5. Consortium for Biomedical Research in Epidemiology and Public Health (CIBERESP), Carlos III Institute of Health, 28029 Madrid, Spain
* Correspondence: alena.kazimirova@szu.sk (A.K.); mdu@nilu.no (M.D.)

Received: 31 January 2020; Accepted: 28 February 2020; Published: 5 March 2020

Abstract: The genotoxicity of anatase/rutile TiO_2 nanoparticles (TiO_2 NPs, NM105 at 3, 15 and 75 $\mu g/cm^2$) was assessed with the mammalian in-vitro Hypoxanthine guanine phosphoribosyl transferase (*Hprt*) gene mutation test in Chinese hamster lung (V79) fibroblasts after 24 h exposure. Two dispersion procedures giving different size distribution and dispersion stability were used to investigate whether the effects of TiO_2 NPs depend on the state of agglomeration. TiO_2 NPs were fully characterised in the previous European FP7 projects NanoTEST and NanoREG2. Uptake of TiO_2 NPs was measured by transmission electron microscopy (TEM). TiO_2 NPs were found in cytoplasmic vesicles, as well as close to the nucleus. The internalisation of TiO_2 NPs did not depend on the state of agglomeration and dispersion used. The cytotoxicity of TiO_2 NPs was measured by determining both the relative growth activity (RGA) and the plating efficiency (PE). There were no substantial effects of exposure time (24, 48 and 72 h), although a tendency to lower RGA at longer exposure was observed. No significant difference in PE values and no increases in the *Hprt* gene mutant frequency were found in exposed relative to unexposed cultures in spite of evidence of uptake of NPs by cells.

Keywords: titanium dioxide nanoparticles; V79 cells; genotoxicity; *Hprt*

---

1. Introduction

Nano-sized or ultrafine titanium dioxide particles (TiO_2 NPs) are among the most widely used nanomaterials. TiO_2 is a poorly soluble particulate material with numerous applications such as food colorant or white pigment in the production of paints, paper, plastics, ink and welding rod-coating material. TiO_2 NPs (<100 nm) are increasingly used in other industrial products, such as cosmetics, skin care products (in sunscreens, as an ultraviolet blocking agent), toothpaste, and pharmaceuticals [1–4]. It can even be used as a food additive, for example to whiten skimmed milk [5]. Therefore, potential widespread exposure may occur during manufacturing and use [6].

Whether TiO_2NPs represent any hazard to humans is a question addressed by various regulatory agencies. Genotoxicity studies of TiO_2NPs have been widely performed detecting different types of DNA damage such as strand breaks and various DNA lesions (using mostly the comet assay), gene mutations in bacteria and in mammalian cells, as well as chromosomal damage representing possible clastogenic or aneugenic effects. However, in-vivo and in-vitro studies have reported conflicting results; some indicate that TiO$_2$ NPs are genotoxic [6–9], whereas others give negative results [8,10–12]. This inconsistency is related to the different particle types used, with different NP sizes and physico-chemical properties, NP dispersion and exposure conditions, as well as to the use of different cell culture media, cellular models, and test methods [13–16]. Most of genotoxic effects are seen in cells derived from the respiratory, and the circulatory systems. Where internal exposure of the lungs can occur, there is a possibility that TiO$_2$ NP may exert genotoxic effects, most probably through secondary mechanisms (e.g. oxidative stress); however, direct interaction with the genetic material cannot be excluded. Overall, the studies indicating that TiO$_2$ NPs are genotoxic outweigh the studies that state otherwise. According to that, TiO$_2$ NPs can be treated as potentially hazardous compounds [5] consistent with the fact that TiO$_2$ itself is classified as a class 2B carcinogen [17].

The mammalian gene mutation tests belong to the set of assays recommended by the regulatory bodies and, in nanomaterial genotoxicity testing, they are preferred since the Ames test is not suitable due to the size of bacteria (comparable with NPs themselves) and the fact that the bacterial wall limits significantly the uptake of NPs [14,18]. The most commonly used target genes for measuring the induction of mutations in mammalian cells are the thymidine kinase (*Tk*) and the hypoxanthine guanine phosphoribosyl transpherase (*Hprt*) genes. Specifically, the *Hprt* mutation assay has already been successfully applied to the evaluation of different nanomaterials [6,18–21].

With regard to studies using TiO$_2$ NPs to induce *Hprt* mutants, previous studies have already been reported, where positive effects were observed in the WIL2-NS human B-cell lymphoblastoid cell line (24 h exposure of 130 µg/mL UF-TiO$_2$) [6], and in V79-4 hamster cells (2 h of short-term treatment of 20 and 100 µg/mL anatase TiO$_2$ NPs [7]. Interestingly, negative results were obtained with anatase TiO$_2$ NPs (10–40 µg/mL) in a long-term (60 days) exposure experiment. In that case, Chinese hamster ovary cells (CHO-K1) cells appear to adapt to chronic exposure to TiO$_2$ NPs and detoxify the excess of reactive oxygen species (ROS), possibly through an up-regulation of super oxide dismutase (SOD), in addition to reducing particle uptake [10].

In this context, the aim of our work is to investigate whether TiO$_2$ NPs induce mutagenic effect in the *Hprt* gene, and whether this effect depends on the dispersion procedure used, e.g. on different states of agglomeration.

2. Material and Methods

2.1. Cells

V79-4 adherent hamster cells isolated from the lung of a normal Chinese hamster (male), were purchased from European Collection of Authenticated Cell Cultures (ECACC, catalogue number 86041102). Cells were cultured in Dulbecco's minimal essential medium (DMEM) D6046 (Sigma, Steinheim, Germany) supplemented with 10% (v/v) heat-inactivated fetal bovine serum (FBS, Gibco, Grand Island, NY, USA) and 1% (v/v) penicillin-streptomycin (Gibco) at 37 °C in a 5% CO$_2$ humidified atmosphere. Cells were thawed and sub-cultured 2–4 times before use in the experiments, at an initial density of 2×10^5 cells/mL in vented T-75 cm^2 flasks. Cultures were maintained with density not exceeding 1×10^6 cells/mL at the time of passage. Cells were seeded 24 h to reach 50–70% confluence before exposure to test substance. Trypan blue assay was used to check cell viability after trypsinization of cells.

2.2. Nanoparticle Characterization, Dispersion and Cell Exposure

TiO$_2$ NP (NM-105), an anatase/rutile nanopowder of nominal size 21 nm (15–60 nm), was received from the EU Joint Research Centre (Ispra, Italy). It was manufactured by Evonik (Essen, Germany), and marketed as Aeroxide TiO$_2$ P-25. TiO$_2$ NPs were fully characterised in previous EU projects [13,22], and results are summarised in Table 1.

Table 1. Summary of primary physical and chemical properties of the used TiO$_2$ NPs NM-105 [13].

Type of Characteristics	Properties of NM-105
Phase	White ultra-fine powder
Shape of particles	Irregular/ellipsoidal
Particle size (nm)	15–60
Crystal structure	Anatase/Rutile in ratio of 70:30 or 80:20
Surface area (m^2/g)	61
Pore volume (mL/g)	0.13
Zeta-potential at pH 7 (mV)	−30.2
Chemical composition of particles	Ti, O
Ti purity of particles	>99%
Surface chemistry	Uncoated
Impurities of concern	Co (920 ppm), Fe (16 ppm)

For the treatment of cells we used TiO$_2$ NP dispersed by two different procedures, either with or without serum in stock solution. This can permit investigations on how the state of aggregation/agglomeration and stability of the dispersion could influence TiO$_2$ NP cytotoxicity and genotoxicity.

Dispersion Procedure DP1

Stock suspensions of TiO$_2$ NPs at 5 mg/mL were freshly prepared for each experiment, using the dispersion procedure DP1 developed as part of the FP7 project NanoTEST. For 1 mL of stock suspension, 5 mg of TiO$_2$ NPs mixed with 1 mL of 10% fetal bovine serum (FBS, Gibco) in PBS (phosphate buffered saline) in a glass tube was sonicated using an ultrasonic probe sonicator (Labsonic, Sartorius, Gottingen Germany) at 100 W for 15 min on ice/water. This suspension was added to cell culture medium. Serial dilutions were made in cell culture medium to obtain the full range of NP suspensions, from 3 to 75 µg/cm^2, which were then immediately added to cells.

Dispersion Procedure DP2

In DP2, 20 mg of TiO$_2$ NPs was suspended in 10 mL of culture medium with 15 mM HEPES buffer and without FBS (the procedure developed at University Paris Diderot France [13]). The suspension was sonicated using the ultrasonic probe sonicator at 60 W for 3 min on ice/water, vortexed for 10 s, and within 2 min of sonication—aliquoted and stored at −20 °C for further use. TiO$_2$ NP suspension aliquots were thawed just before use, vortexed for 10 s, sonicated at 60 W for 1 min on ice/water and added to cell culture medium. Serial dilutions were made in cell culture medium to obtain the full range of TiO$_2$ NP suspensions from 3 to 75 µg/cm^2, which were then immediately added to cells.

2.3. Extrinsic Properties of TiO$_2$ NPs

Particle size, size distribution, state of agglomeration and stability of TiO$_2$ NPs, both in stock solution as well as in culture medium, were characterized by Nanoparticle Tracking Analysis (NTA) using NanoSight NS 500 (NanoSight Limited, Netherhampton, Salisbury, UK). Table 2 shows size, agglomeration state and stability in culture medium measured by Dynamic Light Scattering DLS [22].

Table 2. Average hydrodynamic diameters determined, by Dynamic Light Scattering (DLS), of the obtained TiO$_2$ NPs stock dispersions [22].

Medium	TiO$_2$ Stock Dispersion DP1	TiO$_2$ Stock Dispersion DP2
DMEM +10% FBS	Bimodal distribution, 112 (± 20) nm and 296 (± 55) nm	752 (± 397) nm
Size stability after 48 h	Stable ~2 days 125 (± 27) nm and 366 (± 65) nm	Large Agglomerates

DMEM—Dulbecco's minimal essential medium; FBS—fetal bovine serum.

2.4. Cellular Uptake

Cellular uptake of TiO$_2$ NPs was measured by transmission electron microscopy (TEM). V79-4 cells were grown on 6-well plates at a density of 1.75×10^5 cells/well. Cells were exposed to TiO$_2$ NPs dispersed according to DP1 and DP2 (3, 10, 30 µg/cm^2) for 24 h. At the end of the exposure time, cells were centrifuged, fixed in 2.5% (v/v) glutaraldehyde (EM grade, Merck, Darmstadt, Germany) and 2% (w/v) paraformaldehyde (EMS, Hatfield, PA, USA) in 0.1 M cacodylate buffer at pH 7.4 (PB, Sigma-Aldrich, Steinheim, Germany), and processed following conventional procedures, as previously described [23]. Samples were first post-fixed with osmium tetroxide, dehydrated in acetone, later embedded in Epon, and finally polymerized at 60 °C, and cut with an ultramicrotome Leica EM UC6 using a diamond knife and mounted on copper grids. Before image acquisition, sections were stained using uranyl acetate and Reynolds lead-citrate solutions. All images were examined using a JEOL 1400 (JEOL LTC, Tokyo, Japan) TEM at 120 kV equipped with a CCD GATAN ES1000W Erlangshen camera.

2.5. Relative Growth Activity (RGA)

RGA measurements are based on cell proliferation activity of the cells during a period of treatment or after treatment with the tested compound. Cells were seeded at concentration 1×10^5 cells per well on 12-well plates in 2 mL culture medium and were kept for 24 h under standard conditions at 37 °C in a 5% CO$_2$ humidified atmosphere. Cells were then exposed to different concentrations (ranging from 0.12 to 75 µg/cm^2) of TiO$_2$ NPs lasting for 24, 48, and 72 h. Untreated cells, just with cell culture medium, were used as a negative control and hydrogen peroxide (H$_2$O$_2$, 100 µM, 5 min in PBS) was used as a positive control. Just after exposure, medium was removed from the culture and cells were washed with PBS, trypsinized, and re-suspended in 1 mL of medium. Finally, 10 µL of the final cell suspension was mixed with 10 µL of 0.4% trypan blue (Life Technologies, OR, USA) to determine the percentage of viable cells (unstained) and stained cells with damaged membranes. This determination was carried out using a Countess™ Automated Cell Counter (Invitrogen). RGA was calculated as already published [24].

2.6. Plating Efficiency (PE)

To determine the potential cytotoxic effects of the treatment, after 24 h exposure of V79-4 cells to TiO$_2$ NPs, they were washed, trypsinized and counted, as described above. After that, 50 cells per well were inoculated in 6-well plates (for each concentration tested one plate was used) and incubated at 37 °C for 7 days. Untreated cells, just with cell culture medium, were used as a negative control. Finally, cells were stained by using 1% methylene blue (Sigma) and the number of resulting colonies was counted manually. PE values were calculated according to the formula:

$$PE\ (\%) = \frac{number\ of\ colonies\ in\ exposed\ cultures}{number\ of\ colonies\ in\ unexposed\ cultures} \times 100\%$$

2.7. Hprt Mammalian Gene Mutation Assay

The mammalian in vitro *Hprt* gene mutation test was performed according to the OECD Guidelines for the Testing of Chemicals 476 [25]. V79-4 cells were cultured in 100 mm diameter Petri dishes; 1×10^6 cells were inoculated per dish in 10 mL medium in duplicate for each concentration, and incubated at

37 °C. On the following day, the cells were exposed to TiO$_2$ NPs for 24 h, at concentrations from 3 to 75 µg/cm^2.

Untreated cells cultured in medium for 24 h were used as negative control and cells treated for 3h with 0.1 mM methyl methanesulfonate (MMS; Sigma), served as the positive control.

After exposure, the medium was removed, and cells were washed, trypsinized and re-suspended in 2 mL of medium. They were then seeded in 100 mm diameter Petri dishes at 3×10^5 cells/dish, 3 dishes per concentration. Cells were grown for 8 days, during which they were subcultured three times; duplicate samples were taken at 6 and 8 days after treatment for analysis of mutant frequencies. To detect mutants, cells were inoculated in 100 mm diameter Petri dishes at 2×10^5 cells/dish, 5 dishes per sample giving a total of 10^6 cells per sample and grown in medium containing 6-thioguanine (Sigma) at 5 µg/mL for 10 days to form colonies. 6-Thioguanine is an analogue of guanine, toxic to cells with functioning *Hprt* gene, and so only *Hprt*$^-$ cells survive. Mutant colonies were counted manually after staining with 1% methylene blue; only colonies with at least 50 cells were counted.

For each of the two harvests (6 and 8 day duplicate samples), the frequency of surviving cells was assessed using the PE assay, as described above. Treated and untreated cells were seeded in 6-well plates at 50 cells per well, 1 plate per concentration, and incubated for 7 days at 37 °C to form colonies. Cell viability was calculated for each mutant harvest on the basis of the number of colonies as a percentage of the number of inoculated cells. The mutant frequency was determined as previously described [24].

2.8. Statistical Analysis

One way analysis of variance ANOVA test was used, followed by Dunnett´s multiple comparison test for the post hoc analysis. Prism 7.0 (GraphPad Software, San Diego, CA, USA) and Microsoft Excel 2013 were used for statistics and mathematical analysis. Differences with $P < 0.05$ were considered statistically significant.

3. Results

3.1. TiO$_2$ Characterization, Extrinsic Properties

As NPs change their properties depending on the surrounding environment, we also measured extrinsic properties of TiO$_2$ NPs. We also aimed to identify whether size and stability of dispersion can influence the potential effect. The size distribution, state of agglomeration and stability of the tested TiO$_2$ NPs were analysed in culture medium before the treatment and immediately after the treatment (times 0 and 24 h) by using NTA measured by NanoSight NS 500. The average size of the TiO$_2$ NPs in DMEM at time 0, was 228 ± 3.2 nm, and 184 ± 3.5 nm, for DP1 and DP2, respectively. After 24 h, the mean size of TiO$_2$ NPs prepared by DP1 was 154.1 ± 6.7, while TiO$_2$ NPs prepared by DP2 had an average size of 217 ± 3.6 showing relatively stable dispersion for both DPs, as showed in Figure 1. After 24 h, the TiO$_2$ NPs dispersion DP2 was similar to time 0 h, but when we compare the concentration of particles per mL between time 0 and 24 h, a decrease in the concentration was observed. Extrinsic characteristics of size, size distribution, and the level of agglomeration/aggregation of NPs in dispersions measured by DLS are described in Table 2.

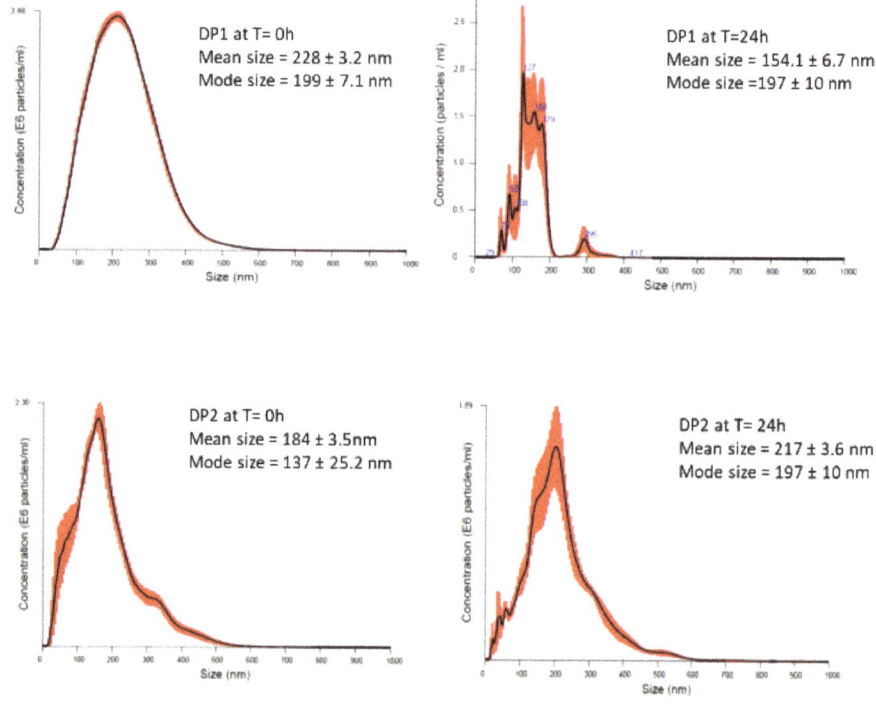

Figure 1. Particle size distribution obtained by (NTA) of TiO$_2$ NPs using the two proposed dispersion procedures (DP1 and DP2) in culture medium at 0 and 24 h. The black line is the mean distribution and the red filling represent standard errors between captured videos.

3.2. Uptake of TiO$_2$ NPs Measured by the TEM

The potential cell uptake of TiO$_2$ NPs was investigated in V79-4 cells after exposures to 3, 10 and 30 µg/cm^2 of the TiO$_2$ NPs prepared using both dispersion procedures. Figure 2 shows that after 24 h of TiO$_2$ NPs exposure they were taken up mostly as agglomerates and these were found in cytoplasm and vesicles. Agglomerates of TiO$_2$ NPs were also detected in contact with the cell nucleus even when low concentrations of TiO$_2$ NPs were used. It seems that the uptake of TiO$_2$ NPs did not depend on the used dispersion since there was no difference in uptake of TiO$_2$ NPs, whichever dispersion procedure was used.

3.3. Cytotoxic Effect of TiO$_2$ NPs on V79-4 Cells

An important endpoint for measuring the effect of NPs on cells is cytotoxicity. In our study the cytotoxicity of TiO$_2$ NPs in V79-4 cells was measured by determining both the RGA and the PE values. RGA measures cytotoxicity in population of cells, while the PE gives information on individual cell toxicity. RGA values were determined as the ratio between the number of living cells, after exposures lasting for 24, 48 and 72 h, versus the number of living cells in the unexposed cultures. Figure 3 shows that, in general, TiO$_2$ NPs exposures were not excessively toxic with rather more marked effects when DP1 was used. In addition, no significant effects of exposure time were seen, although there was a tendency to observe higher effects at longer exposure times.

The PE values were determined as the ratio of the number of colonies observed in the exposed cultures versus those observed in the unexposed cultures. Exposure lasted for 24 h and colonies were counted after 7 days of growth. As shown in Figure 4, no significant differences were observed between the negative control and each of the concentrations used (3, 15 and 75 µg/cm^2). In addition, no differences in PE values were observed between the two dispersion procedures.

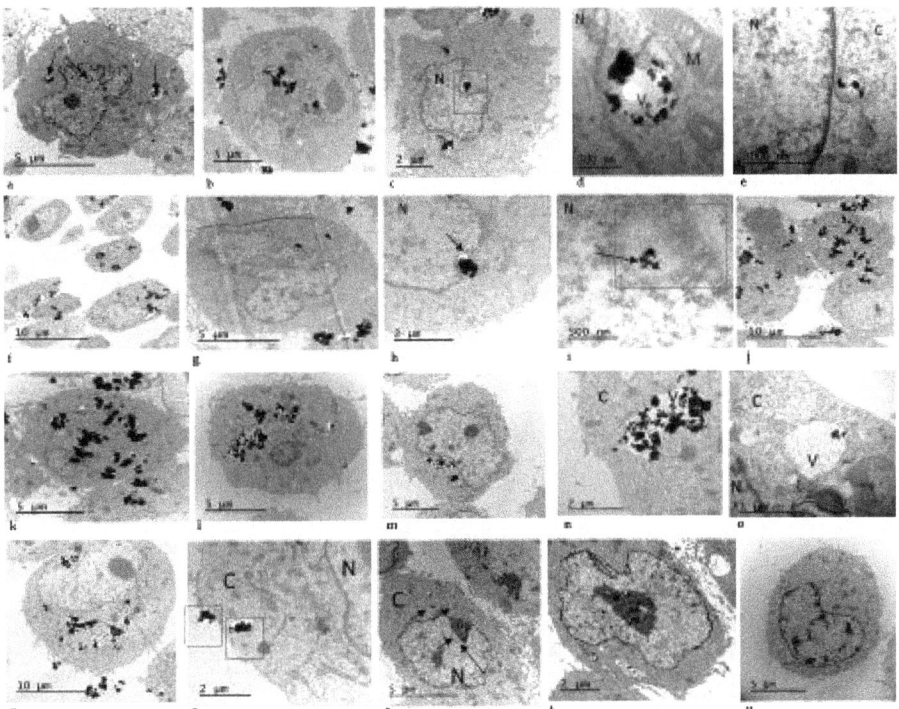

Figure 2. Representative transmission electron microscopy (TEM) figures of titanium dioxide TiO$_2$ NM105 uptake by Chinese hamster lung fibroblast (V79-4) cells exposed to 3, 10 and 30 µg/cm^2 of TiO$_2$ NPs dispersed according to dispersion procedure 1 (DP1) and dispersion procedure 2 (DP2). DP1 3 µg/cm^2 (**a–e**), DP1 10 µg/cm^2 (**f–i**), DP1 30 µg/cm^2 (**j,k**), DP2 3 µg/cm^2 (**l–o**), DP2 10 µg/cm^2 (**p–r**), DP2 30 µg/cm^2 (**s,t**), Negative control untreated V79-4 cells (**u**). N = nucleus; C = cytoplasm; V = vesicle, M = mitochondrion.

3.4. Mammalian Hprt Gene Mutation Assay, the Effect After TiO$_2$ NPs Exposure

Genotoxicity is one of the most crucial effects that should be investigated in assessing safety of chemicals including NPs and it covers several genotoxicity endpoints, namely gene mutations, and structural and numerical chromosome aberrations. In our study we assessed the mutation potential of TiO$_2$ NPs in V79-4 cells in two different experiments for each harvest point. As observed in Figure 5, there were no significant differences between the negative control and any of the three (3, 15 and 75 µg/cm^2) concentrations used. This observed lack of mutagenic effects was independent of the dispersion used. In contrast, the positive control (MMS, 0.1 mM, 3 h) showed a clear induction of *Hprt* mutants, supporting the validity of the assay, and confirming the lack of mutagenic potential of the TiO$_2$ NPs, at least under our experimental conditions.

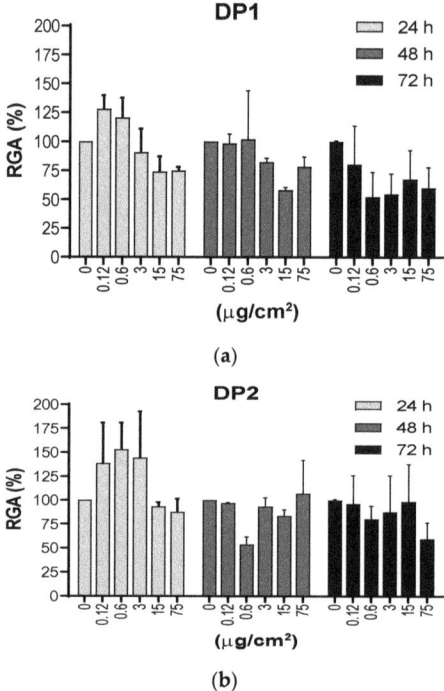

Figure 3. (**a**) and (**b**). Cytotoxic effects measured as the relative growth activity (RGA %) on V79-4 cells exposed to TiO_2 NPs prepared using the two dispersion procedures (DP1 and DP2). Cells were treated with 5 concentrations ($\mu g/cm^2$) of TiO_2 NPs for 24, 48 and 72 h, and the cell numbers were counted at each time point immediately, following trypan blue staining. There were no statistical significances between exposed and unexposed cultures. Cytotoxicity of MMS was not been observed (RGA = 70%). Data are expressed as the means ± SEM of two parallel experiments, according to the used procedures.

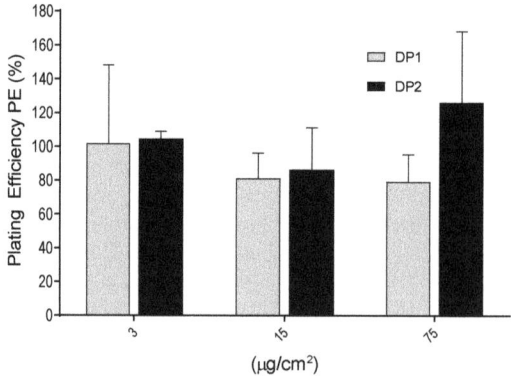

Figure 4. Cytotoxic effects of TiO_2 NPs measured by the plating efficiency (PE %) in V79-4 cells. Bars represent cytotoxicity relative to 100% of untreated cells Data are expressed as the means ± SEM of two parallel seedings for plating efficiency, according to the used procedure. No statistical significances between exposed and unexposed cultures were observed.

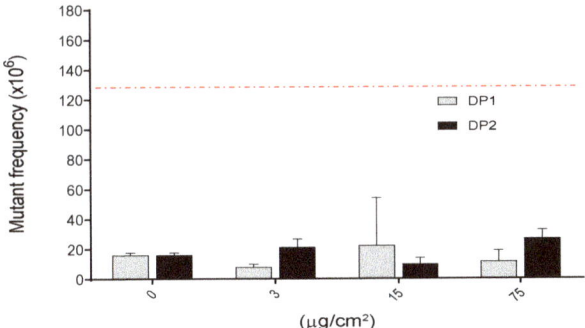

Figure 5. Induction of *Hprt* gene mutants after the exposure of V79-4 cells to different concentrations of TiO$_2$ NPs for 24 h. There were no statistical significances between exposed and unexposed cultures. *Hprt* gene mutant frequency in treated cells with positive control MMS (0.1 mM, 3 h), which gave 131.6 ± 2.30 *Hprt* gene mutants. This value is indicated as a red-dashed line. Data are expressed as the means ± SEM of two parallel seedings for mutation frequency MF1 and MF2, according to the used procedure.

4. Discussion

In-vitro toxicology data, based on well-designed experiments are required for risk assessment strategies designed for the testing of engineered nanomaterials. Until now, while in-vitro tests have been successfully applied in nanotoxicology studies, reference and quality standards are not always included: determination of physico-chemical properties, a range of appropriate controls (including stabilizer controls) and representative cell models, among other aspects, are crucially important.

Furthermore, physical processes in the preparation of the nanomaterials to be tested, such as dissolution, aggregation and sedimentation must be taken into consideration to better understand the mechanism of ENM toxicity [26]. In our study, the effects of TiO$_2$ NPs were compared using two different DPs: one with serum in the stock solution and one without, in order to investigate whether the dispersion procedure and dispersion components could influence NP cytotoxicity and genotoxicity. In addition, we have evaluated the genotoxic potency by detecting their ability to induce gene mutations at the *Hprt* locus. It should be noted that the evaluation of the genotoxic potential of TiO$_2$ NPs has been the subject of different reviews [16,27–30].

The *Hprt* gene mutation assay has been widely used in human biomonitoring and this target seems to be a valuable biomarker to determine the genotoxic/carcinogenic risk of exposures [31]. Accordingly, the mammalian gene mutation test is considered a surrogate in vitro marker for use in cancer risk assessment, together with the micronucleus assay. The use of the *Hprt* forward gene mutation assay allows the quantification of a wide set of genetic changes such as base substitutions, amplifications, or small deletions. This assay has already been used to determine the mutagenicity of TiO$_2$ NPs in different types of cells [6,7,10,32]. Thus, in cultured WIL2-NS cells, a human B-cell lymphoblastoid cell line, ultrafine TiO$_2$ particles (<100 nm in diameter) induced approximately 2.5-fold increases in the mutation frequency, in addition to significant toxicity [6]. However, negative results were obtained when TiO$_2$ NPs were evaluated in Chinese hamster ovary (CHO-K1) cells subject to chronic exposures of up to 60 days [10]. In such cells no cytotoxic effects were apparent using the XTT (2,3-bis(2-methoxy-4-nitro-5-sulfophenyl)22H-tetrazolium-5-caboxyanilide), trypan-blue exclusion, and colony-forming assays for viability and, in addition, no variations in the frequency of *Hprt* mutations were reported. Finally, the *Hprt* assay has also been used in V79 cells to determine the mutagenic potential of TiO$_2$ NPs, showing a clear dose-dependent effect [7,32]. This disparity in the obtained results would support the view that there are many factors affecting the outcome when the genotoxicity of NPs in general, and TiO$_2$ NPs in particular, is evaluated. It is important to point out that, in spite of the reported contradictory data, TiO$_2$ NPs are well taken up by mammalian cells, including V79 cells. In this case, our positive uptake findings have been confirmed by a recent study using flow cytometric analysis and TEM in the same cell line [32]. In this study TEM micrographs showed the internalization (confirmed by SEM/EDX analysis) of TiO$_2$ NPs in the cytoplasm inducing ultra-structural changes such as swollen mitochondria and nuclear membrane disruption.

The ability of TiO$_2$ NPs to produce gene mutants has also been tested using gene targets other than the *Hprt* gene. Thus, the mouse lymphoma assay targeting the *Tk* gene was used to determine the mutagenicity of TiO$_2$ NPs, with negative results [33]. These negative results were obtained independently of the presence/absence of the microsomal S9 fraction in the culture medium.

As previously indicated, the *Hprt* assay has also been used to evaluate the genotoxic potential of other nanomaterials. Thus, by using silver nanomaterials it was shown that such NPs were mutagenic in V79-4 cells and, interestingly, this effect depended on their size [26]. On the other hand, amorphous silica NPs were evaluated for the detection of both *Hprt* mutants and ROS production in V79 cells, with negative results [34]. Furthermore, when multi wall carbon nanotubes were tested in the dose-range of 0.12 to 12 μg/cm^2, significant cellular uptake was observed by using transmission electron microscopy. In addition, a clear concentration-dependent increase in the induction of *Hprt* mutants was seen together with a significant increase in the levels of intracellular reactive oxygen species [20]. Finally, this gene mutation assay has also been used to detect the mutagenic potential of nickel oxide NPs. In that case, a small but statistically significant increase in the frequency of *Hprt* mutations was observed for NiO NPs but only at one of the different tested doses [21].

From our results it appears that the dispersion procedure is not a factor modulating the genotoxicity of TiO$_2$ NPs. Thus, there were no significant increases in the *Hprt* gene mutation frequency when the two different methods in our study were applied. These results would agree with those reported using the same TiO$_2$ NPs, where no increases in the frequency of micronuclei in TK6 cells, rat bone marrow erythrocytes, or human lymphocytes were observed following three different dispersion procedures [35]. In the same study, using the comet assay, TiO$_2$ NPs dispersed in a stable, non-agglomerated state were able to induce DNA strand breaks in human white blood cells, although no increases in levels of DNA oxidation were seen. The overall conclusion of that study is that NPs in an agglomerated state were unable to cause DNA damage. The observed differences in the results obtained with the different assays can be consequences of the differences in the mechanisms underlying the genotoxic effects detected by the different assays [35]. The dispersion procedure not only can affect genotoxicity but also toxicity. The levels of agglomeration/aggregation of NPs and their size distribution depends on the dispersion procedure, and on the use of serum in stock solution. In our case, DP1 using FBS gave a relatively stable dispersion of TiO$_2$ NPs, while with the second procedure DP2, rapid formation of TiO$_2$ NP agglomerates occurred in the testing medium as measured by DLS, as well as by TEM [13]. Our results show also a discrepancy in measurement of size distribution and stability of dispersion in exposure medium between NTA and DLS measurements, implying that DLS gives a more realistic measure of extrinsic properties of NPs, compared with NTA.

Independently of the results obtained in this study, a procedure giving more stable dispersion should be preferred, so as to avoid false negative data that may be caused by the uptake difficulties associated with big agglomerations/aggregations.

Author Contributions: Conceptualization: M.D., A.K., methodology: A.K., L.R., N.E.Y., A.G.-R., M.B., NTA: N.E.Y., TEM analysis: A.G.-R., R.M., statistical analysis: N.E.Y., writing—original draft preparation, A.K., N.E.Y.; writing—review and editing, A.K., M.D., R.M., N.E.Y., funding acquisition: M.D. All authors have read and agree to the published version of the manuscript.

Funding: A. Kazimirova was supported by QualityNano Transnational Access fellowship. This investigation has been supported by the EC FP7 NANoREG (Grant Agreement NMP4-LA-2013-310584), EC FP7 QualityNano (grant agreement INFRA-2010-1.131), by the Research Council of Norway, the project NorNANoREG (239199/O70) and by RiskGONE, contract no H2020-NMBP-TO-IND-2018-814425.

Acknowledgments: We thank Iren Elisabeth Sturtzel for their excellent help with experiments. Authors also thank Andrew Collins for critical reading and language corrections.

Conflicts of Interest: The authors report no conflicts of interest. The authors alone are responsible for the content and writing of the paper.

References

1. Baan, R.; Straif, K.; Grosse, Y.; Secretan, B.; El Ghissassi, F.; Cogliano, V. Carcinogenicity of carbon black, titanium dioxide, and talc. *Lancet Oncol.* **2006**, *7*, 295–296. [CrossRef]
2. Weir, A.; Westerhoff, P.; Fabricius, L.; von Goetz, N. Titanium dioxide nanoparticles in food and personal care products. *Environ. Sci. Technol.* **2013**, *46*, 2242–2250. [CrossRef] [PubMed]
3. Chen, X.X.; Cheng, B.; Yang, Y.X.; Cao, A.N.; Liu, J.H.; Du, L.J.; Liu, Y.F.; Zhao, Y.L.; Wang, H.F. Characterization and preliminary toxicity assay of nano-titaniumdioxide additive in sugar-coated chewing gum. *Small* **2013**, *9*, 1765–1774. [CrossRef] [PubMed]
4. Winkler, H.C.; Notter, T.; Meyer, U.; Naegeli, H. Critical review of the safety assessment of titanium dioxide additives in food. *J. Nanobiotechnol.* **2018**, *16*, 51. [CrossRef]
5. Shi, H.; Magaye, R.; Castranova, V.; Zhao, Z. Titanium dioxide nanoparticles: a review of current toxicological data. *Part. Fibre Toxicol.* **2013**, *10*, 15. [CrossRef]
6. Wang, J.J.; Sanderson, B.J.; Wang, H. Cyto- and genotoxicity of ultrafine TiO_2 particles in cultured human lymphoblastoid cells. *Mutat. Res.* **2007**, *628*, 99–106. [CrossRef]
7. Chen, Z.; Wang, Y.; Ba, T.; Li, Y.; Pu, J.; Chen, T.; Song, Y.; Gu, Y.; Qian, Q.; Yang, J.; et al. Genotoxic evaluation of titanium dioxide nanoparticles in vivo and in vitro. *Toxicol. Lett.* **2014**, *226*, 314–319. [CrossRef]
8. Tavares, A.M.; Louro, H.; Antunes, S.; Quarré, S.; Simar, S.; Temmerman, P.J.D.; Verleysen, E.; Mast, J.; Jensen, K.A.; Norppa, H.; et al. Genotoxicity evaluation of nanosized titanium dioxide, synthetic amorphous silica and multi-walled carbon nanotubes in human lymphocytes. *Toxicol. In Vitro* **2013**, *28*, 60–69. [CrossRef]
9. El Yamani, N.; Collins, A.R.; Rundén-Pran, E.; Fjellsbo, L.M.; Shaposhnikov, S.; Zienolddiny, S.; Dusinska, M. In vitro genotoxicity testing of four reference metal nanomaterials, titanium dioxide, zinc oxide, cerium oxide and silver: towards reliable hazard assessment. *Mutagenesis* **2017**, *32*, 117–126. [CrossRef]
10. Wang, S.; Hunter, L.A.; Arslan, Z.; Wilkerson, M.G.; Wickliffe, J.K. Chronic exposure to nanosized anatase titanium dioxide is not cyto- or genotoxic to Chinese hamster ovary cells. *Environ. Mol. Mutagen.* **2011**, *52*, 614–622. [CrossRef]
11. Guichard, Y.; Schmit, J.; Darne, C.; Gaté, L.; Goutet, M.; Rousset, D.; Rastoix, O.; Wrobel, R.; Witschger, O.; Martin, A.; et al. Cytotoxicity and genotoxicity of nanosized and microsized titanium dioxide and iron oxide particles in Syrian hamster embryo cells. *Ann. Occup. Hyg.* **2012**, *56*, 631–644. [PubMed]
12. Hamzeh, M.; Sunahara, G.I. In vitro cytotoxicity and genotoxicity studies of titanium dioxide (TiO_2) nanoparticles in Chinese hamster lung fibroblast cells. *Toxicol. In Vitro* **2013**, *27*, 864–873. [CrossRef]
13. Magdolenova, Z.; Bilanicova, D.; Pojana, G.; Fjellsbø, L.M.; Hudecova, A.; Hasplova, K.; Marcomini, A.; Dusinska, M. Impact of agglomeration and different dispersions of titanium dioxide nanoparticles on the human related in vitro cytotoxicity and genotoxicity. *J. Environ. Monit.* **2012**, *14*, 455. [CrossRef] [PubMed]
14. Magdolenova, Z.; Collins, A.; Kumar, A.; Dhawan, A.; Stone, V.; Dusinska, M. Mechanisms of genotoxicity. A review of in vitro and in vivo studies with engineered nanoparticles. *Nanotoxicology* **2014**, *8*, 233–278. [CrossRef] [PubMed]
15. Prasad, R.Y.; Wallace, K.; Daniel, K.M.; Tennant, A.H.; Zucker, R.M.; Strickland, J.; Dreher, K.; Kligerman, A.D.; Blackman, C.F.; Demarini, D.M. Effect of treatment media on the agglomeration of titanium dioxide nanoparticles: impact on genotoxicity, cellular interaction, and cell cycle. *ACS Nano* **2013**, *7*, 1929–1942. [CrossRef] [PubMed]
16. Charles, S.; Jomini, S.; Fessard, V.; Bigorgne-Vizade, E.; Rousselle, C.; Michel, C. Assessment of the in vitro genotoxicity of TiO_2 nanoparticles in a regulatory context. *Nanotoxicology* **2018**, *12*, 357–374. [CrossRef]
17. IARC Working Group on the Evaluation of Carcinogenic. Risks to humans: carbon black, titanium dioxide, and talc. *IARC Monogr. Eval. Carcinog. Risks Hum.* **2010**, *93*, 1.
18. Doak, S.H.; Manshian, B.; Jenkins, G.J.S.; Singh, N. In vitro genotoxicity testing strategy for nanomaterials and the adaptation of current OECD guidelines. *Mutat. Res.* **2012**, *745*, 104–111. [CrossRef]
19. Asakura, M.; Sasaki, T.; Sugiyama, T.; Takaya, M.; Koda, S.; Nagano, K.; Arito, H.; Fukushima, S. Genotoxicity and cytotoxicity of multi-wall carbon nanotubes in cultured Chinese hamster lung cells in comparison with chrysotile A fibers. *J. Occup. Health* **2010**, *52*, 155–166. [CrossRef]

20. Rubio, L.; El Yamani, N.; Kazimirova, A.; Dusinska, M.; Marcos, R. Multi-walled carbon nanotubes (NM401) induce ROS-mediated HPRT mutations in Chinese hamster lung fibroblasts. *Environ. Res.* **2016**, *146*, 185–190. [CrossRef]
21. Åkerlund, E.; Cappellini, F.; Di Bucchianico, S.; Islam, S.; Skoglund, S.; Derr, R.; Odnevall Wallinder, I.; Hendriks, G.; Karlsson, H.L. Genotoxic and mutagenic properties of Ni and NiO nanoparticles investigated by comet assay, γ-H2AX staining, *Hprt* mutation assay and ToxTracker reporter cell lines. *Environ. Mol. Mutagen.* **2018**, *59*, 211–222. [PubMed]
22. Dusinska, M.; Boland, S.; Saunders, M.; Juillerat-Jeanneret, L.; Tran, L.; Pojana, G.; Marcomini, A.; Volkovova, K.; Tulinska, J.; Knudsen, L.E.; et al. Towards an alternative testing strategy for nanomaterials used in nanomedicine: Lessons from NanoTEST. *Nanotoxicology* **2015**, *7*, 118–132. [CrossRef] [PubMed]
23. Annangi, B.; Bach, J.; Vales, G.; Rubio, L.; Marcos, R.; Hernández, A. Long-term exposures to low doses of cobalt nanoparticles induce cell transformation enhanced by oxidative damage. *Nanotoxicology* **2015**, *9*, 138–147. [CrossRef] [PubMed]
24. Huk, A.; Izak-Nau, E.; El Yamani, N.; Uggerud, H.; Vadset, M.; Zasonska, B.; Duschl, A.; Dusinska, M. Impact of nanosilver on various DNA lesions and *HPRT* gene mutations -effects of charge and surface coating. *Part. Fibre Toxicol.* **2015**, *12*, 25. [CrossRef]
25. OECD Test, No. 476: In Vitro Mammalian Cell Gene Mutation Tests Using the Hprt and xprt Genes. In *OECD Guidelines for the Testing of Chemicals, Section 4: Health Effects*; OECD: Paris, France, 2016; Available online: https://www.oecd-ilibrary.org/docserver/9789264264809-en.pdf?expires=1582877457&id=id&accname=guest&checksum=AF948B418DF0BC20B908E85A06F87F69 (accessed on 17 August 2016).
26. Huk, A.; Izak-Nau, E.; Reidy, B.; Boyles, M.; Duschl, A.; Lynch, I.; Dušinska, M. Is the toxic potential of nanosilver dependent on its size? *Part. Fibre Toxicol.* **2014**, *11*, 65. [CrossRef]
27. Chen, T.; Yan, J.; Li, Y. Genotoxicity of titanium dioxide nanoparticles. *J. Food Drug Anal.* **2014**, *22*, 95–104. [CrossRef]
28. Zhang, X.; Li, W.; Yang, Z. Toxicology of nanosized titanium dioxide: an update. *Arch. Toxicol.* **2015**, *89*, 2207–2217. [CrossRef]
29. Shakeel, M.; Jabeen, F.; Shabbir, S.; Asghar, M.S.; Khan, M.S.; Chaudhry, A.S. Toxicity of nano-titanium dioxide (TiO_2-NP) through various routes of exposure: a review. *Biol. Trace Elem. Res.* **2016**, *172*, 1–36. [CrossRef]
30. Møller, P.; Jensen, D.M.; Wils, R.S.; Andersen, M.H.G.; Danielsen, P.H.; Roursgaard, M. Assessment of evidence for nanosized titanium dioxide-generated DNA strand breaks and oxidatively damaged DNA in cells and animal models. *Nanotoxicology* **2017**, *11*, 1237–1256. [CrossRef]
31. Albertini, R.J. HPRT mutations in humans: biomarkers for mechanistic studies. *Mutat. Res.* **2001**, *489*, 1–16. [CrossRef]
32. Jain, A.K.; Senapati, V.A.; Singh, D.; Dubey, K.; Maurya, R.; Pandey, A.K. Impact of anatase titanium dioxide nanoparticles on mutagenic and genotoxic response in Chinese hamster lung fibroblast cells (V-79): The role of cellular uptake. *Food Chem. Toxicol.* **2017**, *105*, 127–139. [CrossRef] [PubMed]
33. Du, X.; Gao, S.; Hong, L.; Zheng, X.; Zhou, Q.; Wu, J. Genotoxicity evaluation of titanium dioxide nanoparticles using the mouse lymphoma assay and the Ames test. *Mutat. Res. Genet. Toxicol. Environ. Mutagen.* **2019**, *838*, 22–27. [CrossRef] [PubMed]
34. Guichard, Y.; Fontana, C.; Chavinier, E.; Terzetti, F.; Gaté, L.; Binet, S.; Darne, C. Cytotoxic and genotoxic evaluation of different synthetic amorphous silica nanomaterials in the V79 cell line. *Toxicol. Ind. Health.* **2015**, *32*, 1639–1650. [CrossRef] [PubMed]
35. Kazimirova, A.; Barancokova, M.; Staruchova, M.; Drlickova, M.; Volkovova, K.; Dusinska, M. Titanium dioxide nanoparticles tested for genotoxicity with the comet and micronucleus assays in vitro, ex vivo and in vivo. *Mutat. Res.* **2019**, *843*, 57–65. [CrossRef] [PubMed]

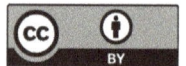

© 2020 by the authors. Licensee MDPI, Basel, Switzerland. This article is an open access article distributed under the terms and conditions of the Creative Commons Attribution (CC BY) license (http://creativecommons.org/licenses/by/4.0/).

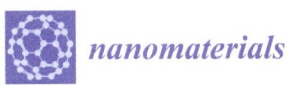

Article

NPs-TiO$_2$ and Lincomycin Coexposure Induces DNA Damage in Cultured Human Amniotic Cells

Filomena Mottola [1], Concetta Iovine [1], Marianna Santonastaso [2], Maria Luisa Romeo [1], Severina Pacifico [1], Luigi Cobellis [2,3] and Lucia Rocco [1,*]

[1] Department of Environmental, Biological and Pharmaceutical Sciences and Technologies, University of Campania "Luigi Vanvitelli", 81100 Caserta, Italy; filomena.mottola@unicampania.it (F.M.); concetta.iovine@unicampania.it (C.I.); maui35@hotmail.it (M.L.R.); severina.pacifico@unicampania.it (S.P.)
[2] Department of Woman, Child and General and Special Surgery, University of Campania "Luigi Vanvitelli", 80138 Napoli, Italy; marianna.santonastaso@unicampania.it (M.S.); luigi.cobellis@unicampania.it (L.C.)
[3] Sant' Anna e San Sebastiano Hospital, 81100 Caserta, Italy
* Correspondence: lucia.rocco@unicampania.it

Received: 29 July 2019; Accepted: 21 October 2019; Published: 23 October 2019

Abstract: Titanium dioxide nanoparticles (NPs-TiO$_2$ or TiO$_2$-NPs) have been employed in many commercial products such as medicines, foods and cosmetics. TiO$_2$-NPs are able to carry antibiotics to target cells enhancing the antimicrobial efficiency; so that these nanoparticles are generally used in antibiotic capsules, like lincomycin, added as a dye. Lincomycin is usually used to treat pregnancy bacterial vaginosis and its combination with TiO$_2$-NPs arises questions on the potential effects on fetus health. This study investigated the potential impact of TiO$_2$-NPs and lincomycin co-exposure on human amniocytes *in vitro*. Cytotoxicity was evaluated with trypan blue vitality test, while genotoxic damage was performed by Comet Test, Diffusion Assay and RAPD-PCR for 48 and 72 exposure hours. Lincomycin exposure produced no genotoxic effects on amniotic cells, instead, the TiO$_2$-NPs exposure induced genotoxicity. TiO$_2$-NPs and lincomycin co-exposure caused significant increase of DNA fragmentation, apoptosis and DNA damage in amniocytes starting from 48 exposure hours. These results contribute to monitor the use of TiO$_2$-NPs combined with drugs in medical application. The potential impact of antibiotics with TiO$_2$-NPs during pregnancy could be associated with adverse effects on embryo DNA. The use of nanomaterials in drugs formulation should be strictly controlled in order to minimize risks.

Keywords: titanium dioxide nanoparticles; lincomycin; human amniotic cells; in vitro genotoxicity; apoptosis; DNA damage

1. Introduction

The toxicology and safe application of the recently developed nanoparticles (NPs) have raised great interest in the last years. There is a growing demand on the use of these NPs in different industries due to some physicochemical properties: small size, large surface area, redox potential, photocatalytic and quantum properties [1–4]. NPs can easily be released and enter human body during the use of commercial products. It has emerged that all types of NPs tested are able to cross the placental barrier [5–7]. Notably, the pregnant women cannot avoid exposing to them. Several studies have shown toxicity and genotoxicity of a wide range of engineered nanoparticles [8–13], consequently this aspect has raised concerns regarding the health of exposed organisms. Among nanomaterials, titanium dioxide nanoparticles (TiO$_2$-NPs) are the most commonly used. TiO$_2$-NPs are applied in medicine as photosensitizer for photodynamic therapy [2,14], drug delivery [15,16] biomedical ceramics [17] and implant biomaterials [18], in foods [19], in cosmetics as sunscreen, toothpaste and personal care products [20–22], in sterilization and in paint industry [23,24]. NPs-TiO$_2$

are inert and poorly soluble nanoparticles that can be absorbed by living organisms generally by oral ingestion, this is the main way of absorption as they are used a food additive, in toothpaste, capsules, and various foods [25]. Regarding the extensive application of TiO_2-NPs in everyday life, the question arises as to whether this nanoparticle has detrimental effects on human health. Human exposure to TiO_2-NPs may also occur through inhalation and ingestion, and then penetrate into the circulatory system and reach other organs (liver, spleen, lungs, brain and testis) [26–28]. TiO_2-NPs exposure causes ovarian and female reproductive system dysfunction in mice [29]. These nanoparticles, like all types of tested NPs, are able to cross the placental barrier and induce damage [6]. TiO_2-NPs prenatal exposure could increase the risk of gestational diabetes, in fact nanoparticles increase maternal fasting blood glucose levels due to gut microbiota alterations [30]. Some studies have also shown that TiO_2-NPs can be transferred from pregnant mice to their offspring and affect mice hippocampus by degeneration, necrosis, and the absence of axonal outgrowth of offspring neurons. This suggested that maternal exposure to TiO_2-NPs caused learning and memory decline in offspring by decreasing the number of neurons and inhibiting axonal and dendritic outgrowth of hippocampal neurons [31]. Furthermore, the TiO_2-NPs induce behavioral deficits related to autism spectrum disorder and neurodevelopmental disorders [32]. The gestational exposure to TiO_2-NPs impairs the growth and development of placenta in mice with a mechanism that seems to be involved in vascularization, proliferation and apoptosis pathways [33]. These alterations cause pregnancy complications, fetal growth retardation and adverse birth outcomes [34], associated with embryonic and bone toxicity due to TiO_2-NPs accumulation in fetal mice. These effects may be due to the direct or indirect role of TiO_2-NPs interfering with Ca, Zn, and other metabolic processes [35]. NPs-TiO_2 induce cytotoxicity and reduce mitotic index in human amniotic fluid cells perturbing cells adhesion ability [36]. One of the most worrying characteristics of NPs-TiO_2, as for all NPs, is their ability to carry any type of substances to the target cells, thus determining a greater effectiveness of the molecule carried, which does not spread throughout the body, but acts directly on the intended target. At the same time, the transport of a toxic substance could improve its toxicity and/or genotoxicity ("Trojan horse" effect) [13,37–40]. The substances, potentially carried by NPs, can be environmental pollutants such as heavy metals or even drugs. This effect is also used in medicine to deliver drugs to target organs. In fact, one approach for increasing the antimicrobial efficacy of antibiotics, without raising the overall dose, is to increase the local targeting concentration by conjugating antibiotics with nanoparticles [41,42]. So, the application of nanoparticles has emerged as an option in the control of bacterial infections in many drugs, that present titanium dioxide as a coloring additive of the capsule, such as lincomycin.

Lincomycin and its derivatives (clindamycin) are antibiotics widely used in clinical practice for the treatment of bacterial infections, in particular those caused by anaerobic species. Lincomycin is bacteriostatic, inhibiting protein synthesis in sensitive bacteria (especially Gram-positive and also protozoans), and bactericidal if used at higher concentrations [43]. Lincomycin and clindamycin are usually used in treatment for bacterial vaginosis in pregnancy, where the normal vaginal microbiota is replaced by a mixed anaerobic microbiota. Bacterial vaginosis may be associated with an increased risk of spontaneous preterm delivery and other complications during pregnancy [44,45], and then the treatment is necessary.

Given the importance of maternal and fetus health during pregnancy, investigation on possible effect of TiO_2-NPs on amniotic fluid cells will give important information about TiO_2-NPs biohazards [36,46]. Therefore, the amniotic cells have been chosen as a model in this study with the aim to assess the effects of titanium dioxide nanoparticles and lincomycin. Lincomycin has been used alone and in combination with TiO_2-NPs to demonstrate the ability of nanoparticles to influence the antibiotic action and also to detect the possible "Trojan horse" effect. Cytological effects and genotoxic damage have been evaluated through the trypan blue vitality test, Comet and Diffusion Assay and the RAPD-PCR technique for two exposure times (48 and 72 h).

2. Materials and Methods

2.1. Chemicals

Titanium dioxide nanoparticles (Aeroxide) were supplied by Evonik Degussa (Essen, Germany; Lot. 614061098). Aeroxide has been 99.9% pure certified and is a blend of 75% rutile and 25% anatase forms with a dimensional average of 21 nm. The preparation of the TiO_2-NPs stock solution (10.0 mg/L) was performed according to literature data [13,38]. Briefly, TiO_2-NPs solution underwent, ultrasonication to disperse nanoparticles and to eliminate agglomeration. Sonication was carried out in medium (Millipore) for 3 h (40 kHz frequency, Dr. Hielscher UP 200S, Germany). UV–Vis spectra were acquired in the range of 200–600 nm by a Shimadzu UV-1700 double beam spectrophotometer. No absorption was detected in the range 300–400 nm, where characteristic peaks for TiO_2-NPs nanoparticles aggregates are known to appear [11,13]. Lincomycin (CAS 7179-49-9, 99% purity) was provided from Sigma-Aldrich. This product was provided as delivered and specified by the issuing Pharmacopoeia. All the substances tested were dissolved in DMSO (dimethylsulfoxide, CAS. 67-68-5).

2.2. Chromatographic Analysis

Chromatographic analysis was carried out using an Agilent 1260 Infinity II HPLC system equipped with 1260 Infinity II VL quaternary pump, and 1260 Infinity II DAD WR diode array detector. CDS LC ChemStation OpenLAB Software was used for data acquisition and analysis.

Separation was achieved using Phenomenex Luna Phenyl-Hexyl, 150 × 2 mm i.d. column (3.0 µm particle size) using a gradient of water (A) and acetonitrile (B), both with 0.1% formic acid. Starting with 10% B, a linear gradient was followed to 25% B in 6.0 min, and held at 25% B for other 1.0 min. Finally, starting conditions were restored and the system re-equilibrated for other 1 min. The total analysis time was 8.0 min, the flow rate was 0.3 mL min^{-1}. Injection volume was 5.0 µL.

2.3. Cell Culture and Exposure Procedure

The human amniotic cells were collected from amniotic fluid of pregnant women undergoing prenatal diagnosis for possible chromosomal abnormalities as a routine procedure during the mid-trimester (15–18 weeks of gestation) at Sant' Anna e San Sebastiano Hospital (Caserta, Italy). Amniotic fluid was collected from pregnant women after written informed consent which was obtained from all participants or their legal guardians, in compliance with the Declaration of Helsinski. Amniotic fluid samples were centrifugate at 1500 rpm for 10 min and suspended into a medium specific for amniocytes growth (Amniomed ®Plus, EuroClone). This medium is a complete medium which contains L-glutamine, FBS, phenol red, sodium bicarbonate, antibiotics and all the necessary growth factors for optimal and selective amniocytes growth. The conditions for the proliferation of amniocyte clones (temperature: 37 °C; pH: between 7.2–7.4; CO_2: 5%) onto a plastic culture flask (surface of 25 cm^2) are selected according to Ascar and collaborator, 2015 [36]. The obtained primary culture amniotic cell was tripsinized, harvested for metaphase spreads and analysed for prenatal diagnosis. After performing prenatal diagnosis, 32 secondary culture amniotic cell (sub-cultures) were then allowed to expand until clones >50 cells formed reaching the cell confluence. Clones were pooled, centrifuged at 1500 rpm for 10 min and suspended into medium and replated on plastic culture flask. When the sub-cultures reached the confluence, the cells were trypsinized with 1 mL of 1 X trypsin-EDTA (Microgem Cat. L0930-100) and divided in four experimental groups: one flask treated with 10 µg/L of TiO_2-NPs, one with 100 mg/L of lincomycin, one with 10 µg/L of TiO_2-NPs plus 100 mg/L of lincomycin, and the last one with 20 µl of DMSO as negative control. As a positive control, 10 mM of H_2O_2 was used. We used a single concentration of TiO_2-NPs antibiotic according to our previous genotoxic studies [11,47]. Time exposure were 48 and 72 h. The same cells pool has been used across all assays and experiments. Incubation was performed as described above. All experiments were performed in triplicate.

2.4. Viability Assay

Amniotic cell viability was assessed by blue trypan assay according to literature data [48]. A cell suspension was mixed with 0.4% dye and examined on a slide with optical microscope to discriminate cells that incorporate the dye from cells that exclude it. A viable cell will have a clear cytoplasm whereas a nonviable cell will have a blue cytoplasm.

2.5. Comet Assay

DNA strand breaks in human amniotic cells have been evaluated by Comet assay [49]. The Comet assay provided the trypsinization of cell samples and then centrifugation at 2000 rpm for 5 min, the pellet was re-suspended in 200 µL of physiological solution. So, the amniotic cells have been mix with the Low Melting Point Agarose (0.5%) and were included into Normal Melting Agarose (1%) layers on slides. After overnight incubation in the cold lysis solution (NaCl 2.5 M, Na_2EDTA 0.1 M, Tris-Base 0.4 M, TRITON-X100 1%, DMSO 10%, pH 10), the slides were site for 10 min in alkaline buffer (NaOH 10N, EDTA 200 mM, pH 12.1), then were exposed to electrophoresis (25V,300 mA) for 15 min. Finally, the slides were fixed in cold methanol, stained with 30% ethidium bromide and observed by the fluorescence microscope with 60X magnification (Nikon Eclipse E-600). Comet assay was performed in triplicate. The images were acquired by means of the "OpenComet" software [50]. The parameter considered was the percentage of damaged DNA present in the comet tail (% Tail DNA). Highly damaged cells, also known as ghost cells or clouds, have been excluded from analysis because they artifactually increase the apparent DNA fragmentation due to actual genotoxicity. In fact, the ghost cells detected after the treatments were due both to the genotoxic damage and to the apoptosis induced by these substances, so they do not allow to discriminate the two processes [51].

2.6. Diffusion Assay

Diffusion assay protocol is the same as the Comet Assay, but the cell slides do not undergo electrophoresis. This assay showed the apoptotic cells that are characterized by irregular contours with nuclei with highly dispersed DNA. The nuclei of the necrotic cells, on the other hand, are larger and not well defined [52]. Diffusion assay was performed in triplicate. The Diffusion assay slides were scored by subdividing the degree of DNA diffusion pattern in five classes of damage as reported by Cantafora and collaborator in 2014 [53] and we considered only class 5 (apoptotic cell).

2.7. RAPD-PCR Technique

Amniotic cell DNA was isolated from 200 µl of all treated cell suspension using the High pure PCR template preparation Kit (ROCHE Diagnostics) according to the manufacturer's instructions to guarantee a sufficiently pure extraction to produce a good quality RAPD-PCR profile. The amplification DNA protocol was conducted through primer 6 (5′-d[CCCGTCAGCA]-3′) [54]. The amplification program provides one first step at 94 °C for 2 min, then 1 min at 95 °C, 1 min at 36 °C and 2 min at 72 °C, for 45 cycles. The reaction products were analysed by means of electrophoresis on 1,5% agarose gel and examined after gel staining with 1% ethidium bromide. The RAPD-PCR profiles have polymorphic patterns that allow the calculation of the template genomic stability (GTS%) as follows:

$$GTS = (1 - a/n) \times 100$$

where a is the average number of polymorphic bands found in each treated sample and n is the total number of bands in the negative control. Appearance of new bands and disappearance of bands are polymorphism detected in RAPD-PCR profiles, which are analysed by comparison to the control sample. The average is calculated for each sample exposed to different molecules. The variations of these values are estimated as a percentage respect to the control set to 100% [13].

2.8. Statistical Analysis

The data were expressed as mean and standard deviation (SD). Differences in the percentage of cell viability, DNA damage and apoptosis genomic stability among the experimental groups were analyzed with the unpaired Student's t-test using GraphPad Prism 6. Only results with p-value ≤ 0.05 were considered statistically significant.

3. Results

3.1. Characterization and Analytical Determinations

Culture media respectively enriched in lincomycin, TiO$_2$-NPs and TiO$_2$-NPs combined with lincomycin underwent chromatographic separation (Figure 1) and UV spectra for chromatographic peaks were extracted. The spectrum of pure lincomycin showed a weak absorbance, with a maximum at 195 nm.

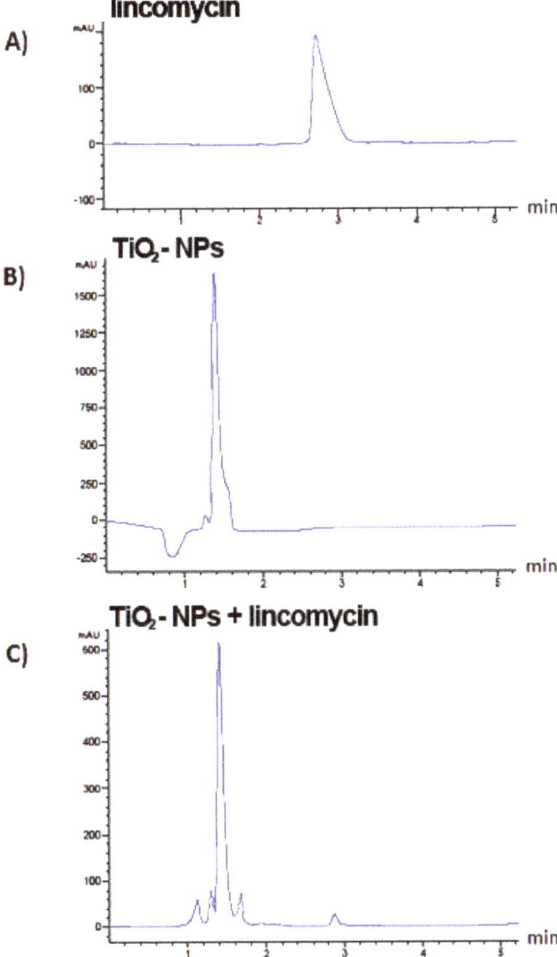

Figure 1. Representative chromatograms of lincomycin, TiO$_2$-NPs and TiO$_2$-NPs + −72h.

In order to verify TiO$_2$-NPs and lincomycin interactions, TiO$_2$-NPs absorbance was also acquired in the range 190–250 nm. Two bands were detected, the first one (herein described as Band I) was at 196 nm, whereas the second (Band II) at 240 nm (Figure 2).

Extracted UV spectra of TiO$_2$-NPs and lincomycin combination showed a hyperchromic effect. In fact, a single peak was detect, with a retention time almost superimposable to that of TiO$_2$-NPs. Indeed, it was observed that a time-dependent increase of TiO$_2$-NPs Band I absorbance (Figure 3).

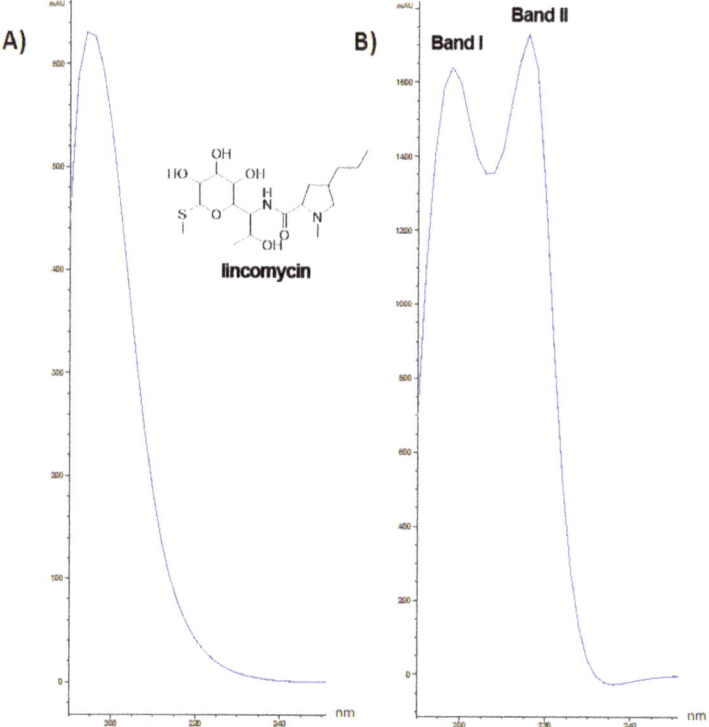

Figure 2. Extracted UV spectra of lincomycin (**A**), and TiO$_2$-NPs (**B**) in the range 190–250 nm.

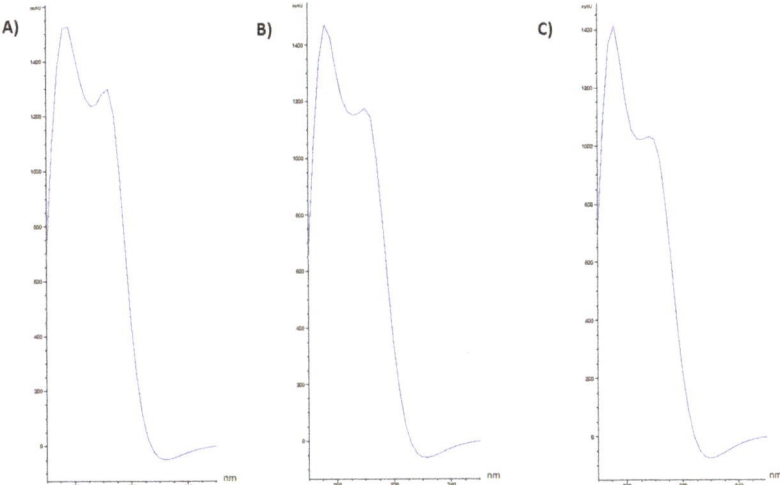

Figure 3. Extracted UV spectra of TiO$_2$-NPs + lincomycin in the range 190–250 nm at (A) t = 0h; (B) t = 48h; (C) t = 72h.

3.2. TiO$_2$-NPs Reduces Amniotic Cells Viability

48 and 72 exposure hours to TiO$_2$-NPs statistically significant reduced amniotic cell viability. The exposure to TiO$_2$-NPs plus lincomycin did not induce a statistically significant changes in viability (Figure 4).

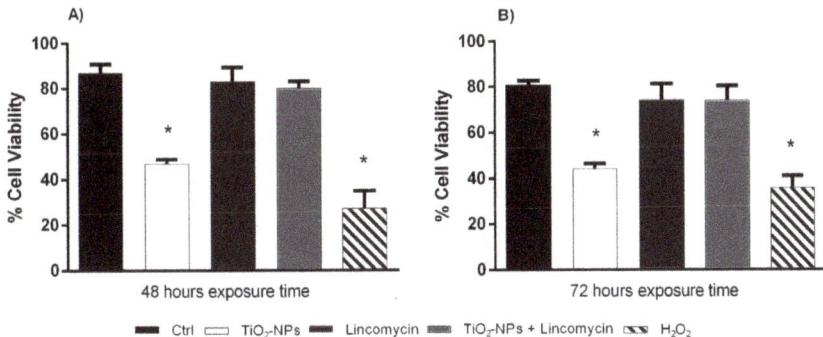

Figure 4. Percentage of alive amniotic cells (ordinate) after 48 h exposure time (**A**) and after 72 h exposure time (**B**) to TiO$_2$-NPs, lincomycin and their combination (abscissa). The dark bar is negative control; the white bar is 10 µg/L TiO$_2$-NPs treated cells; the dark grey bar is 100 mg/L lincomycin treated cells; the light grey bar is 10 µg/L TiO$_2$-NPs + 100 mg/L lincomycin treated cells; the striped bar is 10 mM H$_2$O$_2$ treated cells. * $p \leq 0.05$.

3.3. TiO$_2$-NPs and Lincomycin Co-Exposure Induces an Increase of Amniocyte DNA Fragmentation

The results from Comet Assay showed a statistically significant increase of cell DNA fragmentation after 48 and 72 h exposure to TiO$_2$ nanoparticles alone and in combination with lincomycin. The exposure to lincomycin did not show statistically significant DNA damage (Figure 5).

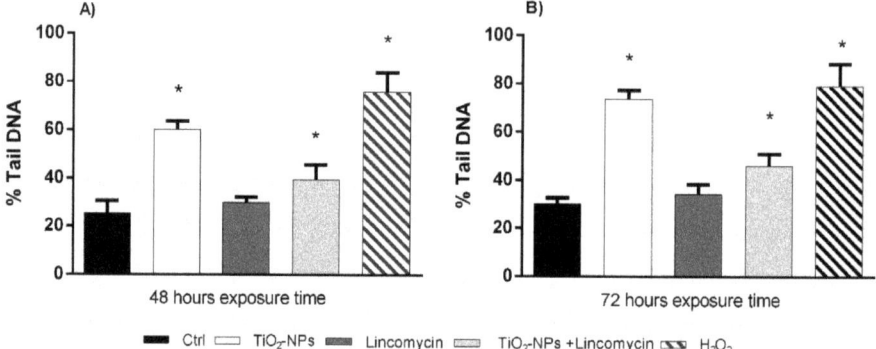

Figure 5. Percentage of DNA in the tail of the comet in amniotic cells (ordinate) after 48 h exposure time (**A**) and after 72 h exposure time (**B**) to TiO$_2$-NPs, lincomycin and their combination (abscissa). The dark bar is negative control; the white bar is 10 μg/L TiO$_2$-NPs treated cells; the dark grey bar is 100 mg/L lincomycin treated cells; the light grey bar is 10 μg/L TiO$_2$-NPs + 100 mg/L lincomycin treated cells; the striped bar is 10 mM H$_2$O$_2$ treated cells. * $p \leq 0.05$.

3.4. TiO$_2$-NPs in Combination with Lincomycin Cause Amniotic Cells Apoptosis

The data from Diffusion assay did not show statistically significant apoptotic damage induced by lincomycin. The exposure to TiO$_2$-NPs and co-exposure to TiO$_2$-NPs and lincomycin after 48 and 72 h induced a statistically significant increase of apoptotic amniotic cells (class 5) with respect to the negative control (Figure 6).

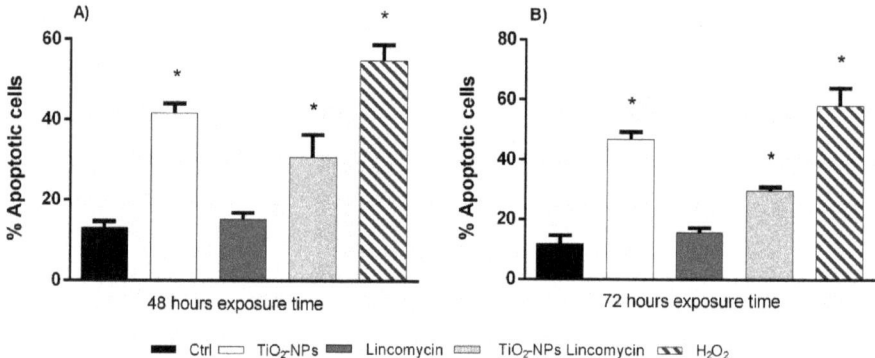

Figure 6. Percentage of apoptotic cells after (ordinate) after 48 h exposure time (**A**) and after 72 h exposure time (**B**) to TiO$_2$-NPs, lincomycin and their combination (abscissa). The dark bar is negative control; the white bar is 10 μg/L TiO$_2$-NPs treated cells; the dark grey bar is 100 mg/L lincomycin treated cells; the light grey bar is 10 μg/L TiO$_2$-NPs + 100 mg/L lincomycin treated cells; the striped bar is 10 mM H$_2$O$_2$ treated cells. * $p \leq 0.05$.

3.5. TiO$_2$-NPs and Lincomycin Determines a Change of DNA Polymorphic Profiles

The RAPD-PCR analysis showed a variation of the polymorphic profiles of the amniotic cell DNA exposed to TiO$_2$-NPs and lincomycin after 48 and 72 exposure hours respect to the DNA of the not-treated amniotic cells. 48 h exposure to lincomycin and TiO$_2$-NPs induced the variation of one and two bands respect to control polymorphic profiles respectively. Co-exposure to lincomycin and TiO$_2$-NPs induced the loss of two bands respect to the control. 72 h exposure to lincomycin determined the gain of a band, instead TiO$_2$-NPs treatment caused three bands variation; lincomycin and TiO$_2$-NPs combination showed the variation of two bands (Table 1).

Table 1. Molecular sizes (bp) of appeared and disappeared bands after amplification with primer P6 in amniotic cell DNA exposed to the TiO$_2$-NPs and lincomycin. *Control bands are at: 200, 300, 320, 400, 500, 520, 700, 950 bp.

Substances Concentration	Hours of Exposure	Gained Bands *	Lost Bands *
TiO2-NPs 10 µg/L	48	850, 530	-
	72	650	320, 400
Lincomycin 100 mg/L	48	-	400
	72	650	-
TiO2-NPs 10 µg/L + Lincomycin 100 mg/L	48	-	400, 520
	72	650	300

3.6. TiO$_2$-NPs and Lincomycin Co-Exposure Decreases Amniotic Cells Genomic Stability

The polymorphic profiles obtained by RAPD-PCR were used to evaluate the percentage of genome stability in human amniotic cells exposed to TiO$_2$-NPs alone and in combination with lincomycin *in vitro*. 48- and 72 h exposure to TiO$_2$ nanoparticles and co-exposure with lincomycin induced a statistically significant reduction in genomic stability (Figure 7).

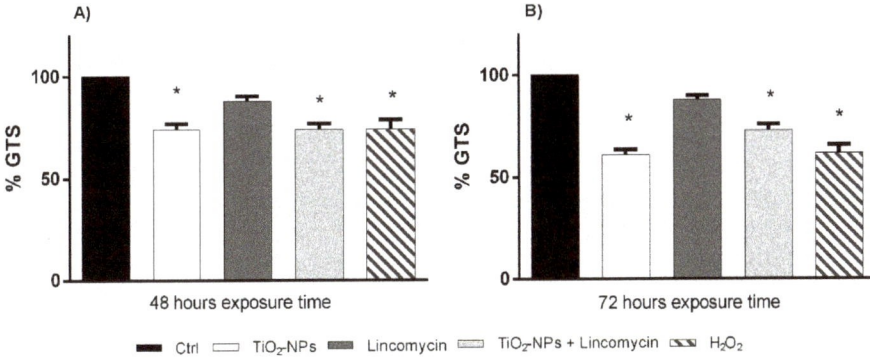

Figure 7. Changes in percentage of Genome Template Stability (ordinate) in amniotic cell DNA after 48 h exposure times (**A**) and after 72 h exposure time (**B**) to TiO$_2$-NPs, lincomycin and their combination (abscissa). The dark bar is negative control; the white bar is 10 µg/L TiO$_2$-NPs treated cells; the dark grey bar is 100 mg/L lincomycin treated cells; the light grey bar is 10 µg/L TiO$_2$-NPs + 100 mg/L lincomycin treated cells; the striped bar is 10 mM H$_2$O$_2$ treated cells. * $p < 0.05$.

4. Discussion

The nanoparticles large-scale application has raised the attention on the possible adverse effects on the exposed organism's health. Titanium dioxide is among the most used nanoparticles in different industrial sectors. NPs-TiO$_2$ can penetrate in different internal organs through inhalation and ingestion and consequently accumulate inducing DNA damage, ROS production, apoptosis and change in cell cycle and nuclear membranes [55–58]. TiO$_2$-NPs are able to diffuse through the protective cellular barriers, such as a placental barrier, and may also involve risks to human health. On that regard it is needed an in-depth investigation of their possible toxicological effects. In an *ex-vivo* human placental perfusion model, Wick and collaborators [59] demonstrated the uptake of nanosized fluorescently labeled polystyrene beads of 50, 80, 240, and 500 nm across the placental barrier. Also, in animal models, the translocation of TiO$_2$-NPs has been reported in brain of prenatally exposed mice. Since the blood barriers are underdeveloped in the fetus, the nanoparticles could easily pass into brain during the early stages of fetal development [60]. In the study conducted by Saquib and collaborators [46], the DLS data revealed the formation of TiO$_2$-NPs aggregates in the RPMI cell culture medium, which were also found to be internalized in the TEM images of the treated human amniotic cell lines. These aggregated NPs, in culture medium, have been reported to enter into cells, such as human amniotic cells, mainly through endocytosis. Their localization in the vacuoles and cell cytoplasm of the exposed cells corresponds well with the observations of Hussain and collaborators [61,62]. In order to safeguard and protect pregnant women and fetus health, the knowledge of the toxic/genotoxic mechanisms of NPs-TiO$_2$ and their association with drugs is very important. The unnecessary supplementation of drugs and commercial products with TiO$_2$-NPs should be restrained during pregnancy until its detrimental effects on embryo development have been clarified. The present work investigated the genotoxic effect of titanium dioxide-NPs and lincomycin on human amniotic fluid cells *in vitro*. The results show that lincomycin exposure has no toxic/genotoxic effects on amniotic cells; differently, TiO$_2$-NPs exposure induced an increase of DNA strand breaks, a reduction of cells viability, a loss of DNA stability and apoptosis for each time tested (48–72 h). Each type of cell has its own vulnerability to NPs; in fact, the metabolic rate, the antioxidant enzyme machinery and DNA repair capabilities of each cell type responded differently based on the concentration of TiO$_2$-NPs, which induced different toxicity levels. Moreover, several crystalline forms of NP-TiO$_2$ and the aggregation of NPs determined a change in their effects due to the increase in their size. Sadhukha and collaborators [63] showed how particle size is a determining factor in biological functions, demonstrating how well-dispersed nanoparticles induce apoptosis while aggregates show different effects.

In order to protect the cell, we suggest that DNA repair activity would be activated as a consequence of DNA damage in cells exposed to TiO$_2$ nanoparticles. This response could be different related to the exposure time and dosage. The results of this study are in accordance with Boland and collaborators [64] who only investigated the effect of short-term exposure to TiO$_2$-NPs and demonstrated how titanium dioxide nanoparticles are harmful to cell survival by activating an exuberant apoptotic response. The latter, to be activated, it requires the internalization of the TiO$_2$ nanoparticles since the accumulation in lysosomes leads to their rupture and to the release of hydrolases such as cathepsins and intracellular ROS production. The primary mechanism of NPs induced toxicity is due to oxidative stress, resulting in damage to cellular membranes and biological macromolecules [65–68]. Our results have demonstrated that the TiO$_2$-NPs induced DNA damage in amniocytes at a concentration of 10 µg/L. Thus, the dose comparison of our study with earlier reports [69,70] suggests the induction of oxidative stress in human amniotic derived fluid cells at relatively lesser concentrations of TiO$_2$-NPs. Furthermore, the nanomaterials released in the cytoplasm allow their access to essential biomolecules causing damage. In addition, the nanoparticles can reach the nucleus, in fact, a high fragmentation was also found by Patel and collaborators in 2017 [71]. The authors showed that exposure to ·OH significantly increases damage to the DNA, which was quantified as a moment and as a percentage of DNA in the tail, in peripheral blood lymphocytes. NPs-TiO$_2$ could induce ·OH radicals which are probably responsible for the DNA damage in the exposed cells [72]. There are contradicting results in literature on exposure with different NPs at different stages of embryo development and also with the differences in experimental models [73–75]. This raises a concern for pregnant women who could be exposed unconsciously due to the environmental spread of these nanoparticles, in fact, one of the main exposures for the general population is through food consumption products, even from food packaging [76]. This study investigation shows that the co-exposure TiO$_2$-NPs and lincomycin induced genotoxic effects without any cytotoxic one; in fact the co-exposure times affected the cell survival and induced changes in genetic material which do not cause cytotoxic effects. However, this mechanism has not been clarified and needs further investigations. Human amniocyte co-treated with TiO$_2$-NPs and lincomycin showed the increase of DNA fragmentation, induction of apoptotic process and DNA damage. The results of Comet Assay demonstrate that the co-exposure induced a statistically significant increase of DNA strand breaks starting from 48 exposure hour. The data obtained by Diffusion assay highlighted the increase of amniotic cell apoptosis from 48 to 72 exposure hours after TiO$_2$-NPs and lincomycin co-exposure. Similarly, the DNA genomic stability was statistically reduced after the co-exposure.

However, we stress that although co-exposure induces genotoxic effects, the latter are still lower than the exposure to TiO$_2$-NPs alone. The results of this work suggested that the combination of TiO$_2$-NPs and lincomycin cause an intermediate level of genotoxicity to amniocytes compared to the exposure of each single compound which by themselves are quite toxic to these cells. Nevertheless, the combination tested produce less toxicity that the same quantity of NPs probably because the co-exposure could affect the bioavailability of the NPs or their biophysical characteristics (e.g., aggregability). In fact, extracted UV spectra of lincomycin and TiO$_2$-NPs showed that when media with TiO$_2$-NPs combined with lincomycin was injected, in each chromatogram, a single peak was detected and its retention time seemed almost superimposable to that of TiO$_2$-NPs. The observation of this hyperchromic effect, together with the disappearance in the HPLC chromatogram of the peak related to pure lincomycin, allowes us to hypothesize the interactions have been established. Therefore, the results demonstrate that the combination of TiO$_2$-NPs and lincomycin leads to the aggregate formation reducing the genotoxcity compared with the dispersed nanoparticles.

The loss or gain of genotoxicity drugs and/or pollutants carried by titanium dioxide nanoparticles could depend on the molecule carried and media, determining or not the "Trojan horse effect". However, the experimental evidence on "Trojan horse effect" is conflicting, in fact, it has been demonstrated no interaction of the TiO$_2$-NPs with organic pollutants (CdCl$_2$ and dioxin) in *Dicentrarchus labrax* in sea water [38,39]. Instead, TiO$_2$-NPs reduced CdCl$_2$-induced effects and DNA damage in *Mytilus galloprovincialis*, whereas, additive effects were no observed [31]. According to these reports, our results suggest the absence of synergistic effect after co-exposure to TiO$_2$-NPs and lincomycin on human amniotic cells, rather co-exposure reduces the TiO$_2$-NPs genotoxicity. Considering that Trojan horse effect is controversial, it could be hypothesized that these nanoparticles could influence the activity of the lincomycin in such a way that could improve its efficacy and thus lead to dosage reduction.

The exposure to TiO$_2$-NPs during pregnancy should be thoroughly investigated and exposure to NPs must be prevented or minimized. Nevertheless, it must be considered that the behavior of the substances tested is relative to an in vitro system that use a single concentration substances, so, it is necessary to complement the in vitro testing by performing a complete genotoxicity assay on a large range of concentrations and by accurately assessing the level of cytotoxicity; then, by performing methodologies able to display relevant genetic events (mutagenesis, chromosomal aberrations). In this way, a complete in vitro genotoxicity profile will be available. As a result, further studies on other in vivo models could be considered to clarify this aspect, so as to carry out prevention interventions on maternal exposure. The data assume that the genotoxicity studies of NPs must be recommended during a comprehensive assessment of the safety of TiO$_2$-NPs and novel types of NPs and nanomaterials.

Author Contributions: F.M. designed the study, acquired and analyzed the data and drafted the manuscript. C.I. carried out Comet and Diffusion Assays. M.S. performed RAPD-PCR experiments. M.L.R. set up cell cultures and different treatments. S.P. performed characterization and analytical determinations. L.C. collected amniotic fluids. L.R. coordinated the study and helped to draft and to revise the manuscript. All authors read and approved the final manuscript.

Funding: This study was supported by Valere project, University of Campania "Luigi Vanvitelli".

Acknowledgments: The authors would like to express their gratitude to Professor Vincenzo Stingo for his valuable advices; his long experience as professor and scientific researcher have been a great help in executing and writing this paper. In addition, we thank Doctor Alessandro Costanzo for his assistance in revising the english of this manuscript.

Conflicts of Interest: The authors declare no conflict of interest.

References

1. Brown, S.C.; Boyko, V.; Meyers, G.; Voetz, M.; Wohlleben, W. Toward advancing nano-object count metrology: A best practice framework. *Environ. Health Perspect.* **2013**, *121*, 1282. [CrossRef] [PubMed]
2. Ackroyd, R.; Kelty, C.; Brown, N.; Reed, M. The history of photodetection and photodynamic therapy. *Photochem. Photobiol.* **2001**, *74*, 656–669. [CrossRef]
3. Colvin, V.L. The potential environmental impact of engineered nanomaterials. *Nat. Biotechnol.* **2003**, *21*, 1166. [CrossRef] [PubMed]
4. Chen, X.; Mao, S.S. Titanium dioxide nanomaterials: Synthesis, properties, modifications, and applications. *Chem. Rev.* **2007**, *107*, 2891–2959. [CrossRef] [PubMed]
5. Yin, F.; Zhu, Y.; Zhang, M.; Yu, H.; Chen, W.; Qin, J. A 3D human placenta-on-a-chip model to probe nanoparticle exposure at the placental barrier. *Toxicol. In vitro* **2019**, *54*, 105–113. [CrossRef]
6. Muoth, C.; Aengenheister, L.; Kucki, M.; Wick, P.; Buerki-Thurnherr, T. Nanoparticle transport across the placental barrier: Pushing the fiel forward! *Nanomedicine* **2016**, *11*, 941–957. [CrossRef]
7. Taylor, U.; Barchanski, A.; Garrels, W.; Klein, S.; Kues, W.; Barcikowski, S.; Rath, D. Toxicity of gold nanoparticles on somatic and reproductive cells. *Adv. Exp. Med. Biol.* **2012**, *733*, 125–133.
8. Jorge de Souza, T.A.; Rosa Souza, L.R.; Franchi, L.P. Silver nanoparticles: An integrated view of green synthesis methods, transformation in the environment, and toxicity. *Ecotoxicol. Environ. Saf.* **2019**, *171*, 691–700. [CrossRef]
9. Singh, S. Zinc oxide nanoparticles impacts: Cytotoxicity, genotoxicity, developmental toxicity, and neurotoxicity. *Toxicol. Mech. Methods* **2019**, *29*, 300–311. [CrossRef]
10. Charles, S.; Jomini, S.; Fessard, V.; Bigorgne-Vizade, E.; Rousselle, C.; Michel, C. Assessment of the in vitro genotoxicity of TiO_2 nanoparticles in a regulatory context. *Nanotoxicology* **2018**, *12*, 357–374. [CrossRef]
11. Santonastaso, M.; Mottola, F.; Colacurci, N.; Iovine, C.; Pacifico, S.; Cammarota, M.; Cesaroni, F.; Rocco, L. In vitro genotoxic effects of titanium dioxide nanoparticles (n-TiO2) in human sperm cells. *Mol. Reprod. Dev.* **2019**. [CrossRef]
12. Wang, R.; Song, B.; Wu, J.; Zhang, Y.; Chen, A.; Shao, L. Potential adverse effects of nanoparticles on the reproductive system. *Int. J. Nanomed.* **2018**, *13*, 8487–8506. [CrossRef] [PubMed]
13. Rocco, L.; Santonastaso, M.; Mottola, F.; Costagliola, D.; Suero, T.; Pacifico, S.; Stingo, V. Genotoxicity assessment of TiO_2 nanoparticles in the teleost Danio rerio. *Ecotoxicol. Environ. Saf.* **2015**, *113*, 223–230. [CrossRef]
14. Ren, W.; Zeng, L.; Shen, Z.; Xiang, L.; Gong, A.N.; Zhang, J.; Mao, C.; Li, A.; Paunesku, T.; Woloschak, G.E.; et al. Enhanced doxorubicin transport to multidrug resistant breast cancer cells via TiO_2 nanocarriers. *RSC Adv.* **2013**, *3*, 20855–20861. [CrossRef]
15. Ortiz-Benítez, E.A.; Velázquez-Guadarrama, N.; Durán Figueroa, N.V.; Quezada, H.; Olivares-Trejo, J.J. Antibacterial mechanism of gold nanoparticles on Streptococcus pneumoniae. *Metallomics* **2019**. [CrossRef]
16. Du, Y.; Ren, W.; Li, Y.; Zhang, Q.; Zeng, L.; Chi, C.; Wu, A.; Tian, J. The enhanced chemotherapeutic effects of doxorubicin loaded PEG coated TiO_2 nanocarriers in an orthotopic breast tumor bearing mouse model. *J. Mater. Chem. B* **2015**, *3*, 1518–1528. [CrossRef]
17. Haugen, H.J.; Will, J.C.O.; Koehler, A.G.; Hopfner, U.; Aigner, J.; Wintermantel, E. Ceramic TiO_2-foams: Characterisation of a potential scaffold. *J. Eur. Ceram. Soc.* **2004**, *24*, 661–666. [CrossRef]
18. Cui, C.; Liu, H.; Li, Y.; Sun, J.; Wanga, R.U.; Liu, S.A.; Greer, L. Fabrication and biocompatibility of nano-TiO_2/titanium alloys biomaterials. *Mater. Lett.* **2005**, *59*, 3144–3148. [CrossRef]
19. Peters, R.J.; Bemmel, V.G.; Herrera-Rivera, Z.; Helsper, H.P.; Marvin, H.J.; Weigel, S.; Tromp, P.C.; Oomen, A.G.; Rietveld, A.G.; Bouwmeester, H. Characterization of titanium dioxide nanoparticles in food products: Analytical methods to define nanoparticles. *J. Agric. Food Chem.* **2014**, *62*, 6285–6293. [CrossRef]
20. Lorenz, C.; Tiede, K.; Tear, S.; Boxall, A.; Von Goetz, N.; Hungerbühler, K. Imaging and characterization of engineered nanoparticles in sunscreens by electron microscopy, under wet and dry conditions. *Int. J. Occup. Environ. Health* **2010**, *16*, 406–428. [CrossRef]
21. Contado, C.; Pagnoni, A. TiO_2 nano-and micro-particles in commercial foundation creams: Field flow-fractionation techniques together with ICP-AES and SQW voltammetry for their characterization. *Anal. Methods* **2010**, *2*, 1112–1124. [CrossRef]
22. Weir, A.; Westerhoff, P.; Fabricius, L.; Hristovski, K.; von Goetz, N. Titanium dioxide nanoparticles in food and personal care products. *Environ. Sci. Technol.* **2012**, *46*, 2242–2250. [CrossRef]

23. Mahmoud, W.M.; Rastogi, T.; Kümmerer, K. Application of titanium dioxide nanoparticles as a photocatalyst for the removal of micropollutants such as pharmaceuticals from water. *Curr. Opin. Green Sustain. Chem.* **2017**, *6*, 1–10. [CrossRef]
24. Rezaei, B.; Mosaddeghi, H. Applications of titanium dioxide nanoparticles. In Proceedings of the Nano-Technology in Environments Conference, Isfahan University of Technology, Isfahan, Iran, 19–20 May 2009.
25. Shi, H.; Magaye, R.; Castranova, V.; Zhao, J. Titanium dioxide nanoparticles: A review of current toxicological data. *Part Fibre Toxicol.* **2013**, *15*, 15. [CrossRef] [PubMed]
26. Shakeel, M.; Jabeen, F.; Shabbir, S.; Asghar, M.S.; Khan, M.S.; Chaudhry, A.S. Toxicity of nano-titanium dioxide (TiO_2-NP) through various routes of exposure: A review. *Biol. Trace Elem. Res.* **2016**, *172*, 1–36. [CrossRef]
27. Elgrabli, D.; Beaudouin, R.; Jbilou, N.; Floriani, M.; Pery, A.; Rogerieux, F.; Lacroix, G. Biodistribution and clearance of TiO_2 nanoparticles in rats after intravenous injection. *PLoS ONE* **2015**, *10*, e012449. [CrossRef] [PubMed]
28. Disdier, C.; Devoy, J.; Cosnefroy, A.; Chalansonnet, M.; Herlin-Boime, N.; Brun, E.; Lund, A.; Mabondzo, A. Tissue biodistribution of intravenously administrated titanium dioxide nanoparticles revealed blood-brain barrier clearance and brain inflammation in rat. *Part Fibre Toxicol.* **2015**, *12*, 27. [CrossRef]
29. Gao, G.; Ze, Y.; Li, B.; Zhao, X.; Zhang, T.; Sheng, L.; Hu, R.; Gui, S.; Sang, X.; Sun, Q.; et al. Ovarian dysfunction and gene-expressed characteristics of female mice caused by long-term exposure to titanium dioxide nanoparticles. *J. Hazard Mater.* **2012**, *243*, 19–27. [CrossRef]
30. Mao, Z.; Li, Y.; Dong, T.; Zhang, L.; Zhang, Y.; Li, S.; Hu, H.; Sun, C.; Xia, Y. Exposure to titanium dioxide nanoparticles during pregnancy changed maternal gut microbiota and increased blood glucose of rat. *Nanoscale Res. Lett.* **2019**, *14*, 26. [CrossRef]
31. Zhou, Y.; Ji, J.; Chen, C.; Hong, F. Retardation of axonal and dendritic outgrowth is associated with the MAPK signaling pathway in offspring mice following maternal exposure to nanosized titanium dioxide. *Agric. Food Chem.* **2019**, *67*, 2709–2715. [CrossRef]
32. Notter, T.; Aengenheister, L.; Weber-Stadlbauer, U.; Naegeli, H.; Wick, P.; Meyer, U.; Buerki-Thurnherr, T. Prenatal exposure to TiO_2 nanoparticles in mice causes behavioral deficits with relevance to autism spectrum disorder and beyond. *Transl. Psychiatr.* **2018**, *8*, 193. [CrossRef] [PubMed]
33. Zhang, L.; Xie, X.; Zhou, Y.; Yu, D.; Deng, Y.; Ouyang, J.; Yang, B.; Luo, D.; Zhang, D.; Kuang, H. Gestational exposure to titanium dioxide nanoparticles impairs the placentation through dysregulation of vascularization, proliferation and apoptosis in mice. *Int. J. Nanomed.* **2018**, *13*, 777–789. [CrossRef] [PubMed]
34. Yamashita, K.; Yoshioka, Y.; Higashisaka, K.; Mimura, K.; Morishita, Y.; Nozaki, M.; Yoshida, T.; Ogura, T.; Nabeshi, H.; Nagano, K.; et al. Silica and titanium dioxide nanoparticles cause pregnancy complications in mice. *Nat. Nanotechnol.* **2011**, *6*, 321–328. [CrossRef] [PubMed]
35. Hong, F.; Zhou, Y.; Zhao, X.; Sheng, L.; Wang, L. Maternal exposure to nanosized titanium dioxide suppresses embryonic development in mice. *Int. J. Nanomed.* **2017**, *12*, 6197–6204. [CrossRef] [PubMed]
36. Ascar, M.S.; Bulut, Z.B.; Ateş, A.; Nami, B.; Koçak, N.; Yıldız, B. Titanium dioxide nanoparticles induce cytotoxicity and reduce mitotic index in human amniotic fluid-derived cells. *Hum. Exp. Toxicol.* **2015**, *34*, 74–82. [CrossRef]
37. Nowack, B.; Bucheli, T.D. Occurrence behavior and effects of nanoparticles in the environment. *Environ. Pollut.* **2007**, *150*, 5–22. [CrossRef]
38. Nigro, M.; Bernardeschi, M.; Costagliola, D.; Della Torre, C.; Frenzilli, G.; Guidi, P.; Lucchesi, P.; Mottola, F.; Santonastaso, M.; Scarcelli, V.; et al. n-TiO_2 and $CdCl_2$ co-exposure to titanium dioxide nanoparticles and cadmium: Genomic, DNA and chromosomal damage evaluation in the marine fish European sea bass (*Dicentrarchus labrax*). *Aquat. Toxicol.* **2015**, *168*, 72–77. [CrossRef]
39. Della Torre, C.; Buonocore, F.; Frenzilli, G.; Corsolini, S.; Brunelli, A.; Guidi, P.; Kocan, A.; Mariottini, M.; Mottola, F.; Nigro, M.; et al. Influence of titanium dioxide nanoparticles on 2,3,7,8-tetrachlorodibenzo-p-dioxin bioconcentration and toxicity in the marine fish European sea bass (*Dicentrarchus labrax*). *Environ. Pollut.* **2015**, *196*, 185–193. [CrossRef]
40. Canesi, L.; Frenzilli, G.; Balbi, T.; Bernardeschi, M.; Ciacci, C.; Corsolini, S.; Della Torre, C.; Fabbri, R.; Faleri, C.; Focardi, S.; et al. Interactive effects of n-TiO2 and 2,3,7,8-TCDD on the marine bivalve *Mytilus galloprovincialis*. *Aquat. Toxicol.* **2014**, *153*, 53–65. [CrossRef]

41. Hussain, S.; Joo, J.; Kang, J.; Kim, B.; Braun, G.B.; She, Z.G.; Kim, D.; Mann, A.P.; Mölder, T.; Teesalu, T.; et al. Antibiotic-loaded nanoparticles targeted to the site of infection enhance antibacterial efficacy. *Nat. Biomed. Eng.* **2018**, *2*, 95–103. [CrossRef]
42. Chen, Y.H.; Li, T.J.; Tsai, B.Y.; Chen, L.K.; Lai, Y.H.; Li, M.J.; Tsai, C.Y.; Tsai, P.J.; Shieh, D.B. Vancomycin-loaded nanoparticles enhance sporicidal and antibacterial efficacy for clostridium difficile Infection. *Front Microbiol.* **2019**, *10*, 1141. [CrossRef] [PubMed]
43. Spížek, J.; Řezanka, T. Lincosamides: Chemical structure, biosynthesis, mechanism of action, resistance, and applications. *Biochem. Pharm.* **2017**, *133*, 20–28. [CrossRef] [PubMed]
44. Haahr, T.; Ersbøll, A.S.; Karlsen, M.A.; Svare, J.; Sneider, K.; Hee, L.; Weile, L.K.; Ziobrowska-Bech, A.; Østergaard, C.; Jensen, J.S.; et al. Treatment of bacterial vaginosis in pregnancy in order to reduce the risk of spontaneous preterm delivery - a clinical recommendation. *Acta Obs. Gynecol. Scand.* **2016**, *95*, 850–860. [CrossRef] [PubMed]
45. Lamont, R.F.; Nhan-Chang, C.L.; Sobel, J.D.; Workowski, K.; Conde-Agudelo, A.; Romero, R. Treatment of abnormal vaginal flora in early pregnancy with clindamycin for the prevention of spontaneous preterm birth: A systematic review and metaanalysis. *Am. J. Obs. Gynecol.* **2011**, *205*, 177–190. [CrossRef]
46. Saquib, Q.; Al-Khedhairy, A.A.; Siddiqui, M.A.; Abou-Tarboush, F.M.; Azam, A.; Musarrat, J. Titanium dioxide nanoparticles induced cytotoxicity, oxidative stress and DNA damage in human amnion epithelial (WISH) cells. *Toxicol. In vitro* **2012**, *26*, 351–361. [CrossRef]
47. Rocco, L.; Peluso, C.; Stingo, V. Micronucleus test and comet assay for the evaluation of zebrafish genomic damage induced by erythromycin and lincomycin. *Environ. Toxicol.* **2012**, *27*, 598–604. [CrossRef]
48. Strober, W. Trypan blue exclusion test of cell viability. *Curr. Protoc. Immunol.* **2001**, *21*, A.3B.1-A.3B.2. [CrossRef]
49. Frenzilli, G.; Nigro, M.; Lyons, B.P. The comet assay for the evaluation of genotoxic impact in aquatic environments. *Mutat. Res. Rev.* **2009**, *681*, 80–89. [CrossRef]
50. Gyori, B.M.; Venkatachalam, G.; Thiagarajan, P.S.; Hsu, D.; Clement, M.V. OpenComet: An automated tool for comet assay image analysis. *Redox Biol.* **2014**, *2*, 457–465.
51. Meintières, S.; Nesslany, F.; Pallardy, M.; Marzin, D. Detection of ghost cells in the standard alkaline comet assay is not a good measure of apoptosis. *Environ. Mol. Mutagen.* **2003**, *41*, 260–269. [CrossRef]
52. Singh, N.P. A simple method for accurate estimation of apoptotic cells. *Exp. Cell Res.* **2000**, *256*, 328–337. [CrossRef] [PubMed]
53. Cantafora, E.; Sean Giorgi, F.; Frenzilli, G.; Scarcelli, V.; Busceti, C.L.; Nigro, M.; Bernardeschi, M.; Fornai, F. Region-specific DNA alterations in focally induced seizures. *J. Neural. Transm.* **2014**, *121*, 1399–1403. [CrossRef] [PubMed]
54. Rocco, L.; Valentino, I.V.; Scapigliati, G.; Stingo, V. RAPD-PCR analysis for molecular characterization and genotoxic studies of a new marine fish cell line derived from Dicentrarchus labrax. *Cytotechnology* **2014**, *66*, 383–393. [CrossRef] [PubMed]
55. Jugan, M.L.; Barillet, S.; Simon-Deckers, A.; Herlin-Boime, N.; Sauvaigo, S.; Douki, T.; Carriere, M. Titanium dioxide nanoparticles exhibit genotoxicity and impair DNA repair activity in A549 cells. *Nanotoxicology* **2012**, *6*, 501–513. [CrossRef]
56. Valdiglesias, V.; Costa, C.; Sharma, V.; Kilic, G.; Pásaro, E.; Teixeira, J.P.; Dhawan, A.; Laffon, B. Comparative study on effects of two different types of titanium dioxide nanoparticles on human neuronal cells. *Food Chem. Toxicol.* **2013**, *57*, 352–361. [CrossRef]
57. Hu, R.; Zheng, L.; Zhang, T.; Gao, G.; Cui, Y.; Cheng, Z.; Cheng, J.; Hong, M.; Tang, M.; Hong, F. Molecular mechanism of hippocampal apoptosis of mice following exposure to titanium dioxide nanoparticles. *J. Hazard Mater.* **2011**, *191*, 32–40. [CrossRef]
58. Petković, J.; Žegura, B.; Stevanović, M. DNA damage and alteration in expression of DNA damage responsive genes induced by TiO_2 nanoparticles in human hepatoma HepG2 cells. *Nanotoxicology* **2011**, *5*, 341–353. [CrossRef]
59. Baranowska-Wójcik, E.; Szwajgier, D.; Oleszczuk, P.; Winiarska-Mieczan, A. Effects of titanium dioxide nanoparticles exposure on human health—A review. *Biol. Trace Elem. Res.* **2019**. [CrossRef]
60. Wick, P.; Malek, A.; Manser, P.; Meili, D.; Maeder-Althaus, X.; Diener, L.; Diener, P.A.; Zisch, A.; Krug, H.F.; Mandach, U.V. Barrier capacity of human placenta for nanosized materials. *Environ. Health Perspect.* **2010**, *118*, 432–436. [CrossRef]

61. Takeda, K.; Suzuki, K.I.; Ishihara, A.; Kubo-Irie, M.; Fujimoto, R.; Tabata, M.; Oshio, S.; Nihei, Y.; Ihara, T.; Sugamata, M. Nanoparticles transferred from pregnant mice to their offspring can damage the genital and cranial nerve systems. *J. Health Sci.* **2009**, *55*, 95–102. [CrossRef]
62. Hussain, S.; Boland, S.; Baeza-Squiban, A.; Hamel, R.; Thomassen, L.C.; Martens, J.A.; Billon-Galland, M.A.; Fleury-Feith, J.; Moisan, F.; Pairon, J.C.; et al. Oxidative stress and proinflammatory effects of carbon black and titanium dioxide nanoparticles: Role of particle surface area and internalized amount. *Toxicology* **2009**, *260*, 142–149. [CrossRef] [PubMed]
63. Hussain, S.; Thomassen, L.C.J.; Ferecatu, I.; Borot, M.C.; Andreau, K.; Martens, J.A.; Fleury, J.; Baeza-Squiban, A.; Marano, F.; Boland, S. Carbon black and titanium dioxide nanoparticles elicit distinct apoptotic pathways in bronchial epithelial cells. *Part. Fiber Toxicol.* **2010**, *7*, 10. [CrossRef] [PubMed]
64. Sadhukha, T.; Wiedmann, T.S.; Panyama, J. Enhancing therapeutic efficacy through designed aggregation of nanoparticles. *Biomaterials* **2014**, *35*, 7860–7869. [CrossRef] [PubMed]
65. Boland, S.; Hussain, S.; Baeza-Squiban, A. Carbon black and titanium dioxide nanoparticles Induce distinct molecular mechanisms of toxicity. *Wiley Interdiscip. Rev. Nanomed. Nanobiotechnol.* **2014**, *6*, 641–652. [CrossRef] [PubMed]
66. Dalton, S.; Janes, P.A.; Jones, N.G.; Nicholson, J.A.; Hallam, K.R.; Allen, G.C. Photocatalytic oxidation of NOx gases using TiO$_2$: A surface spectroscopic approach. *Environ. Pollut.* **2002**, *120*, 415–422. [CrossRef]
67. Donaldson, K.; Stone, V. Current hypotheses on the mechanisms of toxicity of ultrafine particles. *Ann. Ist. Super. Sanità* **2003**, *39*, 405–410.
68. Nel, A.; Xia, T.; Madler, L.; Li, N. Toxic potential of materials at the nanolevel. *Science* **2006**, *311*, 622–627. [CrossRef]
69. Shukla, R.K.; Sharma, V.; Pandey, A.K.; Singh, S.; Sultana, S.; Dhawan, A. ROS-mediated genotoxicity induced by titanium dioxide nanoparticles in human epidermal cells. *Toxicol. In vitro* **2011**, *25*, 231–241. [CrossRef]
70. Kazimirova, A.; Baranokova, M.; Staruchova, M.; Drlickova, M.; Volkovova, K.; Dusinska, M. Titanium dioxide nanoparticles tested for genotoxicity with the comet and micronucleus assays in vitro, ex vivo and in vivo. *Mutat. Res.* **2019**, *843*, 57–65. [CrossRef]
71. Stoccoro, A.; Di Bucchianico, S.; Coppedè, F.; Ponti, J.; Uboldi, C.; Blosi, M.; Delpivo, C.; Ortelli, S.; Costa, A.L.; Migliore, L. Multiple endpoints to evaluate pristine and remediated titanium dioxide nanoparticles genotoxicity in lung epithelial A549 cells. *Toxicol. Lett.* **2017**, *276*, 48–61. [CrossRef]
72. Patel, S.; Patel, P.; Bakshi Sonal, R. Titanium dioxide nanoparticles: An in vitro study of DNA binding, chromosome aberration assay, and comet assay. *Cytotechnology* **2017**, *69*, 245–263. [CrossRef] [PubMed]
73. Reeves, J.F.; Davies, S.J.; Dodd, N.J.F.; Jha, A.N. Hydroxyl radicals (•OH) are associated with titanium dioxide (TiO$_2$) nanoparticle-induced cytotoxicity and oxidative DNA damage in fish cells. *Mutat. Res.* **2008**, *640*, 113–122. [CrossRef] [PubMed]
74. Challier, J.C.; Panigel, M.; Meyer, E. Uptake of colloidal 198Au by fetal liver in rat, after direct intrafetal administration. *Int. J. Nucl. Med. Biol.* **1973**, *1*, 103–106. [PubMed]
75. Bosman, S.J.; Nieto, S.P.; Patton, W.C.; Jacobson, J.D.; Corselli, J.U.; Chan, P.J. Development of mammalian embryos exposed to mixed-size nanoparticles. *Clin. Exp. Obs. Gynecol.* **2005**, *32*, 222–224.
76. Enescu, D.; Cerqueira, M.A.; Fucinos, P.; Pastrana, L.M. Recent advances and challenges on applications of nanotechnology in foodpackaging. A literature review. *Food Chem. Toxicol.* **2019**, *134*, 110814. [CrossRef]

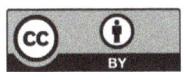 © 2019 by the authors. Licensee MDPI, Basel, Switzerland. This article is an open access article distributed under the terms and conditions of the Creative Commons Attribution (CC BY) license (http://creativecommons.org/licenses/by/4.0/).

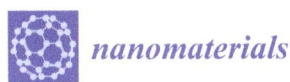

Article

In Vitro Analysis of the Effects of ITER-Like Tungsten Nanoparticles: Cytotoxicity and Epigenotoxicity in BEAS-2B Cells

Chiara Uboldi [1], Marcos Sanles Sobrido [2], Elodie Bernard [3,4], Virginie Tassistro [1], Nathalie Herlin-Boime [5], Dominique Vrel [6], Sébastien Garcia-Argote [7], Stéphane Roche [8], Fréderique Magdinier [8], Gheorghe Dinescu [9], Véronique Malard [4], Laurence Lebaron-Jacobs [4], Jerome Rose [2], Bernard Rousseau [7], Philippe Delaporte [3], Christian Grisolia [10] and Thierry Orsière [1,*]

1. CNRS, IRD, IMBE, Avignon Université, Aix Marseille Université, 13005 Marseille, France
2. CNRS, IRD, INRA, Coll France, CEREGE, Aix Marseille Université, 13545 Aix-en-Provence, France
3. CNRS, LP3, Aix Marseille Université, 13005 Marseille, France
4. CEA, CNRS, BIAM, Aix Marseille Université, 13108 Saint Paul-Lez-Durance, France
5. CEA, IRAMIS UMR NIMBE, Université Paris Saclay, 91191 Gif-sur-Yvette, France
6. LSPM, Université Paris 13, UPR 3407 CNRS, 93430 Villetaneuse, France
7. CEA, SCBM, Université Paris Saclay, 91191 Gif-sur-Yvette, France
8. INSERM, MMG, Aix Marseille Université, 13005 Marseille, France
9. INFLPR, 409 Atomistilor Street, Magurele, 77125 Bucharest, Romania
10. CEA, IRFM, 13108 Saint Paul lez Durance, France
* Correspondence: thierry.orsiere@imbe.fr; Tel.: +33-491-32-45-71

Received: 26 July 2019; Accepted: 26 August 2019; Published: 30 August 2019

Abstract: Tungsten was chosen as a wall component to interact with the plasma generated by the International Thermonuclear Experimental fusion Reactor (ITER). Nevertheless, during plasma operation tritiated tungsten nanoparticles (W-NPs) will be formed and potentially released into the environment following a Loss-Of-Vacuum-Accident, causing occupational or accidental exposure. We therefore investigated, in the bronchial human-derived BEAS-2B cell line, the cytotoxic and epigenotoxic effects of two types of ITER-like W-NPs (plasma sputtering or laser ablation), in their pristine, hydrogenated, and tritiated forms. Long exposures (24 h) induced significant cytotoxicity, especially for the hydrogenated ones. Plasma W-NPs impaired cytostasis more severely than the laser ones and both types and forms of W-NPs induced significant micronuclei formation, as shown by cytokinesis-block micronucleus assay. Single DNA strand breaks, potentially triggered by oxidative stress, occurred upon exposure to W-NPs and independently of their form, as observed by alkaline comet assay. After 24 h it was shown that more than 50% of W was dissolved via oxidative dissolution. Overall, our results indicate that W-NPs can affect the in vitro viability of BEAS-2B cells and induce epigenotoxic alterations. We could not observe significant differences between plasma and laser W-NPs so their toxicity might not be triggered by the synthesis method.

Keywords: tungsten; nanoparticles; tritiated particles; in vitro testing; cytotoxicity; micronuclei formation; DNA damage; epigenetics; DNA methylation; BEAS-2B cells.

1. Introduction

Thermonuclear fusion could potentially represent an unlimited carbon-free source of energy. The International Thermonuclear Experimental fusion Reactor (ITER) project is—at present—exploiting this hypothesis. Based on the current configuration of the ITER fusion plant, tungsten (W) will be the main component of the divertor of the tokamak reactor, the place where the maximum of energy is deposited. Among other materials, W has been chosen thanks to its robustness, its elevated melting point and its resistance to erosion by the tokamak plasma [1]. Nevertheless, tritiated particles will be formed with a theoretical size ranging from tens of nm to tens of micrometers. The safety of reactor's workers and of those living in the nearby area is ensured by High Efficiency Particulate Air (HEPA) filters. Their function is to prevent environmental contamination and occupational or accidental exposure to W particles. However, HEPA filters have a lower retention capability for particles in the 100–500 nm range [2], so a fraction of the ITER-derived W nanoparticles (W-NPs), might escape the reactor in the case of Loss-Of-Vacuum-Accident (LOVA) and disperse into the environment.

Even if W is used in different applications ranging from military use to diagnostics and therapeutic medical devices, from electronics to tanning processes, there is no consensus on its toxicity mechanisms mainly due to its possible redox transformation. Up to now, W has been studied under different forms such as tungsten carbide (WC) alloys doped with cobalt (WC-Co), sodium tungstate (Na_2WO_4), tungsten (VI) oxide nanoparticles (WO_3NPs), and metallic W.

The soluble Na_2WO_4 (W^{6+}) was able to induce apoptosis and cell cycle blockage in human peripheral lymphocytes [3] and, by enhancing the expression of genes related to cancer and inflammation, to alter gene expression in the bronchial human-derived BEAS-2B cell line [4]. WO_3NPs (W^{6+}) impaired the viability of human-derived lung alveolar A549 cells, enhanced DNA damage and micronuclei formation, as well as ROS production and apoptosis [5].

In contrast, more information is available on WC-Co alloys, classified as probably carcinogenic in humans (Group 2A) by the International Agency for Research on Cancer [6]. In BEAS-2B cells, WC-Co was shown to reduce the cellular viability in a time and concentration related manner. When comparing micrometric and nanometric particles, it was observed that only nano-WC-Co caused actin rearrangements and was internalized by BEAS-2B cells [7]. The very same WC-Co particles were reported to impair the cellular viability and increase the secretion of pro-inflammatory cytokines more severely in BEAS-2B than in co-cultures with a monocytic cell line as THP-1 cells or in THP-1 monocultures. These results were explained by suggesting that THP-1 cells might somehow protect the epithelial BEAS-2B cells from the toxic mechanisms exerted by WC-Co [7]. A cell-related effect of WC-Co was also observed in other studies [8–10]. Bastian et al. reported that the A549 cell line was less affected by WC-Co particles than other cell types such as the intestinal Caco-2 and the skin HaCaT cells, and that the presence of cobalt ions enhanced the toxicity of WC particles [8]. Moche et al. showed that WC-Co is a suitable candidate as positive control in genotoxicity assays, but that cell type and exposure length play a key role. In fact, while WC-Co particles did not provide satisfactory positive results in L5178Y mouse lymphoma cells, freshly isolated human lymphocytes were more sensitive, especially at short exposures (4 h) when primary DNA damage was studied, and at long exposures (24 h) when chromosome breakage or loss was considered [9]. Finally, Paget et al. reported that A549 cells underwent less severe cytotoxicity, DNA damage, and cell cycle arrest compared to Caki-1 kidney cell line and Hep3B liver cells, although similar WC-Co internalization was measured [10]. These three above mentioned publications [8–10] suggest that the mechanisms triggering WC-Co cyto- and geno-toxicity are the production of reactive oxidative species (ROS) and the different antioxidant capability in each of the cell types investigated. As previously demonstrated, in fact, Co provides the electrons that deposit on WC particles, thus reducing the oxygen on their surface and generating ROS [11].

The less studied form of W is the metallic one and, to our knowledge, only one publication is available. Machado and coauthors investigated, on A549 lung cells, the effects of mixtures of ballistic debris containing W (W-Ni-Co and W-Ni-Fe) as well as of nanosized and of micrometric metallic W particles [12]. Their results showed that the metallic W nanoparticles exerted severe cytotoxicity but not as significantly as the mixture of ballistic debris, and that the micrometric metallic W did not impair cellular viability [12].

Altogether, the literature suggests that W can impair the integrity and the normal functioning of in vitro cellular systems representative of different organ compartments. Nevertheless, the genotoxic and epigenetic effects of W-NPs have not yet been fully investigated.

In this study, we used the bronchial human-derived epithelial BEAS-2B cell line [13,14] to describe the epigenotoxicity of bench synthesized plasma sputtering and laser ablation ITER-like W-NPs. In order to mimic the particles generated by the ITER fusion reactor, W-NPs produced by plasma sputtering and laser ablation were hydrogenated and tritiated. Moreover, the size of our ITER-like W-NPs resulted in the HEPA filters escape range, further enhancing the importance of our study in an occupational risk perspective. Cell viability, evaluated via the quantification of the adenosine triphosphate (ATP) by luminescence, and cytostasis, evaluated via the cytome version of the Cytokinesis Block MicroNucleus assay (CBMN-cyt), showed that both plasma and laser ITER-like W-NPs are toxic to BEAS-2B cells and that the effect was enhanced upon exposure to hydrogenated/tritiated particles. Laser ablation-derived ITER-like W-NPs seem to exert a slightly enhanced micronuclei formation and primary DNA damage, as shown by CBMN-cyt and alkaline comet assay, respectively. Pancentromeric staining revealed that plasma and laser ITER-like W-NPs induced both clastogenic and aneugenic effects. Epigenetics, in contrast, showed that laser and plasma ITER-like W-NPs had no effects on the DNA methylation of BEAS-2B cells. Finally, oxidative stress, which has been proposed as the factor triggering the cytogenotoxicity of other types of W compounds, has been investigated and a significant alteration of the oxidized/reduced glutathione content was detected. Since more than 50% of W exhibits oxidative dissolution, the role of W^{6+} species must be considered in the biological effects.

2. Materials and Methods

2.1. Reagents

LHC-9 and LHC basal medium, Bovine Serum Albumin (BSA), fibronectin, collagen, PBS, and Trypsin-EDTA were purchased from Thermo Fisher Scientific (Illkirch, France). CellTiter-Glo® Luminescent Cell Viability Assay and GSH-Glo™ Glutathione Assay were purchased from Promega (Charbonnières-les-Bains, France). All other reagents were purchased from Sigma-Aldrich (St. Quentin Fallavier, France).

2.2. Particles Synthesis and Suspensions Preparation

Two synthesis methods were used to produce ITER-like W-NPs with different physico-chemical properties: magnetron plasma sputtering and gas condensation (plasma W-NPs), and laser ablation (laser W-NPs). Detailed description of the production set-up and morphology, composition, and crystalline structure were already described [15–17]. Given the characteristics of the tokamak that will operate at ITER, particles of irregular shape and of smaller size than those produced by other already existing W-based tokamaks are expected. Plasma sputtering and laser ablation were thus believed to be the two synthesis methods that can produce W-NPs that most likely will resemble those generated during ITER operation.

Plasma-derived ITER-like W-NPs were produced in a cluster source by condensation of the metal vapors supplied into argon gas flow by radio-frequency (13.56 MHz) magnetron sputtering discharge [18]. The metallic clusters produced were collected on a dedicated substrate.

Laser-derived ITER-like W-NPs were produced using laser power density deposition on a tungsten target, a dust production technique with relative simplicity and flexibility was developed in preliminary projects [19] and upgraded for the specific requirements of this study. Absorption of the laser energy in the W metallic structure triggers the excitation of free electrons, and this energy is relaxed in the matrix through a thermic wave conveyed by phonons. The brief and intense heat source at the surface of an ITER grade W sample submitted to the laser impulses allows the formation of particles by two processes: ejection of melted material or accretion of particles in the plasma formed in the heated volume. We used a picosecond laser of wavelength 1064 nm, frequency 10 Hz, pulse energy density 5 J/cm^2, and pulse duration 50 ps to produce laser W-NPs [15].

The physical and chemical stability of the W-NPs in biological media were assessed by mean of Dynamic Light Scattering (DLS) using the Mastersizer S (Malvern Panalytical; Orsay, France) and dissolution experiments [17]. The chemical analysis of W in the suspension was performed within inductively coupled plasma mass spectrometry (ICP-MS) (Perkin Elmer Nexion 300; Villebon-sur-Yvette, France). H_2O_2 solutions at room temperature for 24 h were used to digest the solid forms of W solid forms via a total oxidation. The dissolved W species were isolated by combining two filtration stages at 25 and 20 nm [17].

In the facility where radioactive species were manipulated, all the equipment necessary to investigate the physico-chemical properties and the cyto-epi-genotoxic potential of tritiated W-NPs were not available. We therefore included in our study both the pristine and the hydrogenated forms of laser and plasma W-NPs. Pristine is the form in which W-NPs were bench produced; hydrogenated W-NPs were investigated because they are equivalent to the tritiated ones, but not radioactive. Their lack of radioactivity allowed us to thoroughly study them even in the absence of a dedicated facility.

2.3. Cellular Model

The transformed human bronchial epithelial BEAS-2B cell line (ATCC CRL #9609; LGC Standards Sarl, Molsheim, France) was cultured in sterile tissue culture treated flasks or plates pre-coated with LHC basal medium supplemented with BSA (0.01 mg/mL), human fibronectin (0.01 mg/mL), and collagen (0.03 mg/mL). The cultured cells were maintained in LHC-9 medium under standard cell culture conditions (37 °C in 5% CO_2 at 95% humidity) and passaged before confluence by trypsin (0.25%)-EDTA (2.6 mM).

For the experiments with tungsten, BEAS-2B cells were exposed for 2 h and/or 24 h to increasing concentrations (0–150 µg/mL) of plasma and laser ITER-like W-NPs.

2.4. Cytotoxicity Assessment

Intracellular ATP. The viability of BEAS-2B cells was indirectly evaluated via the *in vitro* quantification of intracellular ATP produced by metabolically active cells upon exposure to W-NPs (1–150 µg/mL). The CellTiter-Glo® Luminescence Cell Viability Assay was performed as previously described [20]. Data were acquired using a GloMax® Explorer Multimode Microplate Reader (Promega; Charbonnières-les-Bains, France). For each experimental point, three independent assays were performed, each of them in triplicate ($n = 9$). The percentage of cellular viability was compared to the unexposed control cells.

Cytostasis and cellular replication. By performing the cytome version of the Cytokinesis Block MicroNucleus (CBMN-cyt) assay [21], adapted to the use with nanoparticles [22], cytostasis and cellular replication were also evaluated. To assess cytostasis, the Cytokinesis Block Proliferation Index (CBPI) was calculated by scoring mononucleated, binucleated, and multinucleated cells in the first 500 living cells analyzed in each sample. CBPI, which indicates the average number of cell divisions completed by the cells, was calculated as follows:

$$[(1 \times \text{number binucleated}) + (2 \times \text{number multinucleated}) + (3 \times \text{number multinucleated})]/(500 \text{ viable cells}). \quad (1)$$

The percentage of cytostasis was calculated as recommended by OECD in the test guideline 487 [23]:

$$\{100 - 100 \times [(\text{CBPI exposed cells-1})/(\text{CBPI control cells-1})]\}. \quad (2)$$

The replication index, which represents the proportion of cell division cycles completed in a treated culture during the exposure period and recovery, was calculated as described in the OECD test guideline 487 [23]:

$$[(\text{number of binucleated cells}) + (2 \times \text{number multinucleated cells})]/\text{total exposed cells}/ \\ ([(\text{number binucleated cells}) + (2 \times \text{number multinucleated cells})]/\text{total control cells}) \times 100. \quad (3)$$

2.5. Genotoxicity Studies: Micronucleus and Alkaline Comet Assay

Cytokinesis-Block MicroNucleus assay. To identify chromosome breakage or chromosome loss following exposure W-NPs, the Cytokinesis-Block MicroNucleus assay (CBMN) was performed as described before [20].

Briefly, BEAS-2B cells were seeded onto a two-well Lab-Tek™ II Chamber SlideTM System (Nalgene Nunc International, Villebon sur Yvette, France) and treated with increasing concentrations (0–20 µg/mL) of plasma and laser ITER-like W-NPs. After 24 h exposure, cells were washed and 3 µg/mL cytochalasin B (Sigma Aldrich Chimie Sarl; St. Quentin Fallavier, France) was added to the cultures to block cytokinesis; BEAS-2B cells were kept in culture for an additional 28 h and then cells were fixed with 4% (v/v) paraformaldehyde in PBS. Mitomycin C (MMC, 0.1 µg/mL) served as a positive control, whereas LHC-9 culture medium as the negative one. Upon permeabilization, the cytoskeleton was stained with phalloidin-tetramethylrhodamine B isothiocyanate (Sigma Aldrich Chimie Sarl; St. Quentin Fallavier, France), while nuclei with DAPI ProLong® Gold antifade reagent (Fisher Scientific; Illkirch, France).

CBMN was performed in duplicate, and slides were blindly scored using an Axio Imager. A2 fluorescence microscope (Carl Zeiss S.A.S; Marly Le Roi, France) at 400× magnification. Micronuclei (MN) were only assessed in binucleated (BN) cells that had completed one nuclear division following exposure to the test compounds [20]. For each experimental condition, the number of binucleated micronucleated (BNMN) cells was scored in 1000 BN cells.

Comet assay. To detect the primary DNA damage induced by plasma and laser ITER-like W-NPs in BEAS-2B cells the alkaline comet assay was performed as previously described [20]. BEAS-2B cells, seeded onto pre-coated 12-well plates (BD Falcon; Le Pont de Claix, France), were exposed to W-NPs (1–20 µg/mL) for 2 and 24 h. At the end of the treatment period, cells were washed, trypsinized, resuspended in low melting point agarose, and then spotted onto glass slides pre-coated with 1.6% and 0.8% normal melting point agarose. Cells were then lysed, and the DNA denatured in a MilliQ water solution containing NaOH and EDTA. After electrophoresis (25 V and 300–315 mA), samples were neutralized and dehydrated. Air-dried slides were stained with propidium iodide (PI) right before imaging and data acquisition. Cells incubated only with LHC-9 medium served as negative control, while hydrogen peroxide (110 µM) was used as positive control. Slides, which were prepared in duplicate for each experimental condition, were analyzed under a fluorescence Axio Imager. A2 microscope (Carl Zeiss S.A.S; Marly Le Roi, France) at 400× magnification using the Komet 6.0 software (Andor Bioimaging, Nottingham, UK). DNA damage was expressed as mean % tail DNA ± standard error of the mean (SEM).

2.6. Oxidative Stress Evaluation

The induction of oxidative stress in BEAS-2B cells upon exposure to W-NPs (1–20 µg/mL) was detected by performing the GSH/GSSG-Glo™ Assay (Promega; Charbonnières-les-Bains, France), a luminescence-based system suitable to determine the ratio between the reduced glutathione GSH and its oxidized form GSSG in cultured cells. According to the manufacturer instructions, cells were cultured in a 96-well plate and then exposed for 30 min to plasma or laser W-NPs. After exposure, ITER-like W-NPs solutions were removed, and cells were lysed with total glutathione or oxidized glutathione lysis reagent. Luciferin detection regent was then added, and plates were further incubated for 15 min before luminescence was read at a GloMax® Explorer Multimode Microplate Reader

(Promega; Charbonnières-les-Bains, France). Data were analyzed by subtracting the GSSG reaction signal from the total glutathione to obtain the value of reduced glutathione in the sample. Data were expressed as % GSH/GSSG ratio ± SEM. Exposed cells were compared to the untreated ones.

2.7. Epigenotoxic Effects of W-NPs

We investigated if pristine plasma and laser ITER-like W-NPs induced epigenetic effects, such as variation in the DNA methylation, in BEAS-2B cells. Cells were seeded onto pre-coated T25 flasks and cultivated under standard conditions until they reached 80% confluency. The BEAS-2B cultures were then exposed for 24 h to 1 and 5 µg/mL pristine plasma and laser ITER-like W-NPs, and untreated controls were also included in the experimental set-up. The collection of the samples was performed at different time points (Table 1).

Table 1. Experimental set-up for epigenetic sampling preparation.

Day −1	Cells collected before exposure (generation F0)
Day 0	Cells collected at the time of their exposure to plasma and laser ITER-like W-NPs (generation F0)
Day 1	Cells collected at the end of the 24 h exposure (generation F0)
Day 3	Cells collected 2 days after the end of the exposure (generation F0)
Day 7	Day 3 cells passaged and collected at day 6 after the end of the exposure (generation F1)

BEAS-2B cells were collected as follows: cell culture medium was removed and cells were washed in PBS before being trypsinized and centrifuged (1200 rpm, 5 min, RT). The pellets were dried by aspiration and then stored at −20 °C before DNA methylation was investigated.

We analyzed the methylation of the most frequent repetitive DNA sequences found in the human genome. Alu and LINE are, respectively, short or long interspersed repeats found throughout the genome, i.e., either in highly condensed heterochromatin and transcriptionally inactive loci but also in less condensed regions containing expressed genes. Given this broad distribution, epigenetic status of these two types of repeats is considered as a surrogate marker of the global profile for a given cell. We also analyzed DNA methylation of Satellite 2 and 3 (Sat 2 and Sat 3) repeats, corresponding mainly to heterochromatin associated with centromeric regions and sensitive to exogenous stress. DNA methylation was determined after sodium bisulfite modification of genomic DNA. This method is based on the oxidative desamination of cytosines. Unmethylated cytosines are converted to uraciles while methylation cytosines are not converted, allowing the analysis of individual CGs in any given sequence after PCR amplification and deep sequencing. DNA was extracted from the different types of samples using the Qiagen DNA prep kit following manufacturer's instructions. The DNA methylation protocol, data acquisition, and analysis has already been described [24]. Data are presented as % DNA methylation at different time points.

2.8. Statistical Analysis

Cell viability, primary DNA damage, and oxidative stress were statistically analyzed by one-way ANOVA with Sidak post-hoc test. Cytostasis, cellular replication, and micronuclei frequency were analyzed by Chi-square test. Statistical analysis was performed using GraphPad Prism version 8.1.2 for Windows (GraphPad Software; San Diego, CA, USA).

3. Results

3.1. ITER-Like Plasma and Laser W-NPs Physico-Chemical Characterization

A detailed physico-chemical characterization of the ITER-like plasma and laser W-NPs, in their powder form, was already presented [15,16,19] and is here summarized in Table 2.

Table 2. Summary of the physico-chemical properties of plasma and laser tungsten nanoparticles (W-NPs) powders.

	Plasma W-NPs	
Synthesis	Magnetron Sputtering	
Electron microscopy	Scanning electron microscopy	100–200 nm mean size
	Transmission electron microscopy	Inhomogeneous shape: star-like, squared and round
Crystalline structure	Fourier transform pattern	Beta-phase W metal
	XRD	Beta-phase W metal
Density	Helium pycnometer	14.32 g/cm^3
Surface area	BET	4 m^2/g
W/WO$_x$ ratio (in mass)	Helium pycnometer	90% W metal, 10% WO$_3$
	XAS	90% W metal, 10% WO$_3$
	Laser W-NPs	
Synthesis	High energy laser ablation	
Electron microscopy	Transmission electron microscopy	60–80 nm mean size
Crystalline structure	XRD	Alpha-phase W metal
Density	Helium pycnometer	8.27 g/cm^3
Surface area	BET	43.5 m^2/g
W/WO$_x$ ratio (in mass)	Helium pycnometer	22% W metal, 78% WO$_3$
	XAS	18% W metal, 32% WO$_2$, 50% WO$_3$

The laser W-NPs with a smaller average size were also more oxidized than plasma ones (82% of $W^{4+} + W^{6+}$ compared to 10% of W^{6+} in the case of plasma W-NPs).

The ITER-like plasma and laser W-NPs suspensions were prepared from stock suspension at the initial concentration of 2.5 mg/mL in tris(hydroxymethyl)aminomethane (TRIS) medium. The particle size (Table 3) was determined using Dynamic Light Scattering (DLS). In the case of plasma-derived W-NPs, the particle size in TRIS did not significantly change after hydrogenation and tritiation. When dispersed in LHC-9, plasma-derived W-NPs at t = 0 h showed a slight increase in their mean size and PDI after hydrogenation and tritiation. In the case of laser ITER-like W-NPs dispersed in LHC-9, no significant differences were detected between the three types of laser W-NPs investigated, not in terms of size or in particle stability (PDI and Z pot). While dispersed in TRIS at t = 0, the average size of the pristine laser ITER-like W-NPs is much larger than the TEM size (Table 2). This can suggest an aggregation effect in TRIS medium. The hydrogenation and tritiation tends to decrease the average size of the laser-derived W-NPs. Such size decrease is difficult to interpret but it might be due to a partial oxidative dissolution that, already within 2 h, took place when W-NPs were suspended in LHC-9 culture medium. Indeed, even if it was impossible to quantify the amount of dissolution in the case of laser ITER-like W-NPs due to a low amount of raw material, in the case of pristine plasma ITER-like W-NPs, the dissolved W fraction in mass corresponded to 9%, 23%, 48%, and 58% for t = 0, 2, 4, and 24 h, respectively, for a 100 µg/mL suspension. When diluted at 10 µg/mL, dissolution further increased at 10%, 50%, 60%, and 66% for t = 0, 2, 4, and 24 h, respectively. A detailed W-NPs dissolution protocol (using ICP-MS after filtration at 0.02 µm) and data analysis is available elsewhere [19].

Table 3. Size and zeta potential determination of International Thermonuclear Experimental fusion Reactor (ITER)-like plasma and laser W-NPs in Tris-HCl and in complete BEAS-2B culture medium (LHC-9 medium).

t = 0 h 100 µg/mL	Plasma-Derived W-NPs			Laser-Derived W-NPs		
	Mean Size (nm)	PDI *	Z Pot (mV)	Mean Size (nm)	PDI	Z Pot (mV)
	TRIS buffer					
Pristine	122	0.016	−44	314	0.290	−24
Hydrogenated	107	0.090	−39	265	0.330	−32
Tritiated	126	0.120	−31	284	0.301	−27
	LHC-9 culture medium					
Pristine	103	0.116	−8	162	0.400	−7
Hydrogenated	122	0.250	−10	155	0.350	−11
Tritiated	135	0.210	−13	174	0.500	−10

* PDI: Polydispersity Index.

3.2. Cytotoxic Effects

At 2 h exposure none of the tested particles were able to significantly reduce the viability of BEAS-2B cells, whereas the behavior was different after 24 h incubation (Figure 1).

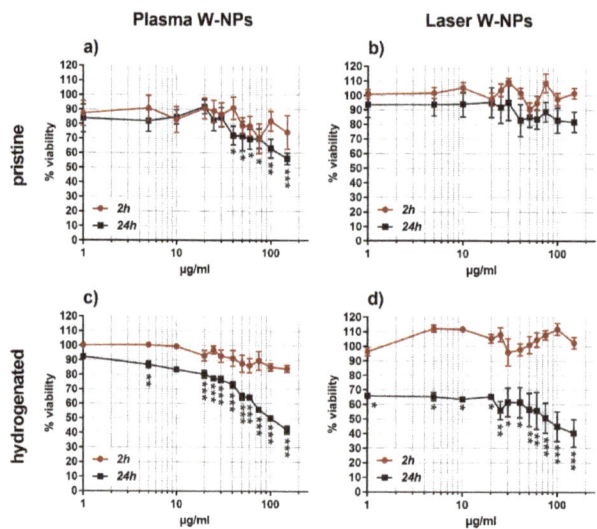

Figure 1. Cytotoxic effects exerted by W-NPs in BEAS-2B cells: (**a**) pristine plasma; (**b**) pristine laser; (**c**) hydrogenated plasma; (**d**) hydrogenated laser. At short exposures (2 h) none of the particles were able to affect the cell viability. After 24 h exposure, in contrast, only pristine laser W-NPs were not cytotoxic. Data are presented as mean % ± SEM of three independent experiments in triplicate. Statistical significance was evaluated by one-way ANOVA with Sidak post-hoc test: * $p < 0.05$; ** $p < 0.01$; *** $p < 0.001$.

Plasma W-NPs, both pristine (Figure 1a) and hydrogenated (Figure 1c), severely affected the metabolic activity of BEAS-2B cells. The cytotoxic effect of pristine plasma W-NPs was statistically significant at concentrations ≥40 µg/mL and increased at the highest tested condition (150 µg/mL).

Hydrogenated plasma W-NPs exhibited a statistically significant impairment of ATP production in BEAS-2B already at 5 µg/mL, which augmented in a concentration related manner.

While upon exposure to pristine laser W-NPs (Figure 1b) no cytotoxic effects were detected neither at 2 h nor at 24 h incubation time, the hydrogenated ones (Figure 1d) severely impaired the metabolism of BEAS-2B at 24 h exposure: 35% cytotoxicity was observed already at the lowest tested concentration of 1 µg/mL, and the effect was increased up to 60% cytotoxicity at 150 µg/mL.

Overall, our results show that at short exposures (2 h) W-NPs do not impair BEAS-2B cell viability, while longer incubations (24 h) have more significant effects. In addition, while at 24 h plasma W-NPs impaired the ATP production in BEAS-2B cells independently of their surface properties, the presence of hydrogen on laser W-NPs is necessary to induce cytotoxic effects. The more severe cytotoxicity observed upon exposure to hydrogenated particles could thus be due to a surface-effect. The presence of hydrogen enhances the cytotoxicity of ITER-like W-NPs and this effect seems time-related, since it does not appear at short exposures (2 h). Tritiated plasma and laser W-NPs could not be tested because of the lack of an appropriate plate reader in the facility where radioactive species are manipulated.

The cytotoxicity data allowed us to select some concentrations of interest for further experiments on the epigenotoxic effects of W-NPs. We thus chose 1–5–10–20 µg/mL as test concentrations because they do induce cytotoxicity without exceeding the levels (55% ± 5%) recommended for the genotoxicity tests [23].

3.3. Effects on Cytostasis and Cellular Replication

Figure 2 shows the cytostasis of BEAS-2B cells in the presence, for 24 h, of plasma (Figure 2a,b) and laser (Figure 2c,d) W-NPs in their pristine, hydrogenated, and tritiated forms. Cytostasis was evaluated via Cytokinesis-Block Proliferation Index (CBPI) and Replication Index (RI).

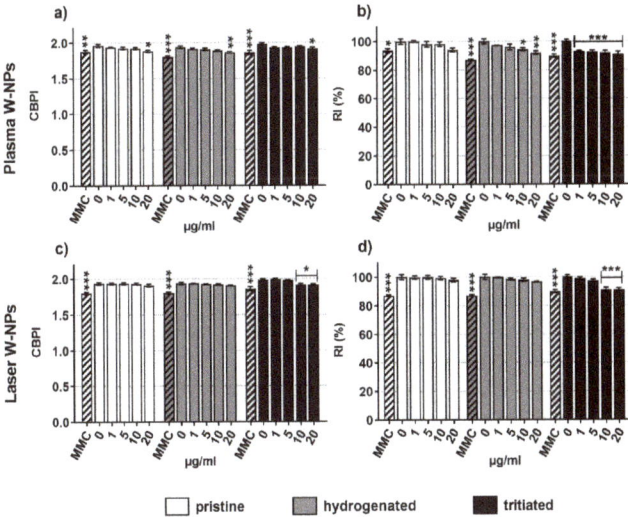

Figure 2. Cytostasis evaluation: (**a**) Cytokinesis Block Proliferation Index (CBPI) upon exposure to plasma W-NPs; (**b**) Replication Index (RI) upon exposure to plasma W-NPs; (**c**) CBPI following incubation with laser W-NPs; (**d**) RI following incubation with laser W-NPs. Independently of the presence or absence of hydrogen and tritium, both plasma and laser W-NPs reduced CBPI and RI of BEAS-2B cells. As expected, the positive control (Mitomycin C (MMC), 0.1 µg/mL) was both cytostatic and cytotoxic. Data are expressed as mean value ± SEM of three independent experiments, each in duplicate. Statistically significant differences from the untreated cells (0 µg/mL) were determined by Chi-square test: * $p < 0.05$, ** $p < 0.01$ and *** $p < 0.001$.

Both types of W-NPs impaired CBPI; nevertheless, no differences were observed comparing the results obtained upon plasma (Figure 2a) and laser (Figure 2c) exposure.

RI was also impaired by plasma and laser W-NPs. Pristine and hygdrogenated plasma (Figure 2b) and laser (Figure 2d) ITER-like W-NPs seem to behave similarly, while tritiated plasma W-NPs seem to exert damage to BEAS-2B cells at lower concentrations than their laser counterparts.

3.4. Micronuclei Formation

The potential chromosomal damage in BEAS-2B cells was evaluated by CBMN assay (Figure 3). Dose-related and statistically significant increased MN frequency was measured following exposure to plasma (Figure 3a) and laser (Figure 3b) W-NPs in their pristine, hydrogenated, and tritiated forms. The presence of hydrogen and tritium did not enhance the genotoxic effect of plasma and laser W-NPs, as already observed for cytostasis and cellular replication (Figure 2).

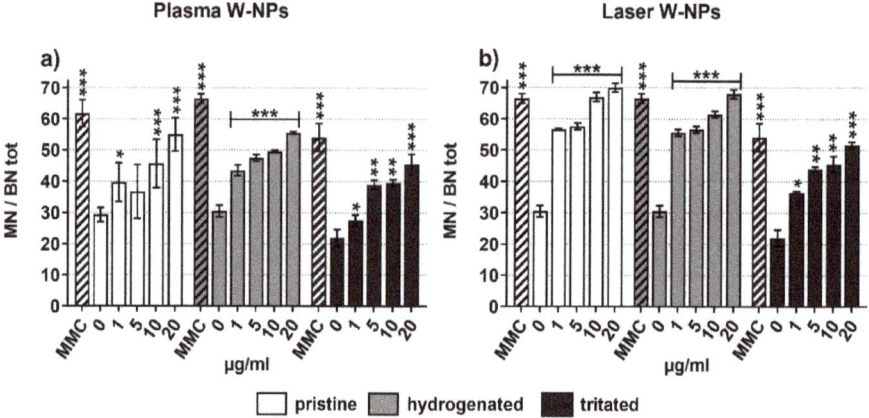

Figure 3. Micronuclei (MN) frequency in BEAS-2B cells exposed to (**a**) plasma W-NPs; (**b**) laser W-NPs. Both plasma and laser W-NPs, independently of the presence/absence of hydrogen and tritium, induced MN formation compared to the untreated cells. MMC (0.1 µg/mL) was used as positive control. Data are expressed as mean value ± SEM of two independent experiments, each in duplicate ($n = 2000$). Statistically significant differences from the untreated cells were determined by Chi-square test: * $p < 0.05$, ** $p < 0.01$ and *** $p < 0.001$.

To investigate more in detail the type of chromosomal damage exerted by the ITER-like plasma and laser W-NPs, a pancentromeric staining was performed (Figure S1). The aim was to distinguish between centromeric positive (CMpos) MN, issued by a whole chromosome loss exerted by an aneugenic compound, and centromeric negative (CMneg) MN, resulting from chromosome fragmentation following exposure to a clastogenic product.

As shown in Figure S1, plasma and laser W-NPs exert both CMpos and CMneg micronuclei. Compared to their respective negative controls, statistically significant CMpos and CMneg MN formation was observed. Since from the graphical representation it was not possible to clearly distinguish and understand which effect (clastogenic or aneugenic) was predominant in laser and plasma W-NPs, the CMpos and CMneg fold increase were calculated. In the presence of plasma W-NPs (Figure S1a,b) CMpos seem to be more induced than CMneg, suggesting a slight but not significant predominant aneugenic potential compared to the clastogenic one. Similarly, a slight predominance of CMpos MN can be observed in BEAS-2B cells upon exposure to laser (Figure S1c,d) W-NPs. Overall, the ITER-like plasma and laser W-NPs display both aneugenic and clastogenic potential.

3.5. DNA Damage Quantification

To evaluate primary DNA lesions, the comet assay was performed following a conventional alkaline protocol. As shown in Figure 4, all the tested ITER-like W-NPs induced DNA fragmentation compared to the untreated BEAS-2B cells. While no differences in the quantification of the DNA damage were observed between tritiated plasma (Figure 4a,b) and laser (Figure 4c,d) at 2 h (Figure 4a,c) and 24 h (Figure 4b,d) exposure, the behavior of pristine and hydrogenated W-NPs was different. In fact, short incubation times generated more severe DNA damage than long exposures. This is very clear in cells exposed to pristine and hydrogenated plasma W-NPs and to pristine laser W-NPs, a bit less pronounced is the difference following incubation with hydrogenated laser W-NPs. The hypothesis to explain these results might be given by the formation of reactive oxidative species (ROS) that participate, as already reported in the literature, in DNA damage.

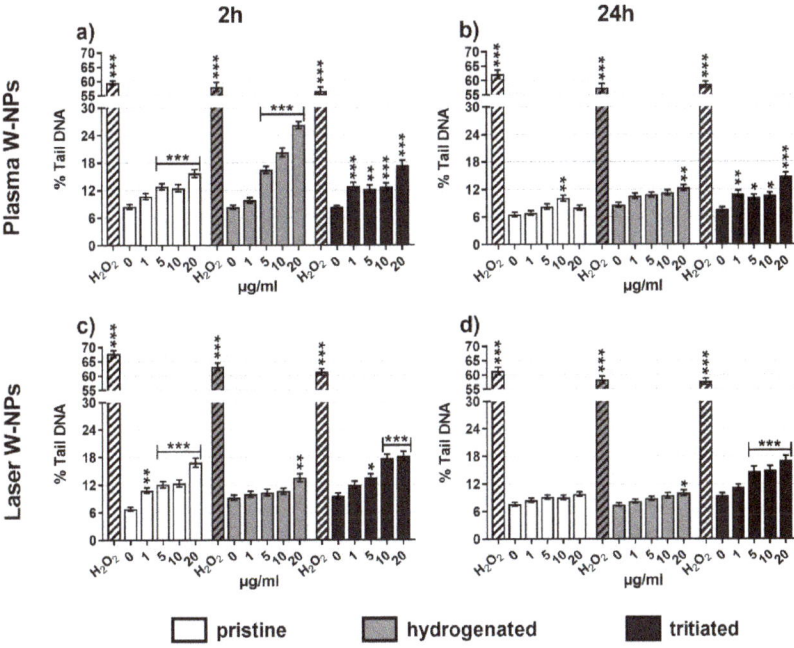

Figure 4. DNA damage by alkaline comet assay: (**a**) 2 h exposure to plasma W-NPs; (**b**) 24 h exposure to plasma W-NPs; (**c**) 2 h exposure to laser W-NPs; (**d**) 24 h exposure to laser W-NPs. Both plasma and laser W-NPs enhanced DNA strand breaks compared to the untreated cells (0 µg/mL) and displayed dose-related behavior. A total of 110 µM hydrogen peroxide (H_2O_2) was used as positive control. Data are presented as mean % tail DNA ± SEM of three independent experiments in triplicate. Statistical significance was evaluated by one-way ANOVA with Holm-Sidak post-hoc test: * $p < 0.05$; ** $p < 0.01$; *** $p < 0.001$.

3.6. Oxidative Stress

To verify our hypothesis that ROS play a role in the induction of DNA damage, we measured oxidative stress in BEAS-2B cells exposed to plasma (Figure 5a) and laser (Figure 5b) W-NPs. Already after 30 min exposure a highly statistically significant imbalance of the GSH/GSSG ratio was detected. With the exception of hydrogenated plasma W-NPs, which exerted the less severe reduction of GSH/GSSG ratio, pristine plasma W-NPs and the two tested types of laser W-NPs showed a dose-related oxidative stress. These data confirmed thus that oxidative stress took place upon exposure to ITER-like W-NPs and that it might trigger DNA damage.

Tritiated plasma and laser W-NPs could not be tested because of the lack of an appropriate plate reader in the radioactive facility. Nevertheless, because the hydrogenated particles can be considered as the non-radioactive equivalent of the tritiated ones, we could suppose that these latter ones have the same behavior than the hydrogenated.

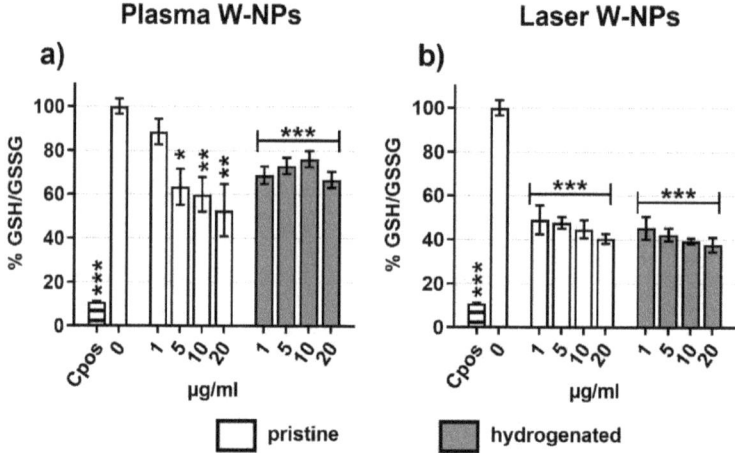

Figure 5. Oxidative stress induced by (**a**) plasma W-NPs; (**b**) laser W-NPs. Compared to the untreated cells (0 µg/mL) both plasma and laser W-NPs induced significant oxidative stress, as evaluated by the GSH/GSSG ratio. Menadione (20 µM) was used as positive control. Data are presented as mean % GSH/GSSG ± SEM of three independent experiments, each in triplicate ($n = 9$). Statistical significance was evaluated by one-way ANOVA with Holm-Sidak post-hoc test: * $p < 0.05$; ** $p < 0.01$; *** $p < 0.001$.

3.7. DNA Methylation Changes Analysis

Epigenetic variations were evaluated at different time points and in different BEAS-2B generations (F0 and F1) upon 24 h exposure to 1–5 µg/mL pristine plasma (Figure 6a) and laser (Figure 6b) ITER-like W-NPs. Compared to the untreated control, for the different sequences analyzed, no significant changes in DNA methylation were observed at any time point tested, with none of the sequences we used in our analysis. Additionally, no differences were observed in the % of methylated DNA in cells exposed to plasma or laser ITER-like W-NPs, confirming again that the biological effects of these two types of particles are similar despite their physico-chemical differences.

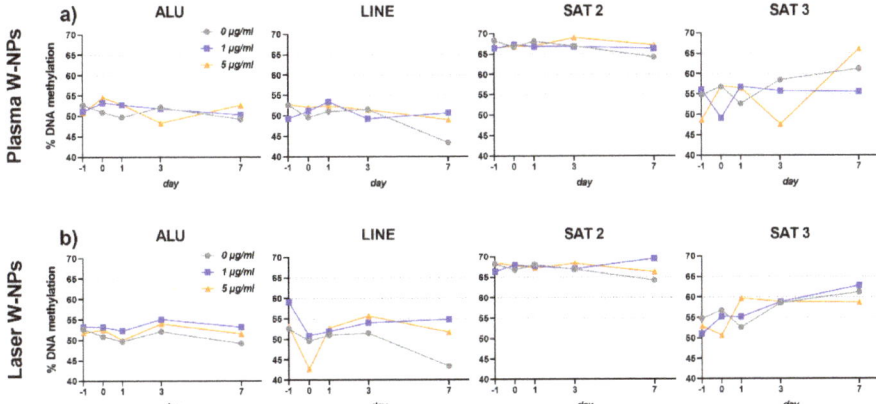

Figure 6. DNA methylation level determined after exposure of BEAS-2B cells to naked induced by pristine (**a**) plasma W-NPs; (**b**) laser W-NPs. No significant differences were observed at any of the time points of any of the BEAS-2B generations investigated. No differences could be observed between the effects exerted by plasma and laser ITER-like W-NPs.

4. Discussion

When thermonuclear fusion reactors become operational, generating tritiated tungsten particles, they could represent a potential risk for the environment and human health as they might be released in case of LOVA. Since the reactor is still under construction, we can only gather preliminary information from the current literature, which is mainly related to different types and forms of W and not to ITER-derived W-NPs.

The aim of our study was thus to provide an evaluation of the cytotoxic, genotoxic, and epigenetic in vitro effects that ITER-like W-NPs might have on human health, in relation with the possible W-NPs transformation in biological media. In particular, we focused our attention to an in vitro 2D model of the lung, the BEAS-2B cell line, that was chosen because inhalation is the main route of exposure to W. Similarly, a significant number of toxicity studies on W were performed on lung-derived cell lines [4,5,7,8,10,12].

The main outcome of the current literature is that W is cytotoxic and induces apoptosis. In addition, W can exert MN formation or DNA damage as well as alter gene expression and arrest the cell cycle. Generally, the production of ROS is considered as the main cause triggering W genotoxicity. Analogously, our data showed that plasma and laser ITER-like W-NPs exert cytotoxic and genotoxic effects in BEAS-2B cells, and the increased oxidative stress might be one of the reasons explaining our results.

Even if we can identify similarities between the outcome of previous studies on W and our data, there are some important differences that we think are pivotal in understanding our results and the mechanisms by which W results toxic. First of all, our bench produced plasma and laser ITER-like W-NPs display peculiar physico-chemical properties [15–17]. More in detail, although they are metallic W-NPs, XAS and helium pycnometer analysis have shown that a significant fraction of tungsten oxide (WO_x) is present and it could participate in the toxicity of the particles. WO_3 represented only a small fraction (10%) of plasma ITER-like W-NPs, while more oxidation was observed on laser ITER-like W-NPs powders (78% WO_3 by helium pycnometer and 50% WO_3 + 32% WO_2 by XAS analysis). Additionally, ITER-like W-NPs are highly soluble. ICP-MS, in fact, revealed that the dissolved W fraction in 100 µg/mL suspensions corresponded, in LHC-9 culture medium, to 9% at t = 0 h and it increased up to 23% and 58% at, respectively, 2 and 24 h incubation [17]. As expected, further dilution of W suspension to 10 µg/mL enhanced their dissolution kinetic: 10% was the soluble W fraction measured at t = 0 h, while 50% and 66% was dissolved at t = 2–24 h [17]. All together these data indicate that the ITER-like W-NPs we investigated were characterized by oxidation and dissolution. These findings bring thus a new perspective on the toxicity of ITER-like W-NPs and they make the plasma and laser particles we investigated unusual.

Not much information is reported in the literature on the solubility of W-containing particles, on their oxidation, and on the involvement of ionic W and W oxides in exerting toxicity. In contrast, studies on the soluble Na_2WO_4 and the on WO_3NP have already been reported. Sodium tungstate was applied to BEAS-2B cells at concentrations ranging from 50 to 250 µM in order to investigate the carcinogenicity of W via several endpoints such as cell transformation, cell migration, and the activation of multiple cancer-related pathways [4]. After 6 weeks of treatment, results clearly showed that Na_2WO_4 increased BEAS-2B colonies formation at all tested doses; in addition, cell migration was tested via the cell scratch assay and the transformed clones were able to heal the wound within less than a day after the scratch was made. Changes in gene expression due to tungstate exposure were observed in BEAS-2B transformed clones: RNA sequencing showed that more than 16,000 genes were altered and the majority of them were related to lung cancer and leukemia, inflammation, and tumor morphology. Overall, the results of Laulicht and coauthors showed that ionic W has carcinogenic in vitro potential [4].

In freshly isolated human peripheral blood lymphocytes (hPBL) Na_2WO_4 was applied in the range 0.1–1–10 mM for 24–96 h and apoptosis, cell cycle, and cytokines secretions were investigated [3]. Early apoptosis increased in tungstate exposed hPBL whereas the number of lymphocytes entering the cell cycle was reduced. Already at relatively low concentration (1 mM), W in its ionic form significantly increased the G_0/G_1 fraction and impaired the number of cells in S- or G_2/M-phase. Moreover, when 5-ethynyl-2′-deoxyuridine (EdU) was used to test DNA synthesis, tungstate was observed to reduce, up to 50%, the EdU-positive cells, also those in G_0/G_1-phase. Likewise, the production of cytokines such as TNF-α, IL-10, and IL-6 resulted significantly lowered, probably due to the high rate of apoptotic hPBL upon exposure to Na_2WO_4. Osterburg and coauthors suggested that the mechanism by which ionic W induces toxic effects depends on its ability to inhibit phosphatase and alter the phosphorylation of some intracellular molecules [3].

From the literature, ionic W seems thus to induce a variety of effects on different in vitro cellular systems. This effect is confirmed by our results on the soluble plasma and laser ITER-like W-NPs that, at least after 24 h exposure, decreased viability and, even if not in a significant manner, the cytostasis of BEAS-2B cells. If we only consider the ionic W released by plasma and laser W-NPs as the key factor triggering cytotoxicity, we should keep in mind that the differences in cell viability observed at 2 and 24 h exposure might depend on the kinetic of dissolution of the particles. In fact, the amount of ionic W measured by ICP-MS was low at 2 h (9%–10%), but much higher (58%–66%) at 24 h. We thus suggest this is one of the reasons that allowed us to observe more cytotoxic effects at long than at short exposures (Figure 1).

Since the presence of WO_2 and WO_3 we detected during powders characterization is not negligible [24], oxidation should also be considered when analyzing plasma and laser ITER-like W-NPs toxicity. Ex vivo bone cells and hepatocytes of 8 weeks old male Sprague-Dawley rats were used to investigate the cytotoxicity, the genotoxicity, and the mutagenic potential of WO_3NPs [25,26]. Upon 30 days of intraperitoneal injections of WO_3NPs at the dose of 25–50–100 mg/kg b.w., bone cells were collected from tibia. While chromosome aberration test did not show any difference in bone cells from exposed rats compared to the untreated controls, mitotic index, a marker for cytotoxicity, and MN frequency, an indicator of genotoxic damage, were affected by WO_3NPs. Mitotic index was significantly decreased at all the tested doses; MN frequency, conversely, was enhanced only in rats exposed to 50–100 mg/kg b.w. [25]. Turkez and coauthors further investigated the effects of WO_3NPs in rat hepatocytes [26]. After performing an ex vivo culture of hepatocytes, cells were exposed for 72 h to WO_3NPs concentrations ranging from 5 to 1000 ppm. The cytotoxic potential was detected by observing a decrease in cell viability, assayed by 3-(4,5-dimethylthiazol-2-yl)-2,5-diphenyltetrazolium bromide (MTT) test, and an increase in the levels of extracellular lactate dehydrogenase at fairly high concentrations (≥300 ppm). Surprisingly, no MN formation was observed at any of the tested WO$_3$NPs concentrations, while oxidative stress and secondary oxidative DNA damage were reported [26]. From the publications of Turkez and coauthors [25,26] it seems that WO$_3$NPs are feebly cytotoxic and could induce chromosome losses. They also generate significant oxidative stress that can cause indirect DNA damage via the formation of adducts, as observed via 8-oxo-2-deoxyguanosine quantification or impair mitotic spindle.

In contrast, plasma and laser ITER-like W-NPs showed significant cytotoxicity on BEAS-2B cultures, they resulted genotoxic by significantly enhancing the MN frequency and by inducing DNA strand breaks. In agreement with previous studies [25,26], we equally observed oxidative stress that might have triggered DNA damage. Nevertheless, the differences between our results and those of Turkez and coauthors [25,26] might be due to the fact that only a fraction of our ITER-like W-NPs was oxidized. We think that both oxidation and dissolution played a synergistic role in the initiation of ITER-like W-NPs toxicity. Since the current literature on WO$_3$NPs does not provide information on the particle dissolution, further comparison cannot be done between the studies of Turkez et al. [25,26] and ours.

While we do not have any physico-chemical information on the WO$_3$NPs used in the Sprague-Dawley ex vivo studies presented just above [25,26], Chinde and colleagues have presented a thorough characterization of the WO$_3$NPs they have tested on the alveolar A549 cell line [5]. In milliQ water, by TEM, the mean size of WO$_3$NPs corresponded to 54 ± 29 nm, while DLS corresponded, respectively, to 170 ± 2 nm and 224 ± 5 nm in milliQ and in DMEM cell culture medium. WO$_3$NPs are thus slightly bigger than the plasma and laser ITER W-NPs we investigated, whose size range, via DLS and in LHC-9 cell culture medium, was set to 103–135 nm and to 155–174 nm, respectively.

Chinde and coauthors have also investigated the dissolution of WO$_3$NPs in cell culture medium. Particles were suspended for 24–48 h in DMEM and the nominal WO$_3$ concentration was compared to total W measured by ICP-MS. While the nominal WO$_3$ concentration of 200 and 300 µg/mL corresponded to 170 and 330 µg/mL total W concentration before ultracentrifugation, only a small fraction of soluble W (0.9 and 2.4 µg/mL) was detected in ultracentrifuged solutions [5]. These results clearly indicate that Chinde et al. used non-soluble WO$_3$NPs; conversely, our ITER-like W-NPs showed a significant dissolved W mass fraction already at t = 0 h in cell culture medium which further increased up to 24 h (Table 2).

Our results on BEAS-2B cells confirm the in vitro lung toxicity of WO$_3$NPs observed by Chinde and coauthors, although some differences in the experimental set-up and in its outcome are noticeable. In A549 cells, the cytotoxicity was observed at high concentrations (≥200 µg/mL WO$_3$NPs; 24–48 h exposure duration) [5], whereas in BEAS-2B cells and at 24 h exposure, plasma and laser ITER-like W-NPs resulted cytotoxic already at 1 µg/mL. Similarly, DNA damage, MN frequency, apoptosis, and oxidative stress were only enhanced in A549 cells exposed at nominal concentrations ≥200 µg/mL WO$_3$NPs [5]. Moreover, WO$_3$NPs uptake quantification showed that only 0.3% of particles were internalized by A549 cells, and that the most significant fraction (70%–75%) of W was diluted in the supernatant.

The nominal concentrations tested and the oxidation state of the particles represent the greater differences between the study of Chinde et al. and ours. Nominal WO$_3$NPs concentrations of at least 200 µg/mL, in fact, differ by 10-fold compared to the maximal plasma and laser ITER-like W-NPs concentration we tested (20 µg/mL). Additionally, plasma and laser ITER-like W-NPs contained, respectively, 10% WO$_3$ and 32% WO$_2$/50% WO$_3$, which further decreases the nominal concentration of WO$_x$ we applied to BEAS-2B cells. Since only a fraction of the plasma and laser ITER-like W-NPs powders is oxidized on their surface, our hypothesis is that the oxidation and the oxidation state are not the unique factors inducing cytotoxic and genotoxic effects in BEAS-2B cells.

To our knowledge, very few epigenetic investigations have been performed on various forms of W. Verma and co-workers investigated by Western blot the posttranslational histone epigenetic modifications, such as acetylation of histone 3 (H3), phosphorylation of Ser10 (H3-Ser10), and the trimethylation of histone H3 on lysine 4 (H3K4me3) in the tail of histone H3 in human embryonic kidney (HEK293), human neuroepithelioma (SKNMC), mouse myoblast (C2C12), and hippocampal primary neuronal cultures exposed to 50–184 μg/mL metal W and W-alloys (91% W, 6% Ni, 3% Co) for 1 day or 1 week, depending on the cell type [27]. H3K4me3 showed no changes in any of the cell cultures following metal exposure, indicating absence of modification in transcriptional activation of genes. Whereas W induced dephosphorylation of H3-Ser10 exclusively in HEK293 cells, tungsten-alloy reduced H3-Ser10 phosphorylation in C2C12 cells and hippocampal primary neuronal cultures, probably taking advantage of the synergistic toxic effects of W with Ni and Co [27]. H3K4me3, as well as the demethylation of histone H3 at lysine residue 9 (H3K9me2), were further investigated in BEAS-2B and A549 cells exposed, in vitro, to 1–2.5–5–10 mM Na_2WO_4 for 48 h [28]. Via Western blot analysis Laulicht-Glick and coauthors observed that global levels of both H3K4me3 and H3K9me2 increased compared to the untreated controls, and that the methylation was not reversible when the treatment solutions were removed and cells further incubated with cell culture medium. Further investigation revealed that the degradation of the demethylases JMJD1A and JARID1A caused the increased H3 methylation in BEAS-2B and A549 [28].

Conversely to Verma et al. [27] and to Laulicht-Glick et al. [28], we quantified the variations in DNA methylation of BEAS-2B cells upon 24 h exposure to 1–5 μg/mL plasma and laser ITER-like W-NPs. Under our experimental conditions we did not detect changes in DNA methylation compared to the control cells, not at any of the days post-exposure nor in sub-cultured BEAS-2B cells (F1 generation). Additional tests might be required, extending the exposure period or increasing the test concentrations, to verify if and at which time point epigenetic effects are induced by ITER-like W-NPs.

5. Conclusions

Despite its use, W still represents a potential occupational or accidental risk. Even if, upon intake, the human body rapidly excretes W, traces could be found in kidney, liver, bones, and spleen [29]. The Occupational Safety and Health Administration (OSHA) has established that 5 and 1 mg/m^3 are the permissible exposure limits for, respectively, insoluble and soluble W compounds employed in the construction and shipyard industries [30,31]. Nevertheless, no information is yet available on ITER-derived W-NPs, their morphology, their physico-chemical properties, and their biological profile. All together, these facts highlight the importance of our study attempting at fulfilling the gap of knowledge on ITER W-NPs. Under our experimental conditions ITER-like plasma and laser W-NPs induced, in a 2D in vitro model of the respiratory compartment, cytotoxic and genotoxic effects as well as strong oxidative potential. Our data represent thus a first, although not exhaustive, multi-endpoint characterization of the biological profile and of the potential risk that ITER-released W-NPs might induce on human health.

Supplementary Materials: The following are available online at http://www.mdpi.com/2079-4991/9/9/1233/s1, Figure S1: Pancentromeric staining in BEAS-2B cells exposed to W-NPs: (**a**) CMpos and CMneg formation upon exposure to plasma W-NPs; (**b**) CMpos and CMneg fold increase compared to untreated cells upon exposure to plasma W-NPs; (**c**) CMpos and CMneg formation upLHCon exposure to laser W-NPs; (**d**) CMpos and CMneg fold increase compared to untreated cells upon exposure to laser W-NPs. Independently of the presence/absence of hydrogen and tritium, ITER-like plasma, and laser W-NPs induced both CMpos and CMneg MN formation compared to the untreated cells (0 μg/mL). MMC (0.1 μg/mL) was used as positive control. Data are expressed as mean value ± SEM of two independent experiments, each in duplicate. Statistically significant differences from the untreated cells were determined by Chi-square test: * $p < 0.05$, ** $p < 0.01$ and *** $p < 0.001$.

Author Contributions: Conceptualization, T.O. and C.G.; methodology, C.U. and T.O.; data analysis, C.U.; data curation, C.U.; writing—original draft preparation, C.U.; writing—review and editing, C.U., T.O., E.B., N.H.-B., D.V., S.R., F.M., V.M., L.L.-J., J.R., P.D., C.G., M.S.S., V.T., S.G.-A., G.D., B.R.; supervision, C.G. and T.O.; project administration, C.G. and T.O.; funding acquisition, T.O. and C.G.

Funding: This research was funded by A*MIDEX, grant number ANR-11-IDEX-0001-02, funded by the "Investissements d'Avenir" French Government program, managed by the French National Research Agency (ANR).

Conflicts of Interest: The authors declare no conflict of interest.

References

1. Davis, J.W.; Barabash, V.R.; Makhankov, A.; Plöchl, L.; Slattery, K.T. Assessment of tungsten for use in the ITER plasma facing components. *J. Nucl. Mater.* **1998**, *258–263*, 308–312. [CrossRef]
2. Huang, S.-H.; Chen, C.-W.; Kuo, Y.-M.; Lai, C.-Y.; McKay, R.; Chen, C.-C. Factors Affecting Filter Penetration and Quality Factor of Particulate Respirators. *Aerosol Air Qual. Res.* **2013**, *13*, 162–171.
3. Osterburg, A.R.; Robinson, C.T.; Schwemberger, S.; Mokashi, V.; Stockelman, M.; Babcock, G.F. Sodium tungstate (Na2WO4) exposure increases apoptosis in human peripheral blood lymphocytes. *J. Immunotoxicol.* **2010**, *7*, 174–182. [PubMed]
4. Laulicht, F.; Brocato, J.; Cartularo, L.; Vaughan, J.; Wu, F.; Kluz, T.; Sun, H.; Oksuz, B.A.; Shen, S.; Peana, M.; et al. Tungsten-induced carcinogenesis in human bronchial epithelial cells. *Toxicol. Appl. Pharmacol.* **2015**, *288*, 33–39. [PubMed]
5. Chinde, S.; Poornachandra, Y.; Panyala, A.; Kumari, S.I.; Yerramsetty, S.; Adicherla, H.; Grover, P. Comparative study of cyto-and genotoxic potential with mechanistic insights of tungsten oxide nano- and microparticles in lung carcinoma cells: Genotoxic potential of tungsten oxide nanoparticles in A549 cells. *J. Appl. Toxicol.* **2018**, *38*, 896–913.
6. WHO International Agency for Research on Cancer. *IARC Monographs on the Evaluation of Carcinogenic Risks to Humans; Cobalt in Hard Metals and Cobalt Sulfate, Gallium Arsenide, Indium Phosphide and Vanadium Pentoxide*; World Health Organization: Geneva, Switzerland, 2006; Volume 86.
7. Armstead, A.L.; Arena, C.B.; Li, B. Exploring the potential role of tungsten carbide cobalt (WC-Co) nanoparticle internalization in observed toxicity toward lung epithelial cells in vitro. *Toxicol. Appl. Pharmacol.* **2014**, *278*, 1–8. [CrossRef]
8. Bastian, S.; Busch, W.; Kühnel, D.; Springer, A.; Meißner, T.; Holke, R.; Scholz, S.; Iwe, M.; Pompe, W.; Gelinsky, M.; et al. Toxicity of Tungsten Carbide and Cobalt-Doped Tungsten Carbide Nanoparticles in Mammalian Cells in vitro. *Environ. Health Perspect.* **2009**, *117*, 530–536. [PubMed]
9. Moche, H.; Chevalier, D.; Barois, N.; Lorge, E.; Claude, N.; Nesslany, F. Tungsten Carbide-Cobalt as a Nanoparticulate Reference Positive Control in In Vitro Genotoxicity Assays. *Toxicol. Sci.* **2014**, *137*, 125–134. [PubMed]
10. Paget, V.; Moche, H.; Kortulewski, T.; Grall, R.; Irbah, L.; Nesslany, F.; Chevillard, S. Human Cell Line-Dependent WC-Co Nanoparticle Cytotoxicity and Genotoxicity: A Key Role of ROS Production. *Toxicol. Sci.* **2015**, *143*, 385–397.
11. Lison, D.; Carbonnelle, P.; Mollo, L.; Lauwerys, R.; Fubini, B. Physicochemical Mechanism of the Interaction between Cobalt Metal and Carbide Particles to Generate Toxic Activated Oxygen Species. *Chem. Res. Toxicol.* **1995**, *8*, 600–606. [CrossRef] [PubMed]
12. Machado, B.; Suro, R.M.; Garza, K.M.; Murr, L. Comparative microstructures and cytotoxicity assays for ballistic aerosols composed of micrometals and nanometals: Respiratory health implications. *Int. J. Nanomed.* **2011**, *6*, 167–178. [CrossRef] [PubMed]
13. Courcot, E.; Leclerc, J.; Lafitte, J.-J.; Mensier, E.; Jaillard, S.; Gosset, P.; Shirali, P.; Pottier, N.; Broly, F.; Lo-Guidice, J.-M. Xenobiotic metabolism and disposition in human lung cell models: Comparison with in vivo expression profiles. *Drug Metab. Dispos. Biol. Fate Chem.* **2012**, *40*, 1953–1965.
14. Forbes, B. Human airway epithelial cell lines for in vitro drug transport and metabolism studies. *Pharm. Sci. Technol. Today* **2000**, *3*, 18–27. [CrossRef]
15. Bernard, E.; Delaporte, P.; Jambon, F.; Rousseau, B.; Grisolia, C.; Chaudanson, D.; Nitsche, S. Tungsten dust in fusion tokamaks: Relevant dust laser production, characterization and behaviour under tritium loading. *Phys. Scr.* **2016**, *T167*, 014071.
16. Bernard, E.; Jambon, F.; Georges, I.; Sanles Sobrido, M.; Rose, J.; Herlin-Boime, N.; Miserque, F.; Beaunier, P.; Vrel, D.; Dine, S.; et al. Design of model tokamak particles for future toxicity studies: Morphology and physical characterization. *Fusion Eng. Des.* **2019**, *145*, 60–65.
17. Sanles Sobrido, M.; Bernard, E.; Angeletti, B.; Malard, V.; Georges, I.; Chaurand, P.; Uboldi, C.; Orsière, T.; Dine, S.; Vrel, D.; et al. Oxidative transformation of Tungsten (W) nanoparticles released in aqueous and biological media in case of Tokamak (nuclear fusion) Lost of Vacuum Accident (LOVA). *Environ. Sci. Nano* **2019**, in press.

18. Acsente, T.; Negrea, R.F.; Nistor, L.C.; Logofatu, C.; Matei, E.; Birjega, R.; Grisolia, C.; Dinescu, G. Synthesis of flower-like tungsten nanoparticles by magnetron sputtering combined with gas aggregation. *Eur. Phys. J. D* **2015**, 69.
19. Vatry, A.; Habib, M.N.; Delaporte, P.; Sentis, M.; Grojo, D.; Grisolia, C.; Rosanvallon, S. Experimental investigation on laser removal of carbon and tungsten particles. *Appl. Surf. Sci.* **2009**, *255*, 5569–5573. [CrossRef]
20. Uboldi, C.; Orsière, T.; Darolles, C.; Aloin, V.; Tassistro, V.; George, I.; Malard, V. Poorly soluble cobalt oxide particles trigger genotoxicity via multiple pathways. *Part. Fibre Toxicol.* **2015**, *13*, 5.
21. Fenech, M. Cytokinesis-block micronucleus cytome assay. *Nat. Protoc.* **2007**, *2*, 1084–1104. [PubMed]
22. Gonzalez, L.; Sanderson, B.J.S.; Kirsch-Volders, M. Adaptations of the in vitro MN assay for the genotoxicity assessment of nanomaterials. *Mutagenesis* **2011**, *26*, 185–191. [PubMed]
23. OECD. *Test No. 487: In Vitro Mammalian Cell Micronucleus Test*; OECD Publishing: Paris, France, 2006.
24. Dion, C.; Roche, S.; Laberthonnière, C.; Broucqsault, N.; Mariot, V.; Xue, S.; Gurzau, A.D.; Nowak, A.; Gordon, C.T.; Gaillard, M.-C.; et al. SMCHD1 is involved in de novo methylation of the *DUX4*-encoding D4Z4 macrosatellite. *Nucleic Acids Res.* **2019**, *47*, 2822–2839. [PubMed]
25. Turkez, H.; Cakmak, B.; Celik, K. Evaluation of the Potential In Vivo Genotoxicity of Tungsten (VI) Oxide Nanopowder for Human Health. *Key Eng. Mater.* **2013**, *543*, 89–92.
26. Turkez, H.; Sonmez, E.; Turkez, O.; Mokhtar, Y.I.; Stefano, A.D.; Turgut, G. The Risk Evaluation of Tungsten Oxide Nanoparticles in Cultured Rat Liver Cells for Its Safe Applications in Nanotechnology. *Braz. Arch. Biol. Technol.* **2014**, *57*, 532–541.
27. Verma, R.; Xu, X.; Jaiswal, M.K.; Olsen, C.; Mears, D.; Caretti, G.; Galdzicki, Z. In vitro profiling of epigenetic modifications underlying heavy metal toxicity of tungsten-alloy and its components. *Toxicol. Appl. Pharmacol.* **2011**, *253*, 178–187. [CrossRef] [PubMed]
28. Laulicht-Glick, F.; Wu, F.; Zhang, X.; Jordan, A.; Brocato, J.; Kluz, T.; Sun, H.; Costa, M. Tungsten exposure causes a selective loss of histone demethylase protein. *Mol. Carcinog.* **2017**, *56*, 1778–1788. [PubMed]
29. Leggett, R.W. A model of the distribution and retention of tungsten in the human body. *Sci. Total Environ.* **1997**, *206*, 147–165. [CrossRef]
30. OSHA. *Occupational Safety and Health Standards for Shipyard Employment. Air Contaminants. Code of Federal Regulations 29 CFR 1915.1000*; Occupational Safety and Health Administration: Washington, DC, USA, 2005.
31. OSHA. *Safety and Health Regulations for Construction. Gases, Vapors, Fumes, Dusts, and Mists. Code of Federal Regulations 29 CFR 1926.55*; Occupational Safety and Health Administration: Washington, DC, USA, 2005.

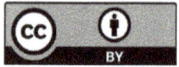

© 2019 by the authors. Licensee MDPI, Basel, Switzerland. This article is an open access article distributed under the terms and conditions of the Creative Commons Attribution (CC BY) license (http://creativecommons.org/licenses/by/4.0/).

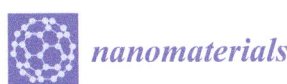

Article

Genotoxicity of Aluminum and Aluminum Oxide Nanomaterials in Rats Following Oral Exposure

Pégah Jalili [1], Sylvie Huet [1], Rachelle Lanceleur [1], Gérard Jarry [1], Ludovic Le Hegarat [1], Fabrice Nesslany [2], Kevin Hogeveen [1] and Valérie Fessard [1,*]

[1] Unité de Toxicologie des Contaminants, Agence Nationale de Sécurité Sanitaire (ANSES), 10 B rue Claude Bourgelat, 35306 Fougères, France; pjalili@uci.edu (P.J.); sylvie.huet@anses.fr (S.H.); rachelle.lanceleur@anses.fr (R.L.); gerard.jarry@anses.fr (G.J.); ludovic.lehegarat@anses.fr (L.L.H.); kevin.hogeveen@anses.fr (K.H.)

[2] Institut Pasteur de Lille, Laboratoire de toxicologie génétique, 1 Rue du Professeur Calmette, 59019 Lille CEDEX, France; fabrice.nesslany@pasteur-lille.fr

* Correspondence: Valerie.fessard@anses.fr; Tel.: +33-(0)2-9994-6685

Received: 9 January 2020; Accepted: 2 February 2020; Published: 11 February 2020

Abstract: Due to several gaps remaining in the toxicological evaluation of nanomaterials (NMs), consumers and public health agencies have shown increasing concern for human health protection. In addition to aluminum (Al) microparticles, Al-containing nanomaterials (Al NMs) have been applied by food industry as additives and contact materials. Due to the limited amount of literature on the toxicity of Al NMs, this study aimed to evaluate the in vivo genotoxic potential of Al^0 and Al_2O_3 NMs after acute oral exposure. Male Sprague-Dawley rats were administered three successive gavages at 6, 12.5 and 25 mg/kg bw. A comparison with $AlCl_3$ was done in order to assess the potential effect of dissolution into Al ions. Both DNA strand breaks and oxidative DNA damage were investigated in six organs/tissues (duodenum, liver, kidney, spleen, blood and bone marrow) with the alkaline and the Fpg-modified comet assays. Concomitantly, chromosomal damage was investigated in bone marrow and colon with the micronucleus assay. The comet assay only showed DNA damage with Al_2O_3 NMs in bone marrow (BM), while $AlCl_3$ induced slight but non-significant oxidative DNA damage in blood. No increase of chromosomal mutations was observed after treatment with the two Al MNs either in the BM or in the colons of rats.

Keywords: genotoxicity; comet assay; micronucleus assay; nanomaterial; aluminum; oral route; gut; liver

1. Introduction

Micro-and nanoscale forms of aluminum (Al) have a great lightness and mechanical resistance, and strong oxidizing power [1]. Due to these unique properties, Al microparticles and Al-containing nanomaterials (Al NMs) have been applied by industry, including in food products [2]. Indeed, they are used as food additives (firming agents, anticaking agents, neutralizing agents, emulsifying agents or texturizers) and in food contact materials, such as cooking tools and food packaging [1–5]. In addition, Al-containing particles are largely used in waste water treatment [6], and in drug vehicles, dental products and other hygiene products, such as toothpaste [1,7–9].

According to the European Food Safety Authority (EFSA) and the Food and Agriculture Organization/World Health of the United Nations (FAO/WHO), provisional tolerable weekly intakes of 1 and 2.3 mg Al/kg/week have been established respectively [1,10]. However, these organizations have raised the fact that this amount can be exceeded to a large extent by some populations, particularly children. As recurrent exposure to micro- and nanoscale Al particles for the general population occurs through foodstuffs, hazard assessment through ingestion should be addressed. Nevertheless, several gaps remain in the toxicological evaluation of Al NMs following oral exposure, which may raise the concern already outlined concerning Al by consumers and public health agencies.

Few in vivo studies are available on the oral toxicity and genotoxicity of Al NMs, most of them focusing on Al_2O_3 NMs. These NMs were shown to accumulate in several organs, including the liver following oral exposure [11–13]. Rodents treated orally with 500 to 2000 mg/kg bw of Al_2O_3 NMs showed deleterious effects in the liver and kidney, and genotoxicity in bone marrow (BM) and oxidative stress in liver [11,14]. According to the ECHA's safety assessment, the data available are inconclusive as to whether or not Al_2O_3 NMs present a genotoxic potential [15]. In contrast, no data on the genotoxicity of Al^0 NMs have been published so far, either in vitro or in vivo.

In vitro studies reported that Al_2O_3 NMs can induce genotoxicity in a variety of mammalian cell lines, including primary human fibroblasts [16], hepatic HepG2 cells [17], human peripheral lymphocytes [18] and Chinese hamster ovary cells (CHO-K1) [19]. These genotoxic effects were found to be associated with oxidative damage [17] although other studies reported no association [16,19].

In addition, there is a lack of information concerning the mechanisms involved, and whether the release of the ionic compound can be the cause of genotoxicity. Indeed, the metal salt $AlCl_3$ has been shown to induce DNA damage in vitro in human peripheral blood lymphocytes, including increases in micronuclei and chromosomal aberrations and positive results in the comet assay [20–22]. In vivo, Paz et al. (2017) reported histopathological lesions in the stomach and the liver, and increased chromosomal damage in BM from 50 mg/kg bw after unique oral exposures to mice [22].

In this study, we aimed to provide new genotoxicity data for Al^0 and Al_2O_3 NMs and to do a comparison with $AlCl_3$. For this purpose, we conducted an in vivo study in rats by gavage. After three oral administrations, the alkaline and Fpg-modified comet assays were performed on several organs to detect DNA breaks and the micronucleus assay to detect if any chromosomal damage could be induced in bone marrow and the colon.

2. Material and Methods

2.1. Chemicals, NMs and Dispersion

$AlCl_3$ (hexahydrate, 231-208-1) was purchased from Sigma Aldrich (Saint Louis, MO, USA).

The selected Al^0 and Al_2O_3 NMs were obtained from IoLiTec (Heilbronn, Germany) and were chosen with a similar primary particle size (approximately 20 nm). The NANOGENOTOX protocol was used for NM dispersion [23,24]. Briefly, particle powder was dispersed in a scintillation vial at a concentration of 2.56 mg/mL in 0.05% BSA in ultra-pure water (dispersion stock solution) by sonication in ice for 16 min at 400 W using a Branson ultrasonic sonicator (Branson Ultrasonics, Eemnes, Netherlands) with a 13 mm probe diameter. Several parameters of physicochemical characterization in the dispersion stock solution and those provided by the suppliers are summarized in Table 1. A more detailed description of the physicochemical characterization of the two NMs was published previously [25,26].

Table 1. Summary of nanomaterial (NM) characteristics.

NM	NM-Code	Average Particle Size [a] (nm)	SSA [b] (m^2/g)	Purity [c]	Bulk Density, True Density [d] (g/cm^3)	Morphology	Pdi [e]	Z-Average Size in the Stock Solution Dispersion at 0 h [e] (nm)	Solubility [f] (24h) (%)
Al^0	NM-0015-HP	18	40–60	>99%	2.7 / 0.008–0.2	Spherical	0.17 ± 0.004	254 ± 4	0.48 ± 0.02
γ-Al$_2$O$_3$	NM-0036-HP	20	<200	99%	- / 0.9	Spherical	0.23 ± 0.015	168 ± 3	0.15 ± 0.01

[a] Average particle size was determined by TEM. [b] Average specific surface area (SSA) was determined by Brunauer-Emmet-Teller (BET). Purity was determined by X-ray powder diffraction (XRD). [d] Density was assessed by normal volumetric test. [e] Pdi and Z-average size were assessed by dynamic light scattering (DLS) using Malvern Zetasizer (Malvern Instruments, Malvern, UK) equipped with a 633-nm laser diode operating at an angle of 173°. [f] Ion release was performed using with a quadrupole inductively coupled plasma mass spectrometry (ICP-MS). [a,b,c,d] Information provided from the supplier. [e,f] Dispersion stock solution.

2.2. Animals and Experimental Design

Male Sprague-Dawley (SD) rats, 8–10 weeks old (around 200 g), were purchased from Janvier (Saint Berthevin, France). Rats were housed in conventional cages and had free access to water and food. Temperature and humidity were kept constant with a light/dark cycle of 12 h/12 h. The animals were treated after at least 5 days of acclimatization. All the experiments were in accordance with the ethical recommendations of the Directive 2010/63/EU of the European Parliament and were validated by the Anses ethical committee (COMETH). Five animals per group were randomly assigned to nine groups including negative and positive controls.

Animals were treated by oral gavage (9.76 mL/kg) at 0, 24 and 45 h. Animals were sacrificed 3 h after the last administration. Al^0 and Al$_2$O$_3$ NMs were given at 6, 12.5 and 25 mg/kg bw, and AlCl$_3$ was given at 25 mg/kg bw. We chose to give a similar mass of compounds to the animals. Nevertheless, the content of Al per animal differed according to the material administered (Table S1). Ultra-pure water with 0.05% BSA was used as vehicle for the negative control group. The positive control was methyl methane sulfonate (MMS from Acros, Geel, Belgium) at 100 mg/kg for the first two oral administrations and at 80 mg/kg for the third. The experimental design was carried out according to the OECD guideline 489 for the comet assay [27].

2.3. Tissue Collection and Sample Preparation

Animals were anesthetized with an intraperitoneal sublethal dose of pentobarbital (60 mg/kg), and the following samples were collected: blood, bone marrow from femur, liver, spleen, kidney, duodenum and colon.

For the comet assay, cells or nuclei were isolated as described in Tarantini et al. (2015) [28]. Briefly, blood was collected directly from the heart before a perfusion step; nuclei of the liver and kidney were mechanically isolated from few small pieces using a Medimachine (BD Biosciences, Le-Pont-de-Claix, France) (5 s in the grinding medium). Spleen cells were harvested by flushing. Sections of duodenum and colon were rinsed with Hank's balanced salt solution (HBSS) medium and epithelial cells were collected by scraping with a coverslip. The rest of the colon and bone marrow cells collected from the two femurs by aspiration with fetal bovine serum were further prepared for the micronucleus assay as described below.

2.4. Alkaline Comet Assay and FpG-Modified Comet Assay

Briefly, after isolation from organs, cells were centrifuged 5 min at 136× g, and the alkaline comet assay and the modified comet assay using the bacterial DNA repair enzyme formamidopyrimidine-DNA glycosylase (Fpg) were performed (2 slides per organ and condition, migration 24 min, 0.7 V/cm and 300 mA) as previously described [28]. FpG (5U/slide) favors the detection of oxidized bases by catalyzing excision of oxidized purines, including the major purine oxidation product 8-oxoguanine, into single-strand breaks [29]. For each tissue and condition (with and without FpG), two slides were prepared. Before scoring, slides were coded, stained with propidium iodide (2.5 µg/mL in PBS) and immediately observed with a fluorescence microscope (Leica DMR, Nanterre, France) equipped with a CCD-200E camera. For each slide, 75 nucleoids were scored using the Comet Assay IV software (Perceptive Instruments, Haverhill, UK). The percentage of DNA in the tail (% Tail DNA) was chosen to evaluate DNA damage. The mean of the median tail intensity value of each slide was calculated for each animal, prior to the calculation of the mean value of each group. When DNA damage was too high to score, the cells were counted as hedgehogs [30,31].

2.5. Bone Marrow Micronucleus Assay (BMMN)

The BMMN assay was carried out following the general principles of the OECD guideline 474 [32]. Briefly, after isolation and centrifugation for 5 min at 210× g, drops of BM cells were spread on a microscope slide and allowed to air dry half a day. After fixation in ethanol 96°, the smears were stained for 3 min with May–Grünwald (MG) reagent, 2 min in MG diluted in Sörensen buffer (50/50V, pH 6.75 ± 0.05), 10 min in 14% Giemsa and 1 min in demineralized water. Duplicate slides were prepared for each animal. At least 2000 polychromatic erythrocytes (PCEs) per slide were examined microscopically to determine the frequency of micronucleated polychromatic erythrocytes (MN-PCEs). For myelotoxicity evaluation, the ratio of PCEs to normochromatic erythrocytes (NCEs) was calculated. Coded slides were analyzed under a bright field microscope and micronuclei were scored by two independent scorers.

2.6. Colon Micronucleus Assay

The "swiss roll" technique was performed as previously described [28]. The whole colon was cut longitudinally prior to a wash with HBSS. The tissue was rolled up from the rectum to the caecum with the mucosa inward, fixed in 4% formaldehyde and embedded in paraffin. Sections were deparaffinized and dehydrated twice in toluene followed by successive baths of ethanol 100%, 95% and 70%. After rinsing and staining with Schiff's reagent (Saint Louis, MO, USA) and fast green, a dehydration step in ethanol 70° and ethanol 96° was performed, and finally, slides were mounted using DPX. Intact colon crypts were chosen, and scoring was done on at least 1000 cells per rat.

2.7. Statistical Analysis

For the in vivo comet assay, the results from the five animals were analyzed using a one-way ANOVA. For the bone marrow and colon MN assays, Pearson's chi square test with Yate's correction was used. Myelotoxicity and hedgehogs over the vehicle control were analyzed with the Mann–Whitney U test (one tailed). Statistical significance was set at $p < 0.05$.

3. Results

3.1. Comet Assay

The results from the alkaline comet assay after three oral treatments with Al^0 NMs and Al_2O_3 NMs at 6, 12.5 or 25 mg/kg bw/day, and $AlCl_3$ at 25 mg/kg bw/day, are shown in Figure 1. Al^0 NMs did not induce an increase in tail intensity irrespective of the organ or tissue investigated compared to the vehicle control group. Al_2O_3 NMs induced a significant increase in tail intensity only in BM at the highest dose (25 mg/kg bw).

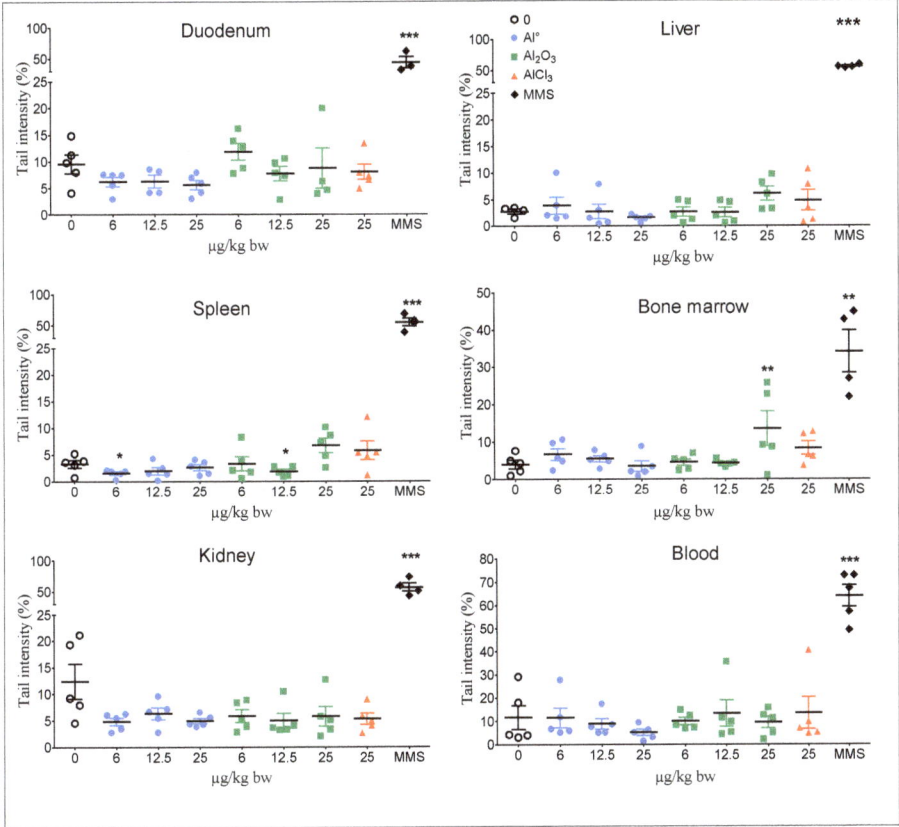

Figure 1. DNA damage in organs/tissues of rats orally exposed to Al^0 NMs, Al_2O_3 NMs or $AlCl_3$. A group treated with the vehicle (0, negative control) and a group treated with a genotoxic agent (MMS, positive control) were included. Significant from control at ** $p < 0.01$, *** $p < 0.001$.

$AlCl_3$ did not induce increases in the DNA tail intensity irrespective of the organ or tissue investigated compared to the vehicle control group.

The data for oxidative DNA damage using the modified Fpg comet assay are shown in Figure 2. No increase in tail intensity was observed in any organ or tissue from rats treated with Al^0 and Al_2O_3 NMs. However, a significant decrease in tail intensity was detected in the duodenums of rats treated with Al^0 NMs for the three doses. An increase in oxidative lesions, although not statistically significant, was observed in the blood of rats treated with $AlCl_3$ at 25 mg/kg bw.

The positive control MMS induced a significant increase in tail intensity for all organs with and without Fpg (*** $p < 0.001$).

With the exception of the positive control MMS, the number of hedgehogs was generally low for all treated groups and tissues in the modified Fpg comet assay except for kidney and spleen (Supplementary Tables S2 and S3).

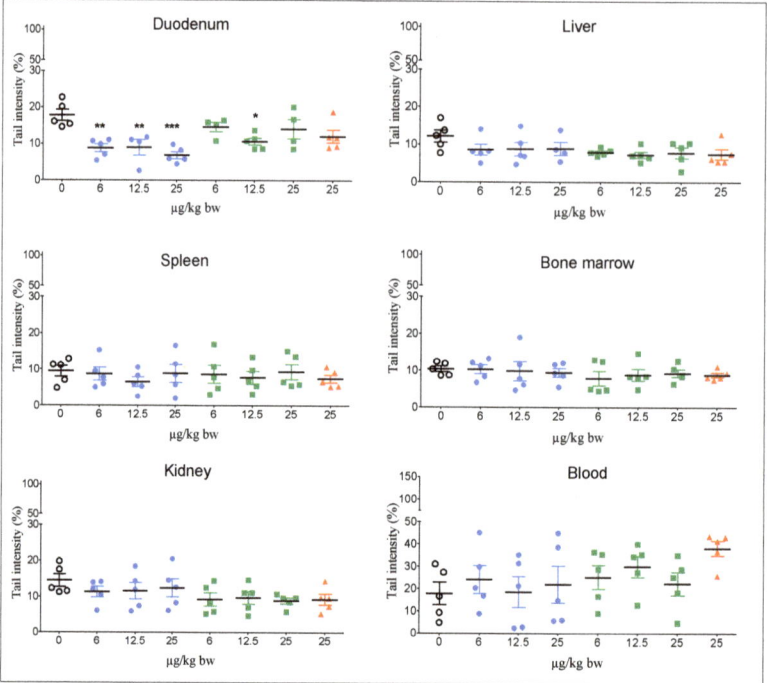

Figure 2. Oxidative DNA damage in different organs/tissues of rats orally exposed to Al^0 NMs, Al_2O_3 NMs or $AlCl_3$. A group treated with the vehicle (0, negative control) was included. Significant from control at * $p < 0.05$, ** $p < 0.01$, *** $p < 0.001$.

3.2. Bone Marrow Micronucleus Assay (BMMN)

The results of the BMMN test conducted after oral exposure to Al^0 NMs and Al_2O_3 NMs at 6, 12.5 or 25 mg/kg bw, and to $AlCl_3$ at 25 mg/kg bw, are presented in Table 2.

Table 2. Genotoxicity of Al^0 NMs, Al_2O_3 NMs and $AlCl_3$ in rats treated orally detected by the micronucleus assay in bone marrow.

		Genotoxicity	Myelotoxicity
		Micronucleated PCE/2 000 PCE	%PCEs
	Doses (mg/kg bw/day)	Mean ± SD	Mean ± SD
Control		1.3 ± 0.91	72.5 ± 26
Al^0	6	2.0 ± 2.0	66.3 ± 13
	12.5	1.5 ± 0.8	71.5 ± 8
	25	2.1 ± 1.0	74.7 ± 16
Al_2O_3	6	1.1 ± 0.7	68.4 ± 18
	12.5	1.6 ± 1.3	65.8 ± 17
	25	0.9 ± 0.8	56.7 ± 17
$AlCl_3$	25	1.5 ± 0.7	65.9 ± 19
MMS	100, 100, 80	16.7 ± 3.7 *	44.5 ± 12

NCE: normochromatic erythrocytes; PCEs: polychromatic erythrocytes; results correspond to mean ± SD, n = 5; * $p < 0.001$ with the Pearson X2 with Yate's correction.

The two Al-NMs did not induce any significant changes in the percentage of MN-PCEs compared to the control group. No significant myelotoxicity was found with either Al-NMs or AlCl$_3$.

The positive control group treated with MMS demonstrated a significant increase in MN-PCEs and a decrease of the percentage of PCEs.

3.3. Micronucleus Assay in Colon

The micronucleus assay in colon (Figure 3) showed that the two Al-NMs and AlCl$_3$ did not induce any significant increase in micronucleated cells compared to control rats. Similarly, no increase in mitosis and apoptosis was detected with the three Al forms. With the positive control MMS, only a significant increase in the level of apoptotic figures was detected.

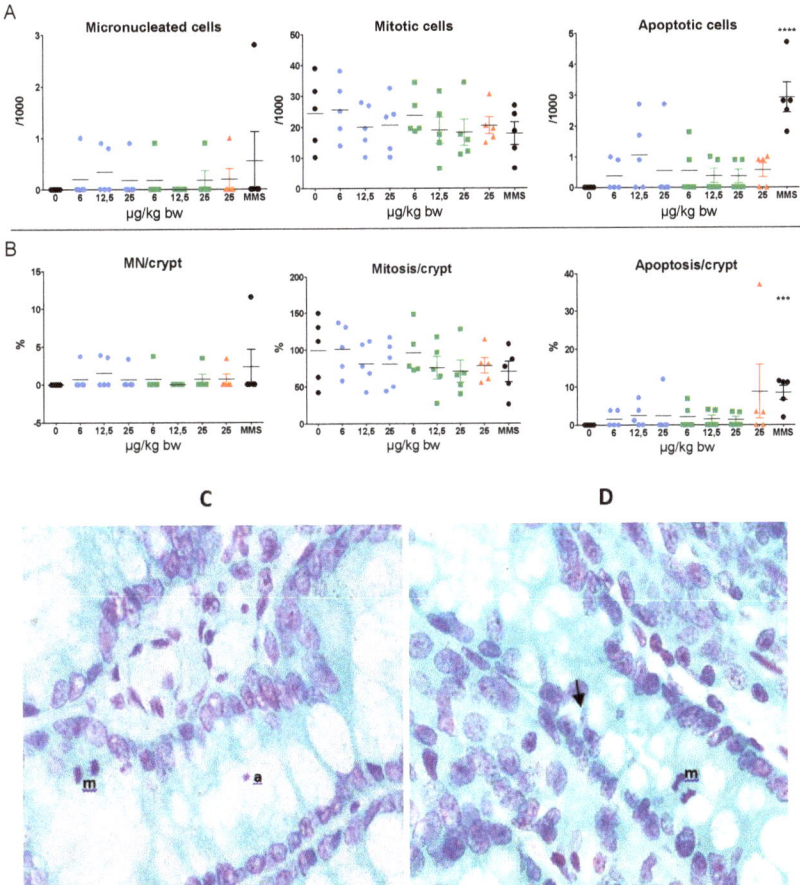

Figure 3. (**A**) MN, mitotic and apoptotic frequencies per 1000 cells in the colon of rats orally exposed to Al NMs and AlCl$_3$ or to the solvent control (0). (**B**) MN, mitosis and apoptosis percentages per crypt. Results correspond to individual values with mean ± SD (n = 5). Significant from control at *** $p < 0.001$, **** $p < 0.0001$ compared to the vehicle control. (**C,D**) Schiff's reagent and fast green counterstained colon sections of rats treated with MMS (**C**) and Al^0 NMs at 12.5 mg/kg bw (**D**). Black arrow indicates micronuclei in cells. a: apoptosis, m: mitosis.

4. Discussion

To date, published data on the oral genotoxicity of Al-containing NMs are scarce. In this study, we investigated the genotoxic potentials of two nanoforms (Al^0 and Al_2O_3) by applying the in vivo OECD guidelines for the comet assay in several key tissues/organs [27], and the micronucleus assay on bone marrow [32] and on colons. In addition, we have compared the responses with the ionic form $AlCl_3$.

The micronucleus assay both on BM and on colon was negative with Al^0 and Al_2O_3 NMs up to 25 mg/kg bw indicating that no chromosome or genome mutations were induced in these two organs. Similarly, a negative response was observed in the blood of rats exposed orally to Al_2O_3 NMs (30 nm and 40 nm) at a unique dose of 500 mg/kg bw. However, doses above 1000 mg/kg bw induced the formation of MN, concomitantly to high levels of Al content in several organs, including blood, liver, spleen and kidney [11]. Nevertheless, such doses are very high and far from human exposure. Intraperitoneal injection of nano- and bulk-Al from 300 to 1200 µg/kg bw in male and female mice did not provoke any increase of MN in BM [33]. In vitro, Al_2O_3 NMs were found to induce MN in a concentration dependent manner after 24 h exposure from 0.5 µg/mL in Chinese hamster cells CHOK1 [19] and in human fibroblasts at 13.3 and 26.6 µg/cm² (50 and 100 µg/mL) [16]. In contrast, no MN increase was found in human blood lymphocytes [34] or RAW 264 macrophages exposed for 72 h to Al_2O_3 NMs [35]. A negative response was also observed with the chromosome aberrations assay in human lymphocytes with Al_2O_3 NMs [18]. Similarly, with the same NMs and dispersion protocol used in our study, we did not detect any increase of MN in human intestinal Caco-2 cells and hepatic HepaRG cells for Al^0 and Al_2O_3 NMs up to 80 µg/cm² and for $AlCl_3$ following 24 h exposure [36].

No DNA damage was observed in the alkaline comet assay in any of the six organs/tissues investigated from rats orally-exposed to Al^0 NMs up to 25 mg/kg bw. Nevertheless, a decrease of the tail intensity was observed in duodenum that may be a result of cross-links induced by NMs, preventing the DNA migration, as described in the literature [37]. In fact, such a cross-linking effect has been recently described in plants treated with $AlCl_3$, and it was suggested that Al may interact with DNA in an electrostatic manner [38]. Further data are necessary to confirm this hypothesis. Due to interference of Al^0 NMs with the assay in vitro, the genotoxic potential of these NMs on hepatic and intestinal cell lines is unclear [36].

In this study we have shown induced DNA damage in BM of rats exposed to 25 mg/kg bw Al_2O_3 NMs but not in the other organs or tissues investigated. Balasubramanyam et al. (2009) observed an increase of DNA damage in blood of rats up to 48 h after a single treatment with 30 and 40 nm Al_2O_3 NMs by gavage; however, this was observed at very high doses (above 1000 mg/kg) [11]. Recently, DNA fragmentation due to cell death (both necrosis and apoptosis) was reported in liver and kidney of rats treated orally for 75 days with 70 mg/kg bw Al_2O_3 NMs [39]. Two other studies have investigated the genotoxic potential of Al_2O_3 NMs after intraperitoneal administration. These have demonstrated DNA damage in blood after 6 weeks of repeated exposure at 1.25 mg/kg bw [40] and in the brains of rats 48 h after a single intraperitoneal administration of Al_2O_3 NMs, although at very high doses (from 4 to 8.5 g/kg bw) which were evaluated as lethal (from 30 to 65% of the LD50) in the same study [41]. In this study, the DNA damage was correlated with Al accumulation in several organs, including the brain.

In vitro, time- and concentration-dependent DNA damage was found in Chinese hamster lung fibroblasts [33] and in liver HepG2 cells [17] exposed to Al_2O_3 NMs from 30 µg/mL. However, other studies have reported negative responses in human peripheral blood cells and human embryonic kidney cells up to 100 µg/mL following a 3 h treatment [42], and in human lymphocytes at 100 µg/mL after a 24 h exposure [18]. Recently, it was shown that Al_2O_3 NMs can inhibit DNA polymerase replication but without affecting mutation rate compared to controls [43].

To investigate if oxidative DNA damage can be increased with Al NMs, we performed the Fpg-modified comet assay. Neither Al^0 nor Al_2O_3 NMs induced oxidative DNA damage in six different organs of rats exposed to 6–25 mg/kg bw. Although in this study we did not observe an increase in oxidative DNA damage with Al_2O_3 NMs, Shah et al. (2015) reported an increase in 8-oxo guanine, an oxidized DNA base, in vivo in the brain of mice treated intraperitoneally with 50 mg/kg Al_2O_3 NMs [44]. Similar results were observed in vitro in mouse neuronal cells treated with Al_2O_3 NMs from 100 to 150 µg/mL [44].

Several metal oxide NMs have been shown to induce oxidative stress [13,14,18,33,45,46] which in some cases was correlated with DNA damage [47]. Several in vivo studies with Al NMs have described a concentration-dependent increase in oxidative stress with Al_2O_3 NMs in several tissues including liver and kidney induced after acute (3 days) and chronic (up to 21 days) oral exposures to rats at doses ranging from 500 to 2000 mg/kg bw [13,14]. Moreover, oxidative stress was observed in several organs of rodents following acute and repeated intraperitoneal exposure [44,48]. Using doses of Al_2O_3 NMs more consistent with daily human exposure (0.5 to 70 mg/kg bw), oxidative stress was detected in rat liver, kidney and erythrocytes after repeated daily oral exposure [39,45,49]. In vitro, some evidence that exposure to Al_2O_3 NMs can induce oxidative stress has been also reported in various cell lines following 24 h exposure [18,33,44,46,47] that can be rapidly repaired depending on the concentration [47]. In contrast, Demir et al. (2015) did not observe any oxidative DNA damage in human peripheral blood cells exposed 3 h to Al_2O_3 NMs up to 10 µg/mL [50]. It was also shown that impairment of mineral homeostasis linked to oxidative stress could be induced by Al_2O_3 NMs in hippocampi of rats after intravenous injections [51].

In agreement with our results for Al^0 and Al_2O_3 NMs, no increase in MN was observed in either in BM or colons of rats exposed to 25 mg/kg bw $AlCl_3$. In other studies, however, $AlCl_3$ was found to increase the number of MN in BM after a unique oral exposure to mice at 50 mg/kg bw [22]. Likewise, increases in MN frequency were observed in rat liver after a 30 day oral exposure [52] or with a 5 mg/kg bw daily intra-peritoneal exposure for 10 weeks [53]. Interestingly, the induction of MN formation following oral exposure could be decreased with an antioxidant treatment (propolis or borax) [52,54] suggesting that the effects of $AlCl_3$ where linked to oxidative stress as described elsewhere [55–57]. Nevertheless, apoptosis has been described as a cause of DNA fragmentation in the liver of mice following acute exposures to $AlCl_3$ (25 mg/kg by ip) [58]. Aluminum acetate (50 mg/kg) was also found to induce chromosome aberrations in BM of mice after both single and seven consecutive day intraperitoneal administration while the MN response was only positive after repeated exposure [59]. In vitro, $AlCl_3$ was reported to increase the number of MN and chromosomal aberrations in peripheral blood lymphocytes after 24 h exposure between 1 and 10 µg/mL [60].

We did not observe any increase in DNA damage with the comet assay in duodenum and liver, in agreement with our in vitro results on liver and intestinal human cells [36]. No DNA damage, with or without Fpg, was detected in the other organs and tissues investigated, with the exception of blood where a slight increase of oxidative DNA damage was observed. Indeed, DNA damage in response to $AlCl_3$ exposure was reported in vitro in human peripheral blood cells [20,21]. Oxidative stress in response to $AlCl_3$ treatment was demonstrated to correlate with oxidative DNA damage induced in human peripheral blood cells [21] and the increase of GSH/GSSG ratio and Hsp70 mRNA levels in human neuroblastoma cells [61].

While a negative response in the MN assay was observed with the three forms of Al both in vitro and in vivo, the comet assay indicated effects of Al_2O_3 NMs on BM and with $AlCl_3$ on blood. No correlation between the in vivo genotoxicity of Al NMs and the ionic salt $AlCl_3$ was observed in our study, and we therefore cannot conclusively determine the potential effect of aluminum ions released from the Al NMs. Although we have previously reported a low solubility of these Al-containing NMs in an in vitro digestion system [25], estimating the solubility of NMs in the intestinal fluid in vivo remains challenging. Therefore, no clear conclusion can be drawn on the role, if any, of metallic ions in the genotoxic effects observed. The differences due to the route of exposure, the Al form tested, the organs studied and the dose of exposure can explain the discrepancies of the responses in the different publications.

5. Conclusions

Our results indicate that Al^0 and Al_2O_3 NMs do not induce chromosomal mutations detected by the micronucleus assay in BM or the colons of rats exposed orally to Al-containing NMs at doses from 6 to 25 mg/kg bw. However, the comet assay showed some increase of DNA damage only in BM with Al_2O_3 NMs, while $AlCl_3$ induced slight oxidative DNA damage in blood. No clear relationship between genotoxic effects and ion release could be determined. Challenges remain in the evaluation of the genotoxicity of Al-containing NMs, and further work is necessary in order to correlate these data with the measurement and characterization of Al NMs in the different organs and body fluids, including data on solubility in vivo.

Supplementary Materials: The following are available online at http://www.mdpi.com/2079-4991/10/2/305/s1. Figure S1: Equivalence between the doses administrated between mass and Al content., Table S1: Percentage of hedgehogs scored on the comet slides without Fpg. Mean ± SD (n = 5 animals per condition except for control duodenum n = 4)., Table S2: Percentage of hedgehogs scored on the comet slides with Fpg. Mean ± SD (n = 5 animals per condition).

Author Contributions: Conceptualization, V.F.; formal analysis, P.J., L.L.H., F.N., K.H. and V.F.; funding acquisition, V.F.; investigation, P.J., S.H., R.L. and G.J.; methodology, P.J., S.H., R.L., G.J. and L.L.H.; project administration, P.J. and V.F.; resources, P.J., S.H., R.L., G.J. and L.L.H.; supervision, F.N., K.H. and V.F.; visualization, P.J.; writing—original draft, P.J.; writing—review and editing, K.H. and V.F. All authors have read and agree to the published version of the manuscript.

Funding: This publication arises from the French-German bilateral project SolNanoTOX funded by the French National Research Agency (ANR, Project ID: ANR-13-IS10-0005) and the German Research Foundation (DFG, Project ID: DFG (FKZ LA 3411/1-1 respectively LA 1177/9-1).

Acknowledgments: The authors would like to thank Jean-Guy Rolland, Gonzague Dourdin and Eulalie Gateau for their technical support.

Conflicts of Interest: The authors declare that there are no conflicts of interest.

References

1. European Food Safety Authority. Safety of aluminium from dietary intake—Scientific Opinion of the Panel on Food Additives, Flavourings, Processing Aids and Food Contact Materials (AFC). *EFSA J.* **2008**, *6*, 754.
2. Willhite, C.C.; Karyakina, N.A.; Yokel, R.A.; Yenugadhati, N.; Wisniewski, T.M.; Arnold, I.M.; Momoli, F.; Krewski, D. Systematic review of potential health risks posed by pharmaceutical, occupational and consumer exposures to metallic and nanoscale aluminum, aluminum oxides, aluminum hydroxide and its soluble salts. *Crit. Rev. Toxicol.* **2014**, *44*, 1–80. [CrossRef] [PubMed]
3. Vignal, C.; Desreumaux, P.; Body-Malapel, M. Gut: An underestimated target organ for Aluminum. *Morphologie* **2016**, *100*, 75–84. [CrossRef] [PubMed]
4. Saiyed, S.M.; Yokel, R.A. Aluminium content of some foods and food products in the USA, with aluminium food additives. *Food Addit. Contam.* **2005**, *22*, 234–244. [CrossRef] [PubMed]
5. Krewski, D.; Yokel, R.A.; Nieboer, E.; Borchelt, D.; Cohen, J.; Harry, J.; Kacew, S.; Lindsay, J.; Mahfouz, A.M.; Rondeau, V. Human health risk assessment for aluminium, aluminium oxide, and aluminium hydroxide. *J. Toxicol. Environ. Health. B Crit. Rev.* **2007**, *10*, 1–269. [CrossRef] [PubMed]
6. Gehrke, I.; Geiser, A.; Somborn-Schulz, A. Innovations in nanotechnology for water treatment. *Nanotechnol. Sci. Appl.* **2015**, *8*, 1–17. [CrossRef] [PubMed]
7. Zhao, J.; Castranova, V. Toxicology of nanomaterials used in nanomedicine. *J. Toxicol. Environ. Health B Crit. Rev.* **2011**, *14*, 593–632. [CrossRef]
8. Frey, A.; Neutra, M.R.; Robey, F.A. Peptomer aluminum oxide nanoparticle conjugates as systemic and mucosal vaccine candidates: Synthesis and characterization of a conjugate derived from the C4 domain of HIV-1MN gp120. *Bioconjug. Chem.* **1997**, *8*, 424–433. [CrossRef]
9. Narayan, R.J.; Adiga, S.P.; Pellin, M.J.; Curtiss, L.A.; Hryn, A.J.; Stafslien, S.; Chisholm, B.; Shih, C.-C.; Shih, C.-M.; Lin, S.-J.; et al. Atomic layer deposition-based functionalization of materials for medical and environmental health applications. *Philos. Trans. R. Soc. A Math. Phys. Eng. Sci.* **2010**, *368*, 2033–2064. [CrossRef]

10. JECFA Summary and Conclusions of the Sixty-Seventh Meeting of the Joint FAO/WHO Expert Committee on Food Additives (JECFA). Available online: http://www.fao.org/3/a-at874e.pdf (accessed on 1 February 2020).
11. Balasubramanyam, A.; Sailaja, N.; Mahboob, M.; Rahman, M.F.; Misra, S.; Hussain, S.M.; Grover, P. Evaluation of genotoxic effects of oral exposure to aluminum oxide nanomaterials in rat bone marrow. *Mutat. Res.* **2009**, *676*, 41–47. [CrossRef]
12. Park, E.J.; Sim, J.; Kim, Y.; Han, B.S.; Yoon, C.; Lee, S.; Cho, M.H.; Lee, B.S.; Kim, J.H. A 13-week repeated-dose oral toxicity and bioaccumulation of aluminum oxide nanoparticles in mice. *Arch. Toxicol.* **2015**, *89*, 371–379. [CrossRef] [PubMed]
13. Shrivastava, R.; Raza, S.; Yadav, A.; Kushwaha, P.; Flora, S.J. Effects of sub-acute exposure to TiO2, ZnO and Al2O3 nanoparticles on oxidative stress and histological changes in mouse liver and brain. *Drug Chem. Toxicol.* **2014**, *37*, 336–347. [CrossRef] [PubMed]
14. Prabhakar, P.V.; Reddy, U.A.; Singh, S.P.; Balasubramanyam, A.; Rahman, M.F.; Indu Kumari, S.; Agawane, S.B.; Murty, U.S.; Grover, P.; Mahboob, M. Oxidative stress induced by aluminum oxide nanomaterials after acute oral treatment in Wistar rats. *J. Appl. Toxicol.* **2012**, *32*, 436–445. [CrossRef] [PubMed]
15. ECHA. Registration dossier Aluminum oxide. Available online: https://echa.europa.eu/fr/registration-dossier/-/registered-dossier/16039/7/7/1 (accessed on 5 January 2020).
16. Tsaousi, A.; Jones, E.; Case, C.P. The in vitro genotoxicity of orthopaedic ceramic (Al2O3) and metal (CoCr alloy) particles. *Mutat. Res.* **2010**, *697*, 1–9. [CrossRef] [PubMed]
17. Alarifi, S.; Ali, D.; Alkahtani, S. Nanoalumina induces apoptosis by impairing antioxidant enzyme systems in human hepatocarcinoma cells. *Int. J. Nanomed.* **2015**, *10*, 3751–3760.
18. Rajiv, S.; Jerobin, J.; Saranya, V.; Nainawat, M.; Sharma, A.; Makwana, P.; Gayathri, C.; Bharath, L.; Singh, M.; Kumar, M.; et al. Comparative cytotoxicity and genotoxicity of cobalt (II, III) oxide, iron (III) oxide, silicon dioxide, and aluminum oxide nanoparticles on human lymphocytes in vitro. *Hum. Exp. Toxicol.* **2016**, *35*, 170–183. [CrossRef]
19. Di Virgilio, A.L.; Reigosa, M.; Arnal, P.M.; Fernandez Lorenzo de Mele, M. Comparative study of the cytotoxic and genotoxic effects of titanium oxide and aluminium oxide nanoparticles in Chinese hamster ovary (CHO-K1) cells. *J. Hazard. Mater.* **2010**, *177*, 711–718. [CrossRef]
20. Lima, P.D.; Leite, D.S.; Vasconcellos, M.C.; Cavalcanti, B.C.; Santos, R.A.; Costa-Lotufo, L.V.; Pessoa, C.; Moraes, M.O.; Burbano, R.R. Genotoxic effects of aluminum chloride in cultured human lymphocytes treated in different phases of cell cycle. *Food Chem. Toxicol.* **2007**, *45*, 1154–1159. [CrossRef]
21. Lankoff, A.; Banasik, A.; Duma, A.; Ochniak, E.; Lisowska, H.; Kuszewski, T.; Gozdz, S.; Wojcik, A. A comet assay study reveals that aluminium induces DNA damage and inhibits the repair of radiation-induced lesions in human peripheral blood lymphocytes. *Toxicol. Lett.* **2006**, *161*, 27–36. [CrossRef]
22. Paz, L.N.; Moura, L.M.; Feio, D.C.; Cardoso, M.S.; Ximenes, W.L.; Montenegro, R.C.; Alves, A.P.; Burbano, R.R.; Lima, P.D. Evaluation of in vivo and in vitro toxicological and genotoxic potential of aluminum chloride. *Chemosphere* **2017**, *175*, 130–137. [CrossRef]
23. Hartmann, N.B.; Jensen, K.A.; Baun, A.; Rasmussen, K.; Rauscher, H.; Tantra, R.; Cupi, D.; Gilliland, D.; Pianella, F.; Riego Sintes, J.M. Techniques and Protocols for Dispersing Nanoparticle Powders in Aqueous Media-Is there a Rationale for Harmonization? *J. Toxicol. Environ. Health B Crit. Rev.* **2015**, *18*, 299–326. [CrossRef] [PubMed]
24. Jensen, K.A.; Kembouche, Y.; Christiansen, E.; Jacobsen, N.R.; Wallin, H.; Guiot, C.; Spalla, O.; Witschger, O. Final Protocol for Producing Suitable Manufactured Nanomaterial Exposure Media. Web-Report. The Generic NANOGENOTOX Dispersion Protocol—Standard Operation Procedure (SOP). Available online: https://www.anses.fr/en/system/files/nanogenotox_deliverable_5.pdf (accessed on 1 February 2020).
25. Sieg, H.; Kastner, C.; Krause, B.; Meyer, T.; Burel, A.; Bohmert, L.; Lichtenstein, D.; Jungnickel, H.; Tentschert, J.; Laux, P.; et al. Impact of an Artificial Digestion Procedure on Aluminum-Containing Nanomaterials. *Langmuir* **2017**, *33*, 10726–10735. [CrossRef] [PubMed]
26. Krause, B.; Meyer, T.; Sieg, H.; Kästner, C.; Reichardt, P.; Tentschert, J.; Jungnickel, H.; Estrela-Lopis, I.; Burel, A.; Chevance, S.; et al. Characterization of aluminum, aluminum oxide and titanium dioxide nanomaterials using a combination of methods for particle surface and size analysis. *RSC Adv.* **2018**, *8*, 14377–14388. [CrossRef]
27. OCDE. *Test No. 489: In Vivo Mammalian Alkaline Comet Assay*; OECD Publishing: Paris, France, 2016.

28. Tarantini, A.; Huet, S.; Jarry, G.; Lanceleur, R.; Poul, M.; Tavares, A.; Vital, N.; Louro, H.; Joao Silva, M.; Fessard, V. Genotoxicity of synthetic amorphous silica nanoparticles in rats following short-term exposure. Part 1: Oral route. *Environ. Mol. Mutagen.* **2015**, *56*, 218–227. [CrossRef]
29. McKelvey-Martin, V.J.; Green, M.H.; Schmezer, P.; Pool-Zobel, B.L.; De Meo, M.P.; Collins, A. The single cell gel electrophoresis assay (comet assay): A European review. *Mutat. Res.* **1993**, *288*, 47–63. [CrossRef]
30. Zeller, A.; Duran-Pacheco, G.; Guerard, M. An appraisal of critical effect sizes for the benchmark dose approach to assess dose-response relationships in genetic toxicology. *Arch. Toxicol.* **2017**, *91*, 3799–3807. [CrossRef]
31. Tice, R.R.; Agurell, E.; Anderson, D.; Burlinson, B.; Hartmann, A.; Kobayashi, H.; Miyamae, Y.; Rojas, E.; Ryu, J.C.; Sasaki, Y.F. Single cell gel/comet assay: Guidelines for in vitro and in vivo genetic toxicology testing. *Environ. Mol. Mutagen.* **2000**, *35*, 206–221. [CrossRef]
32. OCDE. *Test No. 474: Mammalian Erythrocyte Micronucleus Test*; OECD Publishing: Paris, France, 2016.
33. Zhang, Q.; Wang, H.; Ge, C.; Duncan, J.; He, K.; Adeosun, S.O.; Xi, H.; Peng, H.; Niu, Q. Alumina at 50 and 13 nm nanoparticle sizes have potential genotoxicity. *J. Appl. Toxicol.* **2017**, *37*, 1053–1064. [CrossRef]
34. Akbaba, G.B.; Turkez, H. Investigation of the Genotoxicity of Aluminum Oxide, beta-Tricalcium Phosphate, and Zinc Oxide Nanoparticles In Vitro. *Int. J. Toxicol.* **2018**, *37*, 216–222. [CrossRef]
35. Hashimoto, M.; Imazato, S. Cytotoxic and genotoxic characterization of aluminum and silicon oxide nanoparticles in macrophages. *Dent. Mater.* **2015**, *31*, 556–564. [CrossRef]
36. Jalili, P.; Huet, S.; Burel, A.; Krause, B.-C.; Fontana, C.; Gauffre, F.; Guichard, Y.; Laux, P.; Luch, A.; Hogeveen, K.; et al. Genotoxic impact of aluminum-containing nanomaterials in human intestinal and hepatic cells. Manuscript in preparation.
37. McKenna, D.J.; Gallus, M.; McKeown, S.R.; Downes, C.S.; McKelvey-Martin, V.J. Modification of the alkaline Comet assay to allow simultaneous evaluation of mitomycin C-induced DNA cross-link damage and repair of specific DNA sequences in RT4 cells. *DNA Repair* **2003**, *2*, 879–890. [CrossRef]
38. Chen, P.; Sjogren, C.A.; Larsen, P.B.; Schnittger, A. A multi-level response to DNA damage induced by aluminium. *Plant J.* **2019**, *98*, 479–491. [CrossRef] [PubMed]
39. Yousef, M.I.; Mutar, T.F.; Kamel, M.A.E. Hepato-renal toxicity of oral sub-chronic exposure to aluminum oxide and/or zinc oxide nanoparticles in rats. *Toxicol. Rep.* **2019**, *6*, 336–346. [CrossRef] [PubMed]
40. Minigalieva, I.A.; Katsnelson, B.A.; Privalova, L.I.; Sutunkova, M.P.; Gurvich, V.B.; Shur, V.Y.; Shishkina, E.V.; Valamina, I.E.; Makeyev, O.H.; Panov, V.G.; et al. Combined Subchronic Toxicity of Aluminum (III), Titanium (IV) and Silicon (IV) Oxide Nanoparticles and Its Alleviation with a Complex of Bioprotectors. *Int. J. Mol. Sci.* **2018**, *19*, 837. [CrossRef]
41. Morsy, G.M.; El-Ala, K.S.; Ali, A.A. Studies on fate and toxicity of nanoalumina in male albino rats: Lethality, bioaccumulation and genotoxicity. *Toxicol. Ind. Health* **2016**, *32*, 344–359. [CrossRef]
42. Demir, E.; Akca, H.; Turna, F.; Aksakal, S.; Burgucu, D.; Kaya, B.; Tokgun, O.; Vales, G.; Creus, A.; Marcos, R. Genotoxic and cell-transforming effects of titanium dioxide nanoparticles. *Environ. Res.* **2015**, *136*, 300–308. [CrossRef]
43. Gao, C.-H.; Mortimer, M.; Zhang, M.; Holden, P.A.; Cai, P.; Wu, S.; Xin, Y.; Wu, Y.; Huang, Q. Impact of metal oxide nanoparticles on in vitro DNA amplification. *Peer J.* **2019**, *7*, e7228. [CrossRef]
44. Shah, S.A.; Yoon, G.H.; Ahmad, A.; Ullah, F.; Amin, F.U.; Kim, M.O. Nanoscale-alumina induces oxidative stress and accelerates amyloid beta (Aβ) production in ICR female mice. *Nanoscale* **2015**, *7*, 15225–15237. [CrossRef]
45. Canli, E.G.; Atli, G.; Canli, M. Response of the antioxidant enzymes of the erythrocyte and alterations in the serum biomarkers in rats following oral administration of nanoparticles. *Environ. Toxicol. Pharmacol.* **2017**, *50*, 145–150. [CrossRef]
46. Li, X.; Zhang, C.; Zhang, X.; Wang, S.; Meng, Q.; Wu, S.; Yang, H.; Xia, Y.; Chen, R. An acetyl-L-carnitine switch on mitochondrial dysfunction and rescue in the metabolomics study on aluminum oxide nanoparticles. *Part Fibre Toxicol.* **2016**, *13*, 4. [CrossRef]
47. Sliwinska, A.; Kwiatkowski, D.; Czarny, P.; Milczarek, J.; Toma, M.; Korycinska, A.; Szemraj, J.; Sliwinski, T. Genotoxicity and cytotoxicity of ZnO and Al2O3 nanoparticles. *Toxicol. Mech. Methods.* **2015**, *25*, 176–183. [CrossRef] [PubMed]

48. Morsy, G.M.; El-Ala, K.S.; Ali, A.A. Studies on fate and toxicity of nanoalumina in male albino rats: Some haematological, biochemical and histological aspects. *Toxicol. Ind. Health.* **2016**, *32*, 634–655. [CrossRef] [PubMed]
49. Canli, E.G.; Atli, G.; Canli, M. Responses of biomarkers belonging to different metabolic systems of rats following oral administration of aluminium nanoparticle. *Environ. Toxicol. Pharm.* **2019**, *69*, 72–79. [CrossRef] [PubMed]
50. Demir, E.; Burgucu, D.; Turna, F.; Aksakal, S.; Kaya, B. Determination of TiO2, ZrO2, and Al2O3 nanoparticles on genotoxic responses in human peripheral blood lymphocytes and cultured embryonic kidney cells. *J. Toxicol. Environ. Health A* **2013**, *76*, 990–1002. [CrossRef]
51. M'Rad, I.; Jeljeli, M.; Rihane, N.; Hilber, P.; Sakly, M.; Amara, S. Aluminium oxide nanoparticles compromise spatial learning and memory performance in rats. *Excli. J.* **2018**, *17*, 200–210.
52. Turkez, H.; Yousef, M.I.; Geyikoglu, F. Propolis prevents aluminium-induced genetic and hepatic damages in rat liver. *Food Chem. Toxicol.* **2010**, *48*, 2741–2746. [CrossRef]
53. Geyikoglu, F.; Turkez, H.; Bakir, T.O.; Cicek, M. The genotoxic, hepatotoxic, nephrotoxic, haematotoxic and histopathological effects in rats after aluminium chronic intoxication. *Toxicol. Ind. Health* **2013**, *29*, 780–791. [CrossRef]
54. Turkez, H.; Geyikoglu, F.; Tatar, A. Borax counteracts genotoxicity of aluminum in rat liver. *Toxicol. Ind. Health* **2013**, *29*, 775–779. [CrossRef]
55. Cao, Z.; Geng, X.; Jiang, X.; Gao, X.; Liu, K.; Li, Y. Melatonin Attenuates AlCl3-Induced Apoptosis and Osteoblastic Differentiation Suppression by Inhibiting Oxidative Stress in MC3T3-E1 Cells. *Biol. Trace Elem. Res.* **2019**. [CrossRef]
56. Martinez, C.S.; Vera, G.; Ocio, J.A.U.; Pecanha, F.M.; Vassallo, D.V.; Miguel, M.; Wiggers, G.A. Aluminum exposure for 60days at an equivalent human dietary level promotes peripheral dysfunction in rats. *J. Inorg. Biochem.* **2018**, *181*, 169–176. [CrossRef]
57. Yang, X.; Yu, K.; Wang, H.; Zhang, H.; Bai, C.; Song, M.; Han, Y.; Shao, B.; Li, Y.; Li, X. Bone impairment caused by AlCl3 is associated with activation of the JNK apoptotic pathway mediated by oxidative stress. *Food Chem. Toxicol.* **2018**, *116*, 307–314. [CrossRef]
58. Cheng, D.; Zhang, X.; Xu, L.; Li, X.; Hou, L.; Wang, C. Protective and prophylactic effects of chlorogenic acid on aluminum-induced acute hepatotoxicity and hematotoxicity in mice. *Chem. Interact.* **2017**, *273*, 125–132. [CrossRef] [PubMed]
59. D'Souza, S.P.; Vijayalaxmi, K.K.; Naik, P. Assessment of genotoxicity of aluminium acetate in bone marrow, male germ cells and fetal liver cells of Swiss albino mice. *Mutat. Res. Genet. Toxicol. Environ. Mutagen.* **2014**, *766*, 16–22. [CrossRef] [PubMed]
60. Banasik, A.; Lankoff, A.; Piskulak, A.; Adamowska, K.; Lisowska, H.; Wojcik, A. Aluminum-induced micronuclei and apoptosis in human peripheral-blood lymphocytes treated during different phases of the cell cycle. *Environ. Toxicol.* **2005**, *20*, 402–406. [CrossRef] [PubMed]
61. Villarini, M.; Gambelunghe, A.; Giustarini, D.; Ambrosini, M.V.; Fatigoni, C.; Rossi, R.; Dominici, L.; Levorato, S.; Muzi, G.; Piobbico, D.; et al. No evidence of DNA damage by co-exposure to extremely low frequency magnetic fields and aluminum on neuroblastoma cell lines. *Mutat. Res.* **2017**, *823*, 11–21. [CrossRef]

© 2020 by the authors. Licensee MDPI, Basel, Switzerland. This article is an open access article distributed under the terms and conditions of the Creative Commons Attribution (CC BY) license (http://creativecommons.org/licenses/by/4.0/).

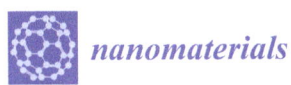

Article

Argovit™ Silver Nanoparticles Effects on *Allium cepa*: Plant Growth Promotion without Cyto Genotoxic Damage

Francisco Casillas-Figueroa [1], María Evarista Arellano-García [2,*], Claudia Leyva-Aguilera [2], Balam Ruíz-Ruíz [3], Roberto Luna Vázquez-Gómez [1], Patricia Radilla-Chávez [1], Rocío Alejandra Chávez-Santoscoy [4], Alexey Pestryakov [5], Yanis Toledano-Magaña [1], Juan Carlos García-Ramos [1,*] and Nina Bogdanchikova [6]

[1] Escuela de Ciencias de la Salud, UABC, Blvd. Zertuche y Blvd., De los Lagos S/N Fracc, Valle Dorado, 22890 Ensenada, Baja California, Mexico; casillas.francisco@uabc.edu.mx (F.C.-F.); cuentarluna@gmail.com (R.L.V.-G.); patyradilla@uabc.edu.mx (P.R.-C.); yanis.toledano@uabc.edu.mx (Y.T.-M.)
[2] Facultad de Ciencias, UABC, Carretera Transpeninsular Ensenada-Tijuana No. 3917 Col. Playitas, 22860 Ensenada, Baja California, Mexico; cleyva@uabc.edu.mx
[3] Facultad de Medicina extensión los Mochis, Universidad Autónoma de Sinaloa, Av. Ángel Flores s/n, Ciudad Universitaria, 81223 Los Mochis, Sinaloa, Mexico; balamruiz@gmail.com
[4] Centro de Biotecnología-FEMSA, Escuela de Ingeniería y Ciencias, ITESM, Monterrey, Eugenio Garza Sada, 2501 Sur, 64849 Monterrey, Nuevo León, Mexico; chavez.santoscoy@tec.mx
[5] Department of Technology of Organic Substances and Polymer Materials, Tomsk Polytechnic University, 634050 Tomsk, Russia; pestryakov2005@yandex.ru
[6] Centro de Nanociencias y Nanotecnología, UNAM, Carretera Tijuana-Ensenada Km 107, 22860 Ensenada, Baja California, Mexico; nina@cnyn.unam.mx
* Correspondence: evarista.arellano@uabc.edu.mx (M.E.A.-G.); juan.carlos.garcia.ramos@uabc.edu.mx (J.C.G.-R.); Tel.: +52-64-6174-5925 (ext. 225) (M.E.A.-G.); +52-64-6175-0707 (ext. 65313) (J.C.G.-R.)

Received: 20 May 2020; Accepted: 13 July 2020; Published: 16 July 2020

Abstract: Due to their antibacterial and antiviral effects, silver nanoparticles (AgNP) are one of the most widely used nanomaterials worldwide in various industries, e.g., in textiles, cosmetics and biomedical-related products. Unfortunately, the lack of complete physicochemical characterization and the variety of models used to evaluate its cytotoxic/genotoxic effect make comparison and decision-making regarding their safe use difficult. In this work, we present a systematic study of the cytotoxic and genotoxic activity of the commercially available AgNPs formulation Argovit™ in *Allium cepa*. The evaluated concentration range, 5–100 µg/mL of metallic silver content (85–1666 µg/mL of complete formulation), is 10–17 times higher than the used for other previously reported polyvinylpyrrolidone (PVP)-AgNP formulations and showed no cytotoxic or genotoxic damage in *Allium cepa*. Conversely, low concentrations (5 and 10 µg/mL) promote growth without damage to roots or bulbs. Until this work, all the formulations of PVP-AgNP evaluated in *Allium cepa* regardless of their size, concentration, or the exposure time had shown phytotoxicity. The biological response observed in *Allium cepa* exposed to Argovit™ is caused by nanoparticles and not by silver ions. The metal/coating agent ratio plays a fundamental role in this response and must be considered within the key physicochemical parameters for the design and manufacture of safer nanomaterials.

Keywords: nongenotoxic silver nanoparticles; genotoxic; cytotoxic; antioxidant activity; silver ions; *Allium cepa*; metal/coating agent ratio

1. Introduction

Silver nanoparticles (AgNPs) are the most widely used nanomaterials worldwide in different areas such as the pharmaceutical, food, biomedical, textile and agricultural industries, due to their high capacity as antimicrobial and antiviral agents [1–3]. Due to the AgNPs diverse areas of application, it is fundamental to know, as much as possible, the toxicological profile of each nanoparticle formulation.

Physicochemical properties of AgNPs, such as size, shape, stability, and the coating agents have been identified as direct modulators of the cytotoxic/genotoxic damage elicited on different cellular systems, e.g., mammals, plants, bacteria [4–9]. Practically all publications identify the release of silver ions and reactive oxygen species (ROS) overproduction as triggers of cellular damage. Additionally, many of them described size-dependent toxicity, as the smaller the nanoparticles, the higher the toxicity found [1,4,9–13].

Conversely, several works associate the cytotoxic damage not to the released silver ions but to the nanoparticle itself [14–18]. Furthermore, it was found that the coating agent could play a significant role in the cytotoxic/genotoxic damage and the cellular uptake by a dependent or independent clathrin/caveolae endocytosis [19–23].

Just a few AgNPs formulations provide a complete characterization, and even fewer have been evaluated on diverse systems, including those recognized as a reference, i.e., primary cultures in the case of mammals [24] and *Allium cepa* for higher plants [25]. The above mentioned makes the task of comparison and decision-making regarding toxicity and safety use of AgNPs very difficult.

Allium cepa is considered one of the most sensitive plant systems to determine the cytotoxic and genotoxic effects of diverse chemical agents. The advantage provided by this system has been widely described in different works and reviews articles [25–28]. Despite all known benefits, the use of this model for nanomaterials still provides controversial results that made hard the task for decision-makers. Most of the problems are not associated with the model itself but to the scarce physicochemical properties of nanomaterials supplied by the authors. Furthermore, in our knowledge, scarce studies reported the physiological response of plants exposed to different concentrations of silver ions and fewer with the coating agent alone.

Diverse biological responses were described when *Allium cepa* was exposed to various formulations of AgNPs. The observed effects were mainly associated with the silver ions released. However, different groups working with very stable AgNPs formulations—most of them coated with polyvinylpyrrolidone (PVP)—showed cytotoxic and genotoxic effects that cannot be associated with the leached silver ions [14,15]. Thus, the biological response must be elicited mainly by the nanoparticle itself and not by its constituents.

Table 1 summarizes the cytotoxic and genotoxic response registered after the exposure of *Allium cepa* to different concentrations of diverse AgNPs formulations from published data. Most of the formulations assessed reported cytotoxic and genotoxic damage, mainly those that lack of coating agent and the biogenically produced nanoparticles [29–37].

It is well known that the coating agent contributes to the stability of AgNPs and, in turn, their toxicity response [3,21,22,38,39]. The use of PVP as a coating agent substantially diminishes the genotoxic damage [40,41]. Minimal effect on root elongation and the mitotic index were found with AgNPs coated with citrate (61.2 nm), PVP (9.4 nm) and CTAB (5.6 nm) [14]. Interestingly, all AgNPs evaluated by Cvjetko [14] produce cytotoxic damage, increasing ROS concentration, and lipoperoxidation with an AgNPs concentration-dependence manner. Although no DNA damage was observed with citrate-AgNPs by comet assay (Table 1).

An essential contribution of the manuscript of Cvjetko is the association of cytotoxic and genotoxic damage to the nanoparticles and not to the released silver ions [14]. Another work by Scherer [15] also reported the cytotoxic and genotoxic effect of PVP-AgNPs with different sizes with no contribution of free Ag^+ ions to cytotoxicity observed. In the mentioned work, the authors describe a cytotoxic and genotoxic effect with a size dependence behavior. Small nanoparticles produce more considerable cytotoxic damage and micronuclei (MN) frequency. All AgNPs studied in this work, no matter the size, produce cytotoxic and genotoxic damage.

Table 1. Comparative analysis of cyto-genotoxicity of Argovit™ AgNPs with other AgNPs formulations described in the literature.

AgNP Source and Physicochemical Characteristics	Shape	Size (nm)	ζ^a (mV)	Ag Content [b]	RP [c] (nm)	[C] [d] (µg/mL)	Exposure Time (h)	Cytotoxic and Genotoxic Damage	Ref.
Commercial Sigma-Aldrich	<100	-	-	99.5%	-	25, 50, 75 and 100 µg/mL	4 h	CA and cell disintegration.	[29]
Commercial Sigma-Aldrich	<100	-	-	99.5%	-	5, 10, 20, 40, 80 µg/mL	2 h of exposure and recovery of 12, 24 and 48 h	20 and 40 µg/mL. Dose-dependence increase in the frequency of cells with MN and CA. ≥10 µg/mL: DNA damage (comet assay)	[37]
Synthesized with male inflorescence of screw pine, *Pandanus odorifer*	-	-	-	-	-	5, 10, 20, 40 and 80 µg/mL	2 h of exposure and recovery of 12, 24 and 48 h	Dose-dependence increase in the frequency of cells with CA. After 2 h of exposure and 48 h of recovery, no differences in cells with MN between control and lower concentrations (5 and 10 µg/mL). ≥20 µg/mL: DNA damage (comet assay)	[37]
Commercial Sigma-Aldrich	-	TEM 70–130, av. ~125; SEM: 90–180, av. 120	−4.86	99.5%	-	25, 50 and 75 µg/mL	24 h	No damage was observed in nuclei isolated from shoots. Nuclei isolated from roots exposed to 25 and 50 µg/mL shown DNA damage determined by comet assay. The major effect was observed with 50 µg/mL. No damage was observed with 75 µg/mL, and the authors suggest agglomeration and precipitation of AgNP.	[42]
Synthesis AgNP-citrate AgNP-PVP AgNP-CTAB	Citrate rod-like PVP spherical CTAB spherical	Citrate 61.2 ± 33.9 (TEM) PVP 9.4 ± 1.3 (TEM) CTAB 5.6 ± 2.1 (TEM)	Citrate −39.8 ± 3.4 PVP −4.8 ± 0.6 CTAB 42.5 ± 2.7	-	-	25, 50, 75, 100 µM (Quantified by ICP-MS) 10 µM AgNO$_3$, 2.5, 5.0, 7.5, 10 µg/mL	72 h	No DNA damage was observed with any of the AgNP-citrate concentrations employed. An increase in tail DNA was recorded after exposure to AgNP-PVP at 100 µM concentration. AgNP-CTAB produces DNA damage only with 50 µM concentration.	[14]
Commercial Nanotech PVP-AgNPs	-	20–30	-	-	-	5, 10, 15 µg/mL	3, 6, 9 h	The decrease in MI and the increase in CA have a dependence on concentration and exposure time	[43]

Table 1. *Cont.*

AgNP Source and Physicochemical Characteristics	Shape	Size (nm)	ζ^a (mV)	Ag Content [b]	RP [c] (nm)	[C] [d] (μg/mL)	Exposure Time (h)	Cytotoxic and Genotoxic Damage	Ref.
AgNPs Synthetized with leaf extract of *Swertia chirata* Commercial Sigma-Aldrich	-	Synthesis 20 Commercial 20	-	-	-	5, 10, 20 μg/mL	4 h	The decrease in MI and the increase in CA have a dependence on concentration. Both AgNPs produce cytotoxic and genotoxic damage similar to $AgNO_3$.	[30]
They were synthesized with *Cola nitida* pod (p), seed (s), and seed shell (ss).	All semi-spherical	p: 12–80 s: 8–50 ss: 5–40	-	-	p: 431 s: 457 ss: 454	0.01, 0.1, 1, 10 and 100 μg/mL	24, 48 and 72 h	Cytotoxic and genotoxic damage have a dependence on concentration and exposure time.	[31]
Synthesized with plant extract	Semi-spherical	25–40	-	-	440	1, 5 and 10 μg/mL	72 h	Produces a reduction in the number and diameter of roots, decreases in MI, and increases the frequency of CA.	[33]
Synthesized AgNPs	-	2–8	-	-	-	1.5 and 15 μg/mL With CMC 1.24 and 12.4 μg/mL	24 h	Cytotoxic and genotoxic effects with concentration-dependence behavior (MI decrease and CA increase). In the presence of CMC, the cytotoxic damage is lower than the observed for AgNPs alone. Genotoxic damage is found only with 12.4 μg/mL.	[34]
Synthesized with Althea officinalis leaf extract (E) and dehydrated root infusion (R)	-	E: 157 ± 11 (DLS), 131 ± 5 (NTA) R: 293 ± 12 (DLS) 227 ± 16 (NTA)	E: 20.1 ± 1 R: 26.0 ± 1	E: 7.2 × 10^{10} NP/mL (NTA); R: 4.6 × 10^{10} NP/mL	E 384 R 380	E: 3 × 10^{10} NP/mL (3.4 μg/mL) R: 3 × 10^8 NP/mL	24 h	An increase in MI and CA observed. AgNPs produce a frequency increase on cells with chromosome damage more than 3-times compared with control, but the extract of *Althea officinalis* produces a frequency increase of nearly 3-times	[35]
Biogenic AgNPs obtained with *Fusarium oxysporum*. Unwashed (AgNPuw) and washed (AgNPw) with water	-	AgNPuw 40.3 ± 3.5 (TEM) 106.2 ± 13 (DLS) AgNPw 40.3 ± 3.5 (TEM) 145.1 ± 4.5 (DLS)	AgNPuw −37.1 ± 2.6 AgNPw −47.8 ± 1.1	-	-	0.5, 1, 5 and 10 μg/mL	24 h	No difference in the MI compared with control, but 5 and 10 μg/mL of AgNPs increase the frequency of CA. No data of lower concentration was provided. Results of genotoxicity at concentrations 5.0 and 10.0 μg/mL show some response, but at concentrations 0.5 and 1.0 μg/mL, the washed and unwashed silver nanoparticles did not present any effect.	[36]

Table 1. Cont.

AgNP Source and Physicochemical Characteristics	Shape	Size (nm)	ζ^a (mV)	Ag Content [b]	RP [c] (nm)	[C] [d] (μg/mL)	Exposure Time (h)	Cytotoxic and Genotoxic Damage	Ref.
Commercial BioPure Silver Nanospheres–PVP (5, 25, 50, 75 nm) PVP: 40 kDa from nanoComposix® Characterization performed by the authors BE: before exposure AE: After exposure	All nanoparticles are spherical	AgNP5 size: 10.4 ± 4.7 nm (TEM). BE d: 42.6 ± 19.2 nm (DLS); AE d: 161.2 ± 55.5 nm (DLS) AgNP25 size: 20.4 ± 7.2 nm (TEM) BE d: 77.1 ± 26.2 nm (DLS); AE d: 94.5 ± 42.9 nm (DLS) AgNP50 size: 51.3 ± 7.4 nm BE d: 80.5 ± 30.4 nm (DLS); AE d: 103.3 ± 46.5 nm (DLS) AgNP75 size: 73.4 ± 4.7 nm BE d: 124.4 ± 48.1 nm (DLS); AE d: 119.8 ± 42.1 nm (DLS)	AgNP5 BE −15.6 AE −8.35 AgNP25 BE −11.2 AE −6.81 AgNP50 BE −16.3 AE −7.53 AgNP75 BE −13.0 AE −6.42	AgNP5 Release of Ag$^+$ from PVP-AgNPs in distilled water: 0.75% AgNP25 Release of Ag$^+$ from PVP-AgNPs in distilled water: 0.29% AgNP50 Release of Ag$^+$ from PVP-AgNPs in distilled water: 0.03% AgNP75 Release of Ag$^+$ from PVP-AgNPs in distilled water: < LOQ	-	100 μg/mL	48 h	The smaller the AgNPs diameter, the more the MI decrease, the MN frequency increases compared to the control group	[15]
Synthesized AgNPs with cocoa pod husk (A = CPHE-AgNPs) and cocoa bean (B = CBE-AgNPs)	A 4–32 (TEM) B 8.9–54.2 (TEM)	-	-	-	A 428 B 438	0.01, 0.1, 1, 10 and 100 μg/mL	24, 48 and 72 h	Cytotoxicity and genotoxicity shown dependence on concentration and time exposure	[32]

[a]: Zeta potential; [b] resonance plasmon; [c] content of silver in the AgNPs formulation; [d] concentration used in the experiments; MI: mitotic index; CA: chromatic aberrations; PVP: polyvinylpyrrolidone; CTAB: cetyltrimethylammonium bromide; CMC: carboxymethylcellulose; LOQ: limit of quantification; BE: before exposure; AE: after exposure.

During the last years, our research group has studied a commercial PVP-AgNPs formulation known as Argovit™ that has shown striking results in agriculture, aquaculture, and human and veterinary medicine [44–51]. These AgNPs have been very useful in disinfection and heal acceleration of diabetic wounds [44], reduction of tumor growth on mice [45], treatment of white spot virus on shrimps without toxic effects [46–52] and distemper on dogs [47], a decrease of the infectivity of Rift Valley fever virus on mice [48], elimination of parasites from fish for human consumption [49], disinfection and promotion of plants growth during micropropagation [50,51], among many others.

In this work, we present the systematic study of *Allium cepa* biological response elicited by the exposure for 24, 48 and 72 h to different concentrations of a fully characterized PVP-AgNPs formulation, silver ions from $AgNO_3$ solution corresponding to the amount of silver contained in the nanoparticles and the corresponding amount of PVP (acting as coating agent of the nanoparticles) for each concentration assessed. The physiological response was evaluated, monitoring the number and length of new roots. The cytotoxic damage was determined considering the mitotic index, the effects on the mitosis cycle, and the evaluation of ROS overproduction, the antioxidant response of the onion, quantification of the total phenol content, and evidence of lipoperoxidation. Finally, the endpoint to determine genotoxic damage was the change in the micronuclei frequency on dividing cells.

2. Materials and Methods

2.1. Materials

The AgNPs formulation used in this work is a stable aqueous suspension that contains 1.2% weight of metallic silver stabilized with 18.8% weight of PVP, commercially available as Argovit™. The final concentration of the suspension is 200 mg/mL (20%) of AgNPs. The AgNPs of this formulation has been described as a spheroidal shape by transmission electron microscopy (TEM) with a diameter distribution between 1 to 90 nm and an average size of 35 ± 12 nm. The hydrodynamic diameter is 70 nm, with a zeta potential of −5 mV and a plasmon resonance found at 420 nm. All determinations performed in distilled water [45]. Silver nanoparticles were donated by Vasily Burmistrov of Vector-Vita Scientific and Production Center (Novosibirsk, Russia). The UV-vis, zeta potential, and hydrodynamic diameter for AgNPs batch used in this work were determined in distilled water. The UV-vis spectra were acquired with an Agilent Cary 60 spectrophotometer (Agilent Technologies, Santa Clara, CA, USA), and the absorption maximum was observed on 424 nm. The zeta potential (−14 mV) and the hydrodynamic diameter (95 nm) were determined with a Zetasizer Nano NS DTS-1060 (Malvern Panalytical Ltd., Worcestershire, UK) The values obtained agree with those reported by the producers.

2.2. Experimental Design

For each treatment, three *Allium cepa* bulbs (2–3 cm of diameter) were used. Roots were removed without primordial destruction. After washing, each bulb was placed in a 50 mL Falcon conical tube. Each tube contained 10 mL of distilled water and the corresponding treatment: AgNPs, $AgNO_3$, or PVP. The final concentrations for AgNPs and $AgNO_3$ were 5, 10, 15, 25, 50, 75 and 100 µg/mL (metallic silver content), while the final PVP concentrations were 78, 156, 235, 391, 783, 1175 and 1566 µg/mL. The PVP concentrations correspond to the maximum amount of polymer used as a coating agent on each AgNPs concentration evaluated, considering that Ag%: PVP% ratio in Argovit™ is 1.2%:18.8%. Distilled water was used as a negative control (C−) and sodium arsenite ($NaAsO_2$) at a concentration of 0.37 µg/mL (2.84 µM) as a positive control (C+). The inclusion of positive genotoxic control is to guarantee that the cyto-genotoxic response observed is a product of the agents studied and not an artifact of the technique. Samples were incubated at 25 °C ± 0.5 °C for 72 h in darkness with the corresponding stimuli, except $NaAsO_2$ samples, which were exposed only for one hour with the stimuli and then placed in distilled water without arsenite to complete the incubation period [53,54]. Due to the high sensitivity of *Allium cepa* to sodium arsenite exposure reported in two studies [55,56], it was decided to use an exposure time of only one hour at 0.37 µg/mL, to prevent masking of genotoxic damage by the cytotoxic effects (induction of apoptosis and necrosis). The onions exposed to sodium arsenite were incubated for 71 h extra in distilled water to resemble the conditions used for AgNPs and AgNO$_3$. Three independent experiments by triplicate were performed for each treatment.

2.3. Sample Preparation

After incubation time, three mm of the root was fixed with MeOH (80% v/v) and then submerged for 2 min in 5 N HCl. After that, samples were rinsed with distilled water to remove the acid excess. Rinsed roots were submerged in the acetic-orcein stain for 30 min and then rinsed with distilled water. Finally, the stained root was placed on a slide with a drop of acetic acid at 45% (v/v). The sample was "squashed" with the help of a coverslip for microscope observation. Observations were performed with a Carl Zeiss Primo Star microscope (Carl Zeiss Microscopy GmbH, Jena, Germany) with a 40× objective.

2.4. Mitotic Index and Genotoxicity

The mitotic index was determined with the ratio of cells in division (P = prophase + M = metaphase + A = anaphase + T = telophase) and the total number of counted cells according to the formula:

$$MI = [(\text{Cells on division (P + M + A + T)})/(\text{Total counted cells})] \times 100 \quad (1)$$

Genotoxicity was determined with the micronuclei frequency present on 1000 cells under division counted to determine the mitotic index [57].

2.5. Determination of Antioxidant Capacity

The antioxidant capacity was determined using the Oxygen Radical Activity Capacity kit (ORAC kit, ab233473, Abcam, Cambridge, MA, USA) according to the method described by [58]. Briefly, one gram of freeze-dried extract (H$_2$O: MeOH, 20: 80 v/v) of *Allium cepa* roots and bulbs were diluted in methanol for quantification. Analyses were performed at 37 °C using a pH 7.4 phosphate buffer. The peroxide radicals were produced by 2,2'-Azobis(2-amidinopropane) dihydrochloride (AAPH), using fluorescein as substrate and Trolox as standard. Fluorescence was measured every 2 min for one hour. A calibration curve of Trolox in the concentration range 10 to 100 µM was used in each plate read. All determinations were done by triplicate.

2.6. Determination of Reactive Oxygen Species (ROS)

The determination of ROS was performed by a direct colorimetric and fluorometric assay that measures hydrogen peroxide (H$_2$O$_2$) as a reactive oxygen metabolic by-product (Hydrogen Peroxide Assay Kit-ab102500, Abcam, Cambridge, MA, USA). The determination was performed following the supplier protocol. Briefly, 5mg of freeze-dried *Allium cepa* roots and bulbs samples were separately homogenized in cold phosphate buffer solution and washed by centrifugation for 2–5 min at 4 °C and 1000× g to remove any insoluble material. The collected supernatant was transferred to a clean tube to keep on ice. Perchloric acid (PCA) 1 M was used for deproteination; the mixture was stirred and incubated on ice for 5 min. PCA was precipitated with 2M KOH. The mixture was centrifuged at 10,000× g for 20 min at 4 °C, and the supernatant was collected. Deproteinized samples were used to determine ROS with Hydrogen Peroxide Assay Kit (Abcam, Cambridge, MA, USA). All determinations were performed by triplicate.

2.7. Determination of Total Phenolic Content (TPC)

Samples from roots and bulbs from the different experimental conditions were extracted for three hours at 250 rpm with a solvent mixture H$_2$O: MeOH (50:50 v/v) at 30 °C. The obtained extracts were filtered under vacuum and concentrated in a rotary evaporator. The concentrated extract was lyophilized, and the obtained freeze-dried powder was stored at −80 °C. The TPC was determined using the Folin–Ciocalteu method previously described by [50]. The absorbance was measured at 760 nm, and TPC was calculated from a calibration curve of gallic acid (10–150 µg/mL) and expressed as milligrams of gallic acid equivalents (GAE) per gram of sample. All assays were carried out in triplicate.

2.8. Determination of Lipoperoxidation (LPO)

Lipid peroxidation was determined indirectly by the quantification of malondialdehyde (MDA) produced by the decomposition of unsaturated fatty acids. 200 mg of freeze-dried roots and bulbs samples were homogenized in 4 mL of 0.1% Trichloroacetic acid (TCA). The extract was centrifugated at $10,000 \times g$ for 15 min. 1 mL of supernatant was collected and mixed with 2 mL of 20% TCA and 2 mL of 0.5% Thiobarbituric acid (TBA). The mixture was heated for 30 min at 95 °C, then cooled on ice. The produced malondialdehyde was quantified reading at 532 and 600 nm. All determinations were performed by triplicate.

2.9. Statistical Analysis

GraphPad Prism 8.4 was used to analyze data, which are expressed as the means ± standard error. One-way ANOVA statistical analysis was performed, followed by Tukey's test to identify significant differences among groups. Significant differences were considered with $p < 0.05$. A Bartlett test [59] was performed before conduct each analysis of variance to probe the null hypothesis that variances in all groups are the same. The results showed $p \geq 0.05$ for all variables considered in this study. We assume normality based on the Bartlett test sensitivity for normal distributions [60].

3. Results and Discussion

Figure 1 shows changes in *Allium cepa* root length with time. After 24 h of exposure, AgNPs with concentrations of 5, 10, 25, and 50 µg/mL, as well as 156 µg/mL for PVP, promoted root elongation compared with the negative control. For this exposure time, the most important elongation was observed for 5 µg/mL of AgNPs. The lowest concentrations of PVP (78 µg/mL) and AgNO$_3$ (5 µg/mL) seem to make root elongation slower. Root elongation increase was observed with the concentration increase of both PVP and AgNO$_3$, but to less degree than the obtained for AgNPs. The minimal root elongation was found in onions exposed to 1175 and 50 µg/mL of PVP and AgNO$_3$, respectively (Figure 1). Most significant changes in root elongation were observed on plants exposed to AgNPs for 48 h, being the most impressive one reached in onion exposed to 5 µg/mL of AgNPs, 3.5-times higher elongation compared with the negative control (Figure 1). PVP and silver nitrate showed similarly or slightly superior elongation values than the negative control, albeit never more than double. After 72 h of exposure, the highest root elongation was still produced by the lowest concentrations of AgNPs assayed, 5 µg/mL and 10 µg/mL.

The number of new roots found after the exposure to AgNPs increases for all assessed concentrations compared with the negative control (Figure 2). As in the case of root elongation, the concentration of 5 µg/mL was the most effective. Interestingly, the number of new roots found for 10, and 15 µg/mL rapidly drops compared with those seen for 5 µg/mL. Then it increases again for concentrations of 25 and 50 µg/mL, but not so impressive as for 5 µg/mL. The number of roots found for 75 and 100 µg/mL drops again.

On the other hand, PVP only promoted the emergence of new roots with the highest concentration assessed, 1566 µg/mL. Meanwhile, AgNO$_3$ shows the changing pattern found for different concentrations of AgNPs but, in this case, involving the concentrations from 15 (maximum root numbers) to 100 µg/mL. For both agents, PVP, and AgNO$_3$, the lowest concentration assessed presents the smaller number of new roots, even lower than for the negative control (Figure 2).

The mitotic index shown in Figure 3 is the primary biomarker used to determine the cytotoxic effect of different substances and provides strong arguments to explain the root elongation and increase of root number elicited by exposure of *Allium cepa* to AgNPs. In our experimental conditions, the MI value for the negative control (C−) was 12.5 ± 1.5. This value is similar to the reported by Dizdari [61] and Cvjetko [14] with IM values of 15 ± 0.32 and 9 ± 0.5, respectively.

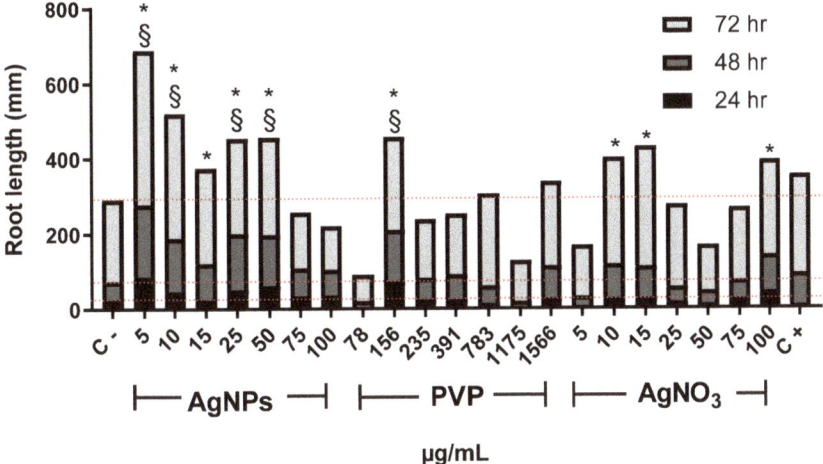

Figure 1. Root elongation of *Allium cepa* exposed to AgNPs, PVP, and AgNO$_3$ with different concentrations after 24 (black), 48 (dark gray), and 72 h (gray) of exposure. The negative control (C−) was distilled water, and 0.37 µg/mL of sodium arsenite was used as a positive control (C+). Dotted lines were included for comparative purposes that show the elongation observed for negative control on each evaluated time. * Indicates significative differences with the negative control ($p < 0.05$); § indicates significative differences with the positive control ($p < 0.05$) after 72 h of exposure.

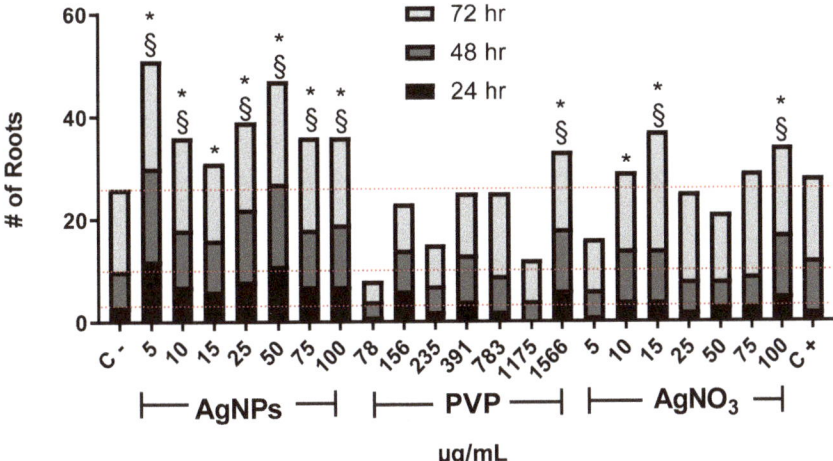

Figure 2. The number of new roots counted on *Allium cepa* exposed to AgNPs, PVP, and AgNO$_3$ with different concentrations after 24 (black), 48 (dark gray), and 72 h (gray) of exposure. Negative control (C−) was distilled water. 0.37 µg/mL of sodium arsenite was used as a positive control (C+). Red dotted lines were included for comparative purposes that show the number of roots observed for negative control on each evaluated time. * Indicates significative differences with the negative control ($p < 0.05$); § indicates significative differences with the positive control ($p < 0.05$) after 72 h of exposure.

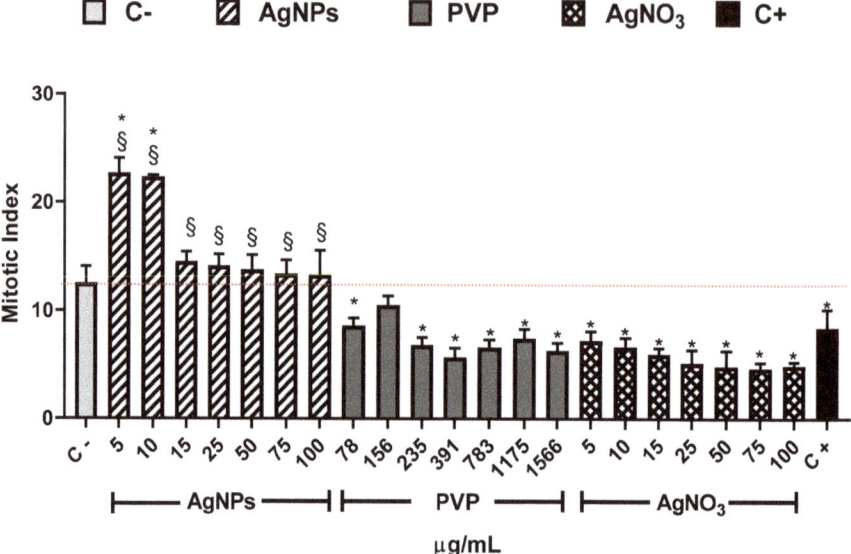

Figure 3. Mitotic index obtained after 72 h of exposure to the corresponding stimuli, AgNPs (lined), PVP (dark gray), and AgNO$_3$ (grid). The concentrations assessed are indicated in the figure. C− corresponds to untreated plants (light gray) and C+ to those exposed to 0.37 µg/mL of sodium arsenite (black). * Indicates significative differences with the negative control ($p < 0.05$); § indicates significative differences with the positive control ($p < 0.05$).

The AgNPs concentrations of 5 and 10 µg/mL showed higher MI values for all the series. Meanwhile, the other concentrations (15–00 µg/mL) showed a MI value similar to the negative control, but never below. On the contrary, for all PVP and AgNO$_3$ concentrations, the MI values are beneath the negative control. MI value ranges are within 8.6 ± 0.7–6.3 ± 0.7 for PVP and 7.2 ± 0.8–4.7 ± 0.5 for AgNO$_3$. MI value for sodium arsenite is close to the MI value of PVP (8.43 ± 1.66). From 5 to 25 µg/mL of silver nitrate, the MI decreases in a concentration-dependent manner; for 50 µg/mL and higher concentrations, the MI keeps practically constant (Figure 3). It is clear from Figure 3 that lower concentrations of this AgNPs formulation promote cellular division, contrary to silver ions that affect cell division starting from the lower concentration assessed. A detailed analysis of cell populations demonstrates that the exposure to AgNPs with concentrations of 5 and 10 µg/mL elicits a critical percentage of cells found in prophase–more than three times in comparison with the negative control (Figure 4). Additionally, a small increase in the frequency of cells in telophase is observed with these concentrations. With higher concentrations of AgNPs (75 and 100 µg/mL), the frequency of cells on prophase is still above the observed for the negative control.

Conversely, PVP and AgNO$_3$ decrease the cell count in all phases compared with the negative control, except for the interphase. Both agents present a cell counting decrease on prophase with a dose-concentration behavior. For the rest of the phases, no dose-dependence behavior was found, but in all of them, a significant reduction in cell counting compared with the negative control was observed, even most important than the produced by sodium arsenite (C+).

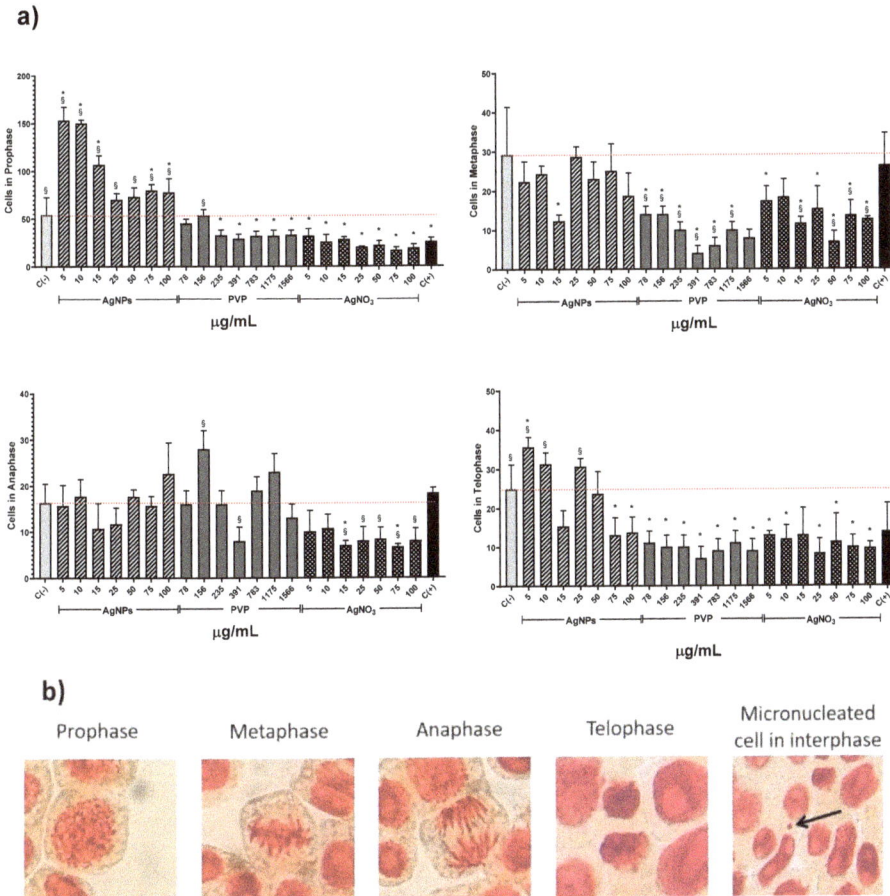

Figure 4. Effects elicited by AgNPs, PVP, and AgNO$_3$ on mitosis of *Allium cepa* root cells. (**a**) Cell population in each phase of mitosis after 72 h of exposure to several concentrations of AgNPs (lined), PVP (dark gray), and AgNO$_3$ (grid). C− corresponds to untreated plants (light gray) and C+ to those exposed to 0.37 µg/mL of sodium arsenite (black). * Indicates significative differences with the negative control ($p < 0.05$); § indicates significative differences with the positive control ($p < 0.05$). (**b**) Representative photographs of cells at different stages of mitosis. Images were obtained with a digital camera adapted to the microscope using a 40× objective.

Exploring the factors that could contribute to cytotoxicity and, in turn, to the decrease of MI values, we quantify the concentration of reactive oxygen species (ROS) within the cells. It is important to note that only PVP at 78 µg/mL and AgNO$_3$ at 75 and 100 µg/mL produce an increase of ROS statistically significant compared with the negative control (Figure 5a). On the other hand, AgNPs provide a significate upsurge of ROS starting from the concentration of 15 µg/mL.

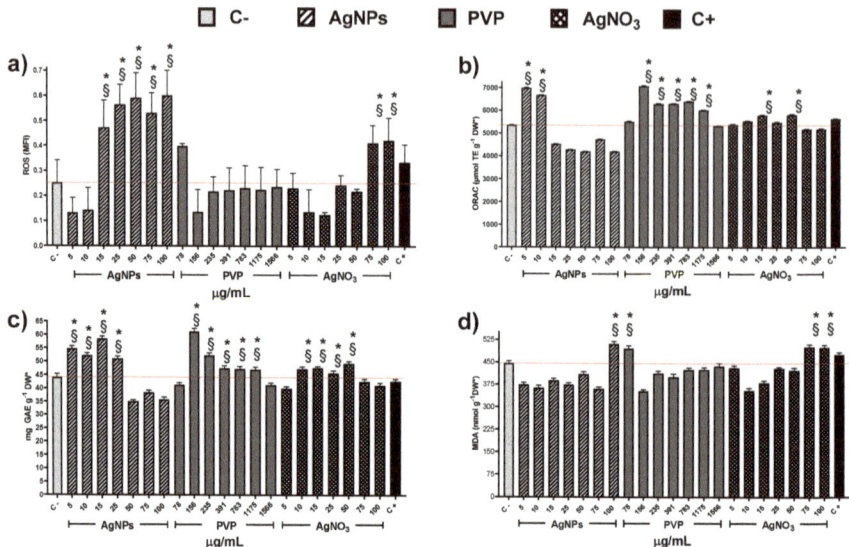

Figure 5. Antioxidant response of *Allium cepa* roots exposed to different stimuli. (**a**) Reactive Oxygen Species, (**b**) Oxygen Radical Absorption Capacity assay, (**c**) Total Phenolic Content, and (**d**) Lipoperoxidation recorded on the onion roots after 72 h for different concentrations of AgNPs (lined), PVP (dark gray), and AgNO$_3$ (grid). C− corresponds to untreated plants (light gray) and C+ to those exposed to 0.37 µg/mL of sodium arsenite (black). * Indicates significative differences with the negative control ($p < 0.05$); § indicates significative differences with the positive control ($p < 0.05$).

The oxygen radical absorbance capacity registered on plants exposed to AgNPs shows an increase compared with negative control only for concentrations of 5 and 10 µg/mL (Figure 5b), despite the ROS underproduced by these concentrations (Figure 5a). Contrariwise, PVP increases the presence of antioxidant agents for the concentration range of 156 to 1175 µg/mL. Silver ions present practically no changes, except for the concentrations 15 and 50 µg/mL (Figure 5b). Figure 5c shows total phenol content (TPC) as a part of the antioxidant response of the onions to the application of the chemical agents. The TPC uprate for AgNPs was observed in the concentration range 5–25 µg/mL, while for PVP and silver ions in a broader range, 156–1175 and 10–75 µg/mL, respectively. The lipoperoxidation (Figure 5d) only show differences in comparison with the negative control for the high concentrations of AgNPs (100 µg/mL) and Ag$^+$ (75 and 100 µg/mL).

Indeed, these results suggest different cytotoxic mechanisms exerted by the substances evaluated in this work. The MI drop registered in onions exposed to Ag$^+$ or PVP did not show a direct association with the overproduction of ROS. On the other hand, the ROS overproduction elicited by AgNPs does not produce changes on the mitotic index compared with the negative control (Figures 3 and 5a).

Essential differences in the antioxidant response of the plant support the proposal of different cytotoxic mechanisms exerted by these agents. The low concentrations of AgNPs cause an upper production of TPC that helps the enzymatic response to fight ROS overproduction. Meanwhile, at 50 to 100 µg/mL, the TPC decreases 20% compared with the negative control, suggesting that from here on, the antioxidant activity ultimately falls on the enzymatic systems. Nevertheless, even at higher AgNPs concentrations, the onion antioxidant response is still useful because the mitotic index presents no changes, and the frequency of cells on prophase and telophase increases compared with the negative control.

Only the higher concentration of AgNPs evaluated, 100 µg/mL, produces an increase of malondialdehyde that can be considered as the beginning of lipoperoxidation compared with the negative control. So, for low concentrations of AgNPs, no ROS overproduction was observed, but an increase in the antioxidant response was found (increase in ORAC and TPC compared with C-), while for Ag$^+$ no changes neither in ROS concentration nor in the antioxidant response was observed. These could explain the drastic root growth activation caused by AgNPs compared with Ag$^+$. For high concentrations of AgNPs and Ag$^+$, two biomarkers associated with phytotoxicity increase compared with C-: ROS increases by 200% and 120%, respectively, and lipoperoxidation increase 12–14% (Figure 4). Nevertheless, antioxidant mechanisms, measured by ORAC and TPC, show a small decrease with AgNPs and has not been modified for Ag$^+$, supporting the hypothesis of different cytotoxic mechanism exerted.

The results obtained with the onion agree with the hormetic effect produced by the same AgNPs formulation on sugar cane [62], vanilla [50], and stevia [63] through ROS overproduction. Besides, this is important to detect the concentration where growth promotion without adverse effects is observed in onions, and the differences in the antioxidant response compared with other plants already exposed to this type of AgNPs. For onions, cytotoxic damage apparently begins with 100 µg/mL of AgNPs because only a small increase of malondialdehyde is observed (Figure 5c). While on the other plants, with this concentration, the damage is quite evident not only at the molecular level but also physiologically, due to different antioxidant response of these plants [50,62,63].

The ROS overproduction and the antioxidant response on the onion bulb are quite similar to those observed on the roots. The main difference consists of TPC production. In the case of the bulb, silver ions enlarge a little bit TPC with the concentration range 5–50 µg/mL. Meanwhile, PVP does it with the range 156–1175 µg/mL, being the latter one of the most significant TPC values registered here. Therefore, no damage was registered on the bulb with any of the AgNPs concentrations evaluated, considering that MDA registered with exposure to 100 µg/mL of AgNPs is just the beginning of cell damage (Figure S1).

Thus, at low AgNPs concentrations factors increasing plant growth (oxygen radical absorption capacity, Figure 5b, and total phenolic content, Figure 5c) are maximum with no evidence of cellular damage. The antioxidant response could explain the increase in the number and length of roots and the mitotic index (Figures 1–3).

It is known that one of the consequences of ROS overproduction is reversible or irreversible nuclear material damage [64]. In order to complete the phytotoxic influence of these compounds on *Allium cepa*, the AgNPs genotoxic potency was determined though the recording of micronuclei (MN) frequency. Figure 6 shows the MN frequency observed after 72 h of exposure to the different agents. *Allium cepa* is one of the most sensitive systems for genetic damage assessment. Moreover, the number of chromosomes provides an essential advantage for tracking genetic damage due to the reduced number of chromosomes [25].

Several authors reported that MN frequency on basal conditions for *Allium cepa* is between 1 and 2 [65–67]. In our experimental conditions, MN counting (1.3 ± 0.5) agrees with those values previously reported.

As expected, the known genotoxic agent sodium arsenite, exhibited the most significant MN frequency, ten-times higher (13 ± 3.6 MN) than the observed for negative control (1.3 ± 0.5 MN). Contrariwise, exposure to AgNPs at any of the concentrations assayed showed lower values than the recorded for the negative control. Interestingly, no increase in MN frequency was recorded on the samples exposed to AgNPs neither with the low (5 and 10 µg/mL) nor the higher concentration (25–100 µg/mL), despite the latter elicit the highest ROS overproduction (Figure 5b). All assessed PVP concentrations show low MN frequency similar to AgNPs and the negative control. (Figure 6). Contrastively, silver ions duplicate MN frequency (2.6 ± 1.1 MN) compared with negative control (1.3 ± 0.5) starting from the lowest concentration (5 µg/mL). For 100 µg/mL of AgNO$_3$, MN frequency reached 11.6 ± 1.5, response quite similar to sodium arsenite (13 ± 3.6 MN). The MN frequency increases with Ag$^+$ concentration demonstrating that silver ions display a concentration-dependent behavior.

It has been reported that low concentrations of silver ions can unidirectionally affect the K$^+$ flux decreasing its intracellular concentration, while higher concentrations produce the same effect but damaging cellular membrane [68]. Additionally, silver ions can block the recognition sites of ethylene, avoiding the completeness of the signaling route [69]. The above could explain the decrease in MI and the diminish of cells in prophase and telophase observed in roots exposed to silver ions.

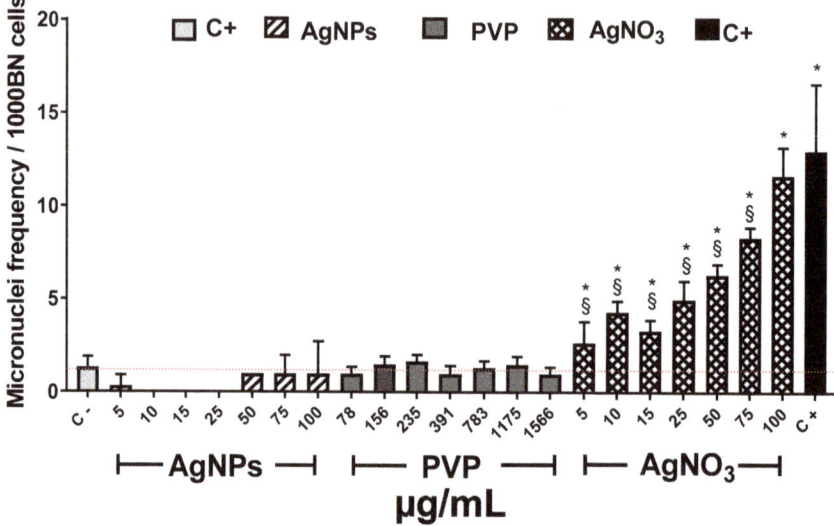

Figure 6. Micronuclei frequency (MN) on *Allium cepa* root exposed to different stimuli. The MNi frequency was recorded after 72 h exposure to different concentrations of AgNPs (lined), PVP (dark gray), and $AgNO_3$ (grid). C− corresponds to untreated plants (light gray) and C+ to those exposed to 0.37 µg/mL of sodium arsenite (black). * Indicates significative differences with the negative control ($p < 0.05$); § indicates significative differences with the positive control ($p < 0.05$).

The results obtained in this work with Ag^+ ions agree with the concentration-dependent phytotoxic effects described by Panda [37] and Yekeen [32] in *Allium cepa*. Panda found a significant decrease in the mitotic index and a substantial increase in the frequency of cells with MN with low concentrations of Ag^+ ions (5 µg/mL) and only 2 h of exposure [37]. The literature data and the different responses from Allium cepa root cells exposed to silver ions and AgNPs support our proposal of different mechanisms of actions elicited by both agents.

On the other hand, the cytotoxic and genotoxic response of *Allium cepa* roots after exposure to sodium arsenite show concentration- and time-dependence behavior. It was demonstrated that micronuclei frequency and mitotic index are directly dependent on sodium arsenite exposure time. Both parameters show an opposite trend with prolonged exposure, that is, as longer the exposure time, lower the mitotic index, and higher the micronuclei frequency recorded [55,56]. Sodium arsenite concentrations of 0.3 to 1 µg/mL after 1h of exposure produce a significant statistical difference in the micronuclei frequency with lower affectation in the mitotic index compared with negative control [55,56]. These results show the tremendous cytotoxic and genotoxic damage produced by low concentrations and short exposure times of sodium arsenite in *Allium cepa* root cells.

In our experimental conditions (0.37 µg/mL and 1 h of exposure), a similar trend than that previously described for sodium arsenite was observed. The length of the roots and appearance of new ones after 24 h (Figures 1 and 2) is lower compared with the negative control, which is consistent with the rapid cytotoxic damage previously described. Moreover, after 72 h, the cytotoxic and genotoxic damage on the root cells exposed to this low concentration of arsenite for a very short time is still measurable, showing a decrease on the mitotic index (Figure 3), a significant reduction of cells in prophase (Figure 4) and a meaningful increase in the micronuclei frequency (Figure 6). All of this is without a considerable difference elicited by arsenite in the antioxidant response, ROS overproduction, total phenol content, or evidence of lipoperoxidation compared with the negative control after 72 h (Figure 5). It is very important to bear in mind that the damage caused by the arsenite must have occurred during the first hours of exposure, but it was so great that even after 72 h of exposure, it is still measurable in parameters such as mitotic index and micronucleus frequency.

On the other hand, low concentrations of AgNPs (5 and 10 µg/mL) produce a rise in the root length promote the appearance of new ones (Figures 1 and 2), increase in the mitotic index (Figure 3) and cells in prophase (Figure 4). These concentrations do not lead to ROS overexpression but increase the total phenol content and the antioxidant response, suggesting that plants grow in order to cut down the possible damage. As the AgNPs concentration increase, noticeable increase the ROS overproduction and the total phenolic content and the antioxidant response decrease. Nevertheless, no differences were observed in the number and length of roots, mitotic index, or the micronuclei frequency compared with the negative control.

These results suggest that *Allium cepa* root cells are better able to handle the possible damage caused by higher concentrations of AgNPs after longer exposure times than the damages caused by a 13 to 270 times lower concentration of arsenite with 72 times less of exposure time than ones applied for AgNPs. In the employed experimental conditions, the damage produced by AgNPs is meager considering the significant damage generated by a low concentration of sodium arsenite after the very short exposure time. However, further experiments must be performed to confirm the lack of cytotoxic and genotoxic damage of the AgNPs formulation evaluated in this work.

All PVP-AgNPs formulations listed in Table 1 produce chromatic aberrations. PVP-AgNPs formulation studied by Cvjetko at a concentration of 10 µg/mL of metallic silver (100 µM) produces DNA damage evidenced by the increase of the comet tail [14]. This concentration, 10 µg/mL, represents only one-tenth of the maximum concentration evaluated for Argovit™ in this work, but the latter did not produce cytotoxic or genotoxic damage even when 100 µg/mL of metallic silver was used. Other PVP-AgNPs with sizes 5, 25, 50, and 75 nm were studied by Scherer at concentrations of 100 µg/mL of the complete nanoparticle formulation observing that the smaller the AgNPs diameter, the more the MI decrease and the MN frequency increases compared to the control group. The concentration of 100 µg/mL of the complete nanoparticle formulation represents the sixteenth part of the Argovit™ concentration used in this work. For Argovit™, 83–666 µg/mL of the complete AgNPs formulation corresponds to 5–100 µg/mL considering the content of metallic silver.

Until this work, all the AgNPs formulations evaluated had shown phytotoxicity on *Allium cepa*. Results obtained in this work show that cytotoxic and genotoxic responses of Argovit™ PVP-AgNPs are less than the effect produced by AgNPs formulations listed on Table 1. The shape, size, and coating agent of the nanoparticles from Table 1 and the evaluated in this work are quite similar, but the latter did not generate phytotoxic damage. The Ag/coating agent ratio is the only factor that could explain the main differences in the toxicological response observed in this work with those previously reported since there are no such dramatic toxicological differences associated with the difference in size, shape or silver content [21,22,38–41,70,71]. Considering dried nanoparticles, the [Ag]/[PVP] ratio expressed in % of weight in the formulation studied here is 6:94. Meanwhile, NanoComposix is 34:66, and the synthesized by Cvjetko is 40:60 [20]. Unfortunately, we have not found information about Nanotech Ltd.'s formulation.

Hence, even though the concentration of AgNPs studied in this work was at least 10–17 times higher than those for previously reported PVP-AgNPs formulations, no cytotoxic nor genotoxic damage for *Allium cepa* was observed. Lack of damage under the experimental conditions assessed could be a good sign regarding their environmental impact, but further experiments with more extended exposure periods must be performed to determine chronic toxicity effects.

4. Conclusions

In this work, the cytotoxic and genotoxic effect of AgNPs formulation Argovit™ for *Allium cepa* (onion), a recognized reference system for higher plants, were studied. Our results allow us to conclude that this AgNPs formulation produces no cytotoxic nor genotoxic damage at the concentrations assessed on *Allium cepa* compared with other PVP-AgNPs formulations reported on literature. Comparative analysis of the behavior of Argovit™ AgNPs and $AgNO_3$ showed that the primary biological effect of Argovit™ is not associated with the released silver ions but to AgNPs themselves. Furthermore, our results show the relevance of evaluating the cyto-genotoxic response of the coating agent since the PVP considered as non-toxic and, therefore, frequently used, caused a significant decrease in the mitotic index of onions exposed to this agent.

The concentrations used in this work for Argovit™ (5–100 µg/mL of metallic silver content or 83–1666 µg/mL of the complete formulation) are 10–17 times higher than the previously reported. It was suggested that the lack of damage elicited by Argovit™ is due to the high proportion of PVP used during their synthesis. A large amount of coating agent could provide to this formulation higher stability and a completely different biological response compared either with other PVP-AgNPs formulations previously reported or to the silver ions.

In the employed experimental conditions and considering the significant damage generated by a low concentration of sodium arsenite after a very short exposure time, the damage produced by AgNPs is meager. This response could be useful for many applications, particularly low concentrations of Argovit™ that stimulate the growth of onions with minimal cytotoxic or genotoxic damage to the roots or the bulb, also increasing the total phenolic content.

Results obtained in this work provide valuable information regarding safer nanomaterials design for therapeutic, biomedical, agrochemical, food, and daily use products by modifying the metal/coating agent ratio. These results will be beneficial for widely used nanomaterials design, such as silver nanoparticles and many other nanoparticles whose production begins to increase nowadays due to their full applications.

Supplementary Materials: The following are available online at http://www.mdpi.com/2079-4991/10/7/1386/s1, Figure S1. Antioxidant response of *Allium cepa* bulbs exposed to different stimuli.

Author Contributions: Conceptualization, M.E.A.-G.; methodology, F.C.-F., B.R.-R. and R.A.C.-S.; validation, R.L.V.-G. and P.C.R.; formal analysis, M.E.A.-G., Y.T.-M., C.L.-A. and J.C.G.-R.; investigation, F.C.-F., B.R.-R. and R.A.C.-S.; resources, M.E.A.-G., N.B. and P.R.-C.; data curation, M.E.A.-G., F.C.-F. and J.C.G.-R.; writing—original draft preparation, J.C.G.-R., Y.T.-M. and F.C.-F.; writing—review and editing, M.E.A.-G., Y.T.-M. and J.C.G.-R.; visualization, M.E.A.-G., J.C.G.-R.; supervision, M.E.A.-G and C.L.-A.; project administration, M.E.A.-G. and N.B.; funding acquisition, A.P. and N.B. All authors have read and agreed to the published version of the manuscript.

Funding: This research was funded by CONACyT, grant number 293417, Red Internacional de Bionanotecnología con impacto en Bionanotecnología, Alimentación y Bioseguridad and Competitiveness Enhancement Program of Tomsk Polytechnic University, project VIU-RSCBMT-197/2020. The APC was funded by Universidad Autónoma de Baja California.

Acknowledgments: Y.T.M. and J.C.G.R. thank CONACyT (294727 Red Farmoquímicos) for the continuous technical support.

Conflicts of Interest: The authors declare no conflict of interest. The funders had no role in the design of the study; in the collection, analyses, or interpretation of data; in the writing of the manuscript, or in the decision to publish the results.

References

1. Liao, C.; Li, Y.; Tjong, S.C. Bactericidal and cytotoxic properties of silver nanoparticles. *Int. J. Mol. Sci.* **2019**, *20*, 449. [CrossRef] [PubMed]
2. Yan, A.; Chen, Z. Impacts of silver nanoparticles on plants: A focus on the phytotoxicity and underlying mechanism. *Int. J. Mol. Sci.* **2019**, *20*, 1003. [CrossRef] [PubMed]

3. Burduşel, A.C.; Gherasim, O.; Grumezescu, A.M.; Mogoantă, L.; Ficai, A.; Andronescu, E. Biomedical Applications of Silver Nanoparticles: An Up-to-Date Overview. *Nanomaterials* **2018**, *8*, 681. [CrossRef] [PubMed]
4. Ahlberg, S.; Antonopulos, A.; Diendorf, J.; Dringen, R.; Epple, M.; Flöck, R.; Goedecke, W.; Graf, C.; Haberl, N.; Helmlinger, J.; et al. PVP-coated, negatively charged silver nanoparticles: A multi-center study of their physicochemical characteristics, cell culture and in vivo experiments. *Beilstein J. Nanotechnol.* **2014**, *5*, 1944–1965. [CrossRef]
5. Butler, K.S.; Peeler, D.J.; Casey, B.J.; Dair, B.J.; Elespuru, R.K. Silver nanoparticles: Correlating nanoparticle size and cellular uptake with genotoxicity. *Mutagenesis* **2015**, *30*, 577–591. [CrossRef] [PubMed]
6. Kedziora, A.; Speruda, M.; Krzyzewska, E.; Rybka, J.; Lukoviak, A.; Bugla-Ploskonska, G. Similarities and Differences between Silver Ions and Silver in Nanoforms as Antibacterial Agents. *Int. J. Mol. Sci.* **2018**, *19*, 444. [CrossRef]
7. Rafique, M.; Sadaf, I.; Rafique, M.S.; Tahir, M.B. A review on green synthesis of silver nanoparticles and their applications. *Artif. Cells Nanomed. Biotechnol.* **2017**, *45*, 1272–1291. [CrossRef]
8. Hadrup, N.; Lam, H.R. Oral toxicity of silver ions, silver nanoparticles and colloidal silver—A review. *Regul. Toxicol. Pharmacol.* **2014**, *68*, 1–7. [CrossRef]
9. Akter, M.; Sikder, M.T.; Rahman, M.M.; Ullah, A.K.M.A.; Hossain, K.F.B.; Banik, S.; Hosokawa, T.; Saito, T.; Kurasaki, M. A systematic review on silver nanoparticles-induced cytotoxicity: Physicochemical properties and perspectives. *J. Adv. Res.* **2018**, *9*, 1–16. [CrossRef]
10. Milić, M.; Leitinger, G.; Pavičić, I.; Zebić Avdičević, M.; Dobrović, S.; Goessler, W.; Vinković Vrček, I. Cellular uptake and toxicity effects of silver nanoparticles in mammalian kidney cells. *J. Appl. Toxicol.* **2015**, *35*, 581–592. [CrossRef]
11. Antony, J.J.; Sivalingam, P.; Chen, B. Toxicological effects of silver nanoparticles. *Environ. Toxicol. Pharmacol.* **2015**, *40*, 729–732. [CrossRef]
12. Liu, W.; Wu, Y.; Wang, C.; Li, H.C.; Wang, T.; Liao, C.Y.; Cui, L.; Zhou, Q.F.; Yan, B.; Jiang, G.B. Impact of silver nanoparticles on human cells: Effect of particle size. *Nanotoxicology* **2010**, *4*, 319–330. [CrossRef] [PubMed]
13. Levard, C.; Hotze, E.M.; Lowry, G.V.; Brown, G.E. Environmental transformations of silver nanoparticles: Impact on stability and toxicity. *Environ. Sci. Technol.* **2012**, *46*, 6900–6914. [CrossRef] [PubMed]
14. Cvjetko, P.; Milošić, A.; Domijan, A.M.; Vinković Vrček, I.; Tolić, S.; Peharec Štefanić, P.; Letofsky-Papst, I.; Tkalec, M.; Balen, B. Toxicity of silver ions and differently coated silver nanoparticles in *Allium cepa* roots. *Ecotoxicol. Environ. Saf.* **2017**, *137*, 18–28. [CrossRef] [PubMed]
15. Scherer, M.D.; Sposito, J.C.V.; Falco, W.F.; Grisolia, A.B.; Andrade, L.H.C.; Lima, S.M.; Machado, G.; Nascimento, V.A.; Gonçalves, D.A.; Wender, H.; et al. Cytotoxic and genotoxic effects of silver nanoparticles on meristematic cells of *Allium cepa* roots: A close analysis of particle size dependence. *Sci. Total Environ.* **2019**, *660*, 459–467. [CrossRef]
16. Foldbjerg, R.; Jiang, X.; Micləuş, T.; Chen, C.; Autrup, H.; Beer, C. Silver nanoparticles—Wolves in sheep's clothing? *Toxicol. Res.* **2015**, *4*, 563–575. [CrossRef]
17. Yin, L.; Cheng, Y.; Espinasse, B.; Colman, B.P.; Auffan, M.; Wiesner, M.; Rose, J.; Liu, J.; Bernhardt, E.S. More than the ions: The effects of silver nanoparticles on lolium multiflorum. *Environ. Sci. Technol.* **2011**, *45*, 2360–2367. [CrossRef] [PubMed]
18. Li, Y.; Qin, T.; Ingle, T.; Yan, J.; He, W.; Yin, J.J.; Chen, T. Differential genotoxicity mechanisms of silver nanoparticles and silver ions. *Arch. Toxicol.* **2017**, *91*, 509–519. [CrossRef]
19. Behzadi, S.; Serpooshan, V.; Tao, W.; Hamaly, M.A.; Alkawareek, M.Y.; Dreaden, E.C.; Brown, D.; Alkilany, A.M.; Farokhzad, O.C.; Mahmoudi, M. Cellular uptake of nanoparticles: Journey inside the cell. *Chem. Soc. Rev.* **2017**, *46*, 4218–4244. [CrossRef]
20. Vinković Vrček, I.; Pavičić, I.; Crnković, T.; Jurašin, D.; Babič, M.; Horák, D.; Lovrić, M.; Ferhatović, L.; Ćurlin, M.; Gajović, S. Does surface coating of metallic nanoparticles modulate their interference with in vitro assays? *RSC Adv.* **2015**, *5*, 70787–70807. [CrossRef]
21. Jurašin, D.D.; Ćurlin, M.; Capjak, I.; Crnković, T.; Lovrić, M.; Babič, M.; Horïk, D.; Vrček, I.V.; Gajović, S. Surface coating affects behavior of metallic nanoparticles in a biological environment. *Beilstein J. Nanotechnol.* **2016**, *7*, 246–262. [CrossRef]

22. Nallanthighal, S.; Chan, C.; Bharali, D.J.; Mousa, S.A.; Vásquez, E.; Reliene, R. Particle coatings but not silver ions mediate genotoxicity of ingested silver nanoparticles in a mouse model. *NanoImpact* **2017**, *5*, 92–100. [CrossRef] [PubMed]
23. Pareek, V.; Gupta, R.; Panwar, J. Do physico-chemical properties of silver nanoparticles decide their interaction with biological media and bactericidal action? A review. *Mater. Sci. Eng. C* **2018**, *90*, 739–749. [CrossRef] [PubMed]
24. OCDE. *OECD 474 Guideline For The Testing Of Chemicals: Mammalian Erythrocyte Micronucleous Test*; OECD Publishing: Paris, France, 2016.
25. Leme, D.M.; Marin-Morales, M.A. *Allium cepa* test in environmental monitoring: A review on its application. *Mutat. Res. Rev. Mutat. Res.* **2009**, *682*, 71–81. [CrossRef] [PubMed]
26. Barreto, M.R.; Aleixo, N.A.; Silvestre, R.B.; Fregonezi, F.; Barud, S.; Dias, S.; Ribeiro, C.A.; Resende, R.A. Genotoxicological safety assessment of puree-only edible films from onion bulb (*Allium cepa* L.) for use in food packaging-related applications. *J. Food Sci.* **2019**. [CrossRef]
27. De Souza, C.P.; de Guedes, T.A.; Fontanetti, C.S. Evaluation of herbicides action on plant bioindicators by genetic biomarkers: A review. *Environ. Monit. Assess.* **2016**, *188*. [CrossRef]
28. Stapulionytė, A.; Kleizaitė, V.; Šiukšta, R.; Žvingila, D.; Taraškevičius, R.; Česnienė, T. Cyto/genotoxicological evaluation of hot spots of soil pollution using *Allium* bioassays in relation to geochemistry. *Mutat. Res. Genet. Toxicol. Environ. Mutagen.* **2019**, *842*, 102–110. [CrossRef] [PubMed]
29. Kumari, M.; Mukherjee, A.; Chandrasekaran, N. Genotoxicity of silver nanoparticles in *Allium cepa*. *Sci. Total Environ.* **2009**, *407*, 5243–5246. [CrossRef]
30. Saha, N.; Dutta Gupta, S. Low-dose toxicity of biogenic silver nanoparticles fabricated by Swertia chirata on root tips and flower buds of *Allium cepa*. *J. Hazard. Mater.* **2017**, *330*, 18–28. [CrossRef]
31. Yekeen, T.A.; Azeez, M.A.; Akinboro, A.; Lateef, A.; Asafa, T.B.; Oladipo, I.C.; Oladokun, S.O.; Ajibola, A.A. Safety evaluation of green synthesized *Cola nitida* pod, seed and seed shell extract-mediated silver nanoparticles (AgNPs) using an *Allium cepa* assay. *J. Taibah Univ. Sci.* **2017**, *11*, 895–909. [CrossRef]
32. Yekeen, T.A.; Azeez, M.A.; Lateef, A.; Asafa, T.B.; Oladipo, I.C.; Badmus, J.A.; Adejumo, S.A.; Ajibola, A.A. Cytogenotoxicity potentials of cocoa pod and bean-mediated green synthesized silver nanoparticles on *Allium cepa* cells. *Caryologia* **2017**, *70*, 366–377. [CrossRef]
33. Debnath, P.; Mondal, A.; Hajra, A.; Das, C.; Mondal, N.K. Cytogenetic effects of silver and gold nanoparticles on *Allium cepa* roots. *J. Genet. Eng. Biotechnol.* **2018**, *16*, 519–526. [CrossRef] [PubMed]
34. Becaro, A.A.; Siqueira, M.C.; Puti, F.C.; de Moura, M.R.; Correa, D.S.; Marconcini, J.M.; Mattoso, L.H.C.; Ferreira, M.D. Cytotoxic and genotoxic effects of silver nanoparticle/carboxymethyl cellulose on *Allium cepa*. *Environ. Monit. Assess.* **2017**, *189*. [CrossRef]
35. Rheder, D.T.; Guilger, M.; Bilesky-José, N.; Germano-Costa, T.; Pasquoto-Stigliani, T.; Gallep, T.B.B.; Grillo, R.; dos Carvalho, C.S.; Fraceto, L.F.; Lima, R. Synthesis of biogenic silver nanoparticles using *Althaea officinalis* as reducing agent: Evaluation of toxicity and ecotoxicity. *Sci. Rep.* **2018**, *8*, 1–11. [CrossRef] [PubMed]
36. Lima, R.; Feitosa, L.O.; Ballottin, D.; Marcato, P.D.; Tasic, L.; Durán, N. Cytotoxicity and genotoxicity of biogenic silver nanoparticles. *J. Phys. Conf. Ser.* **2013**, *429*. [CrossRef]
37. Panda, K.K.; Achary, V.M.M.; Krishnaveni, R.; Padhi, B.K.; Sarangi, S.N.; Sahu, S.N.; Panda, B.B. In vitro biosynthesis and genotoxicity bioassay of silver nanoparticles using plants. *Toxicol. Vitr.* **2011**, *25*, 1097–1105. [CrossRef] [PubMed]
38. Yan, J.; Zhou, T.; Cunningham, C.K.; Chen, T.; Jones, M.Y.; Abbas, M.; Li, Y.; Mei, N.; Guo, X.; Moore, M.M.; et al. Size- and coating-dependent cytotoxicity and genotoxicity of silver nanoparticles evaluated using in vitro standard assays. *Nanotoxicology* **2016**, *10*, 1373–1384. [CrossRef]
39. Andreani, T.; Nogueira, V.; Pinto, V.V.; Ferreira, M.J.; Rasteiro, M.G.; Silva, A.M.; Pereira, R.; Pereira, C.M. Influence of the stabilizers on the toxicity of metallic nanomaterials in aquatic organisms and human cell lines. *Sci. Total Environ.* **2017**, *607*, 1264–1277. [CrossRef] [PubMed]
40. Nymark, P.; Catalán, J.; Suhonen, S.; Järventaus, H.; Birkedal, R.; Clausen, P.A.; Jensen, K.A.; Vippola, M.; Savolainen, K.; Norppa, H. Genotoxicity of polyvinylpyrrolidone-coated silver nanoparticles in BEAS 2B cells. *Toxicology* **2013**, *313*, 38–48. [CrossRef]
41. Panda, K.K.; Achary, V.M.M.; Phaomie, G.; Sahu, H.K.; Parinandi, N.L.; Panda, B.B. Polyvinyl polypyrrolidone attenuates genotoxicity of silver nanoparticles synthesized via green route, tested in Lathyrus sativus L. root bioassay. *Mutat. Res. Genet. Toxicol. Environ. Mutagen.* **2016**, *806*, 11–23. [CrossRef]

42. Ghosh, M.; Manivannan, J.; Sinha, S.; Chakraborty, A.; Mallick, S.K.; Bandyopadhyay, M.; Mukherjee, A. In vitro and in vivo genotoxicity of silver nanoparticles. *Mutat. Res. Genet. Toxicol. Environ. Mutagen.* **2012**, *749*, 60–69. [CrossRef] [PubMed]
43. Fouad, A.S.; Hafez, R.M. The effects of silver ions and silver nanoparticles on cell division and expression of cdc2 gene in *Allium cepa* root tips. *Biol. Plant.* **2018**, *62*, 166–172. [CrossRef]
44. Almonaci Hernández, C.A.; Juarez-Moreno, K.; Castañeda Juarez, M.E.; Almanza-Reyes, H.; Pestryakov, A.; Bogdanchikova, N. Silver Nanoparticles for the Rapid Healing of Diabetic Foot Ulcers. *Int. J. Med. Nano Res.* **2017**, *4*, 19. [CrossRef]
45. Valenzuela-Salas, L.M.; Girón-Vázquez, N.G.; García-Ramos, J.C.; Torres-Bugarín, O.; Gómez, C.; Pestryakov, A.; Villarreal-Gómez, L.J.; Toledano-Magaña, Y.; Bogdanchikova, N. Antiproliferative and antitumor effect of non-genotoxic silver nanoparticles on melanoma models. *Oxid. Med. Cell. Longev.* **2019**, *2019*, 4528241. [CrossRef]
46. Ochoa-Meza, A.R.; Álvarez-Sánchez, A.R.; Romo-Quiñonez, C.R.; Barraza, A.; Magallón-Barajas, F.J.; Chávez-Sánchez, A.; García-Ramos, J.C.; Toledano-Magaña, Y.; Bogdanchikova, N.; Pestryakov, A.; et al. Silver nanoparticles enhance survival of white spot syndrome virus infected *Penaeus vannamei* shrimps by activation of its immunological system. *Fish Shellfish Immunol.* **2019**, *84*, 1083–1089. [CrossRef]
47. Bogdanchikova, N.; Vázquez-Muñoz, R.; Huerta-Saquero, A.; Peña-Jasso, A.; Aguilar-Uzcanga, G.; Picos-Díaz, P.L.; Pestryakov, A.; Burmistrov, V.A.; Martynyuk, O.; Luna-Vázquez-Gómez, R.; et al. Silver nanoparticles composition for treatment of distemper in dogs. *Int. J. Nanotechnol.* **2016**, *13*, 227–237. [CrossRef]
48. Borrego, B.; Lorenzo, G.; Mota-Morales, J.D.; Almanza-Reyes, H.; Mateos, F.; López-Gil, E.; de la Losa, N.; Burmistrov, V.A.; Pestryakov, A.N.; Brun, A.; et al. Potential application of silver nanoparticles to control the infectivity of Rift Valley fever virus in vitro and in vivo. *Nanomed. Nanotechnol. Biol. Med.* **2016**, *12*, 1185–1192. [CrossRef]
49. Pimentel-Acosta, C.A.; Morales-Serna, F.N.; Chávez-Sánchez, M.C.; Lara, H.H.; Pestryakov, A.; Bogdanchikova, N.; Fajer-Ávila, E.J. Efficacy of silver nanoparticles against the adults and eggs of monogenean parasites of fish. *Parasitol. Res.* **2019**, *118*, 1741–1749. [CrossRef]
50. Spinoso-Castillo, J.L.; Chavez-Santoscoy, R.A.; Bogdanchikova, N.; Pérez-Sato, J.A.; Morales-Ramos, V.; Bello-Bello, J.J. Antimicrobial and hormetic effects of silver nanoparticles on in vitro regeneration of vanilla (*Vanilla planifolia* Jacks. ex Andrews) using a temporary immersion system. *Plant Cell. Tissue Organ Cult.* **2017**, *129*, 195–207. [CrossRef]
51. Bello-Bello, J.; Spinoso-Castillo, J.; Arano-Avalos, S.; Martínez-Estrada, E.; Arellano-García, M.; Pestryakov, A.; Toledano-Magaña, Y.; García-Ramos, J.; Bogdanchikova, N. Cytotoxic, Genotoxic, and Polymorphism Effects on *Vanilla planifolia* Jacks ex Andrews after Long-Term Exposure to Argovit®Silver Nanoparticles. *Nanomaterials* **2018**, *8*, 754. [CrossRef]
52. Juarez-Moreno, K.; Mejía-Ruiz, C.H.; Díaz, F.; Reyna-Verdugo, H.; Re, A.D.; Vazquez-Felix, E.F.; Sánchez-Castrejón, E.; Mota-Morales, J.D.; Pestryakov, A.; Bogdanchikova, N. Effect of silver nanoparticles on the metabolic rate, hematological response, and survival of juvenile white shrimp *Litopenaeus vannamei*. *Chemosphere* **2017**, *169*, 716–724. [CrossRef] [PubMed]
53. Fiskesjö, G. Mercury and selenium in a modified *Allium* test. *Hereditas* **1979**, *91*, 169–178. [CrossRef]
54. Fiskesjö, G. The *Allium* test as a standard in environmental monitoring. *Hereditas* **1985**, *102*, 99–112. [CrossRef] [PubMed]
55. Wu, L.; Yi, H.; Yi, M. Assessment of arsenic toxicity using *Allium*/*Vicia* root tip micronucleus assays. *J. Hazard. Mater.* **2010**, *176*, 952–956. [CrossRef]
56. Yi, H.; Wu, L.; Jiang, L. Genotoxicity of arsenic evaluated by *Allium*-root micronucleus assay. *Sci. Total Environ.* **2007**, *383*, 232–236. [CrossRef]
57. Grant, W.F. Chromosome aberrations in plants as a monitoring system. *Environ. Health Perspect.* **1978**, *27*, 37–43. [CrossRef]
58. Huang, D.; Ou, B.; Hampsch-Woodill, M.; Flanagan, J.A.; Prior, R.L. High-throughput assay of oxygen radical absorbance capacity (ORAC) using a multichannel liquid handling system coupled with a microplate fluorescence reader in 96-well format. *J. Agric. Food Chem.* **2002**, *50*, 4437–4444. [CrossRef]
59. Bartlett, M.S. Properties of sufficiency and statistical tests. *Proc. R. Soc. Lond. Ser. A Math. Phys. Sci.* **1937**, *160*, 268–282. [CrossRef]

60. NIST/SEMATECH e-Handbook of Statistical Methods. Available online: http://www.itl.nist.gov/div898/handbook/ (accessed on 11 May 2020).
61. Dizdari, A.M.; Kopliku, D. Cytotoxic and Genotoxic Potency Screening of Two Pesticides on *Allium cepa* L. *Procedia Technol.* **2013**, *8*, 19–26. [CrossRef]
62. Bello-Bello, J.J.; Chavez-Santoscoy, R.A.; Lecona-Guzmán, C.A.; Bogdanchikova, N.; Salinas-Ruíz, J.; Gómez-Merino, F.C.; Pestryakov, A. Hormetic response by silver nanoparticles on in vitro multiplication of sugarcane (*Saccharum* spp. Cv. Mex 69-290) using a temporary immersion system. *Dose Response* **2017**, *15*, 1–9. [CrossRef]
63. Castro-González, C.G.; Sánchez-Segura, L.; Gómez-Merino, F.C.; Bello-Bello, J.J. Exposure of stevia (*Stevia rebaudiana* B.) to silver nanoparticles in vitro: Transport and accumulation. *Sci. Rep.* **2019**, *9*, 10372. [CrossRef] [PubMed]
64. Cox, A.; Venkatachalam, P.; Sahi, S.; Sharma, N. Reprint of: Silver and titanium dioxide nanoparticle toxicity in plants: A review of current research. *Plant Physiol. Biochem.* **2017**, *110*, 33–49. [CrossRef] [PubMed]
65. Bianchi, J.; Mantovani, M.S.; Marin-Morales, M.A. Analysis of the genotoxic potential of low concentrations of Malathion on the *Allium cepa* cells and rat hepatoma tissue culture. *J. Environ. Sci.* **2015**, *36*, 102–111. [CrossRef] [PubMed]
66. Batista, N.J.C.; de Carvalho Melo Cavalcante, A.A.; de Oliveira, M.G.; Medeiros, E.C.N.; Machado, J.L.; Evangelista, S.R.; Dias, J.F.; dos Santos, C.E.I.; Duarte, A.; da Silva, F.R.; et al. Genotoxic and mutagenic evaluation of water samples from a river under the influence of different anthropogenic activities. *Chemosphere* **2016**, *164*, 134–141. [CrossRef]
67. Leme, D.M.; Marin-Morales, M.A. Chromosome aberration and micronucleus frequencies in *Allium cepa* cells exposed to petroleum polluted water-A case study. *Mutat. Res. Genet. Toxicol. Environ. Mutagen.* **2008**, *650*, 80–86. [CrossRef]
68. Coskun, D.; Britto, D.T.; Jean, Y.K.; Schulze, L.M.; Becker, A.; Kronzucker, H.J. Silver ions disrupt K^+ homeostasis and cellular integrity in intact barley (*Hordeum vulgare* L.) roots. *J. Exp. Bot.* **2012**, *63*, 151–162. [CrossRef]
69. Schaller, G.; Binder, B. Inhibitors of Ethylene Biosynthesis and Signaling. In *Methods in Molecular Biology 1573. Ethylene Signaling. Methods and Protocols*; Binder, B., Schaller, G., Eds.; Humana Press: New York, NY, USA, 2017; pp. 223–236.
70. Vecchio, G.; Fenech, M.; Pompa, P.P.; Voelcker, N.H. Lab-on-a-chip-based high-throughput screening of the genotoxicity of engineered nanomaterials. *Small* **2014**, *10*, 2721–2734. [CrossRef]
71. Ghosh, M.; Ghosh, I.; Godderis, L.; Hoet, P.; Mukherjee, A. Genotoxicity of engineered nanoparticles in higher plants. *Mutat. Res. Genet. Toxicol. Environ. Mutagen.* **2019**, *842*, 132–145. [CrossRef]

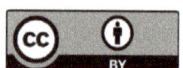

© 2020 by the authors. Licensee MDPI, Basel, Switzerland. This article is an open access article distributed under the terms and conditions of the Creative Commons Attribution (CC BY) license (http://creativecommons.org/licenses/by/4.0/).

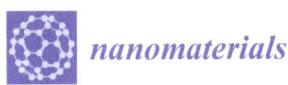

Article

Thermal Reduction of Graphene Oxide Mitigates Its In Vivo Genotoxicity Toward *Xenopus laevis* Tadpoles

Lauris Evariste [1,*], Laura Lagier [1], Patrice Gonzalez [2], Antoine Mottier [1], Florence Mouchet [1], Stéphanie Cadarsi [1], Pierre Lonchambon [3], Guillemine Daffe [4], George Chimowa [3], Cyril Sarrieu [3], Elise Ompraret [3], Anne-Marie Galibert [3], Camélia Matei Ghimbeu [5], Eric Pinelli [1], Emmanuel Flahaut [2] and Laury Gauthier [1]

1. EcoLab, Université de Toulouse, CNRS, INPT, UPS, 31400 Toulouse, France; laura.lagier@hotmail.com (L.L.); antoine.mottier@ensat.fr (A.M.); florence.mouchet@ensat.fr (F.M.); stephaniecad@gmail.com (S.C.); pinelli@ensat.fr (E.P.); laury.gauthier@univ-tlse3.fr (L.G.)
2. Univ. Bordeaux, UMR EPOC CNRS 5805, Aquatic ecotoxicology team, 33120 Arcachon, France; patrice.gonzalez@u-bordeaux.fr (P.G.); emmanuel.flahaut@univ-tlse3.fr (E.F.)
3. CIRIMAT, Université de Toulouse, CNRS, INPT, UPS, UMR CNRS-UPS-INP N°5085, Université Toulouse 3 Paul Sabatier, Bât. CIRIMAT, 118 route de Narbonne, 31062 Toulouse CEDEX 9, France; lonchambon@chimie.ups-tlse.fr (P.L.); gchimowa11@gmail.com (G.C.); cyril.sarrieu@gmail.com (C.S.); eompraret@gmail.com (E.O.); galibert@chimie.ups-tlse.fr (A.-M.G.)
4. CNRS, Universite de Bordeaux, Observatoire Aquitain des Sciences de l'Univers, UMS 2567 POREA, Allee Geoffroy Saint Hilaire, F-33615 Pessac, France; guillemine.daffe@u-bordeaux.fr
5. Institut de Science des Matériaux de Mulhouse (IS2M), UMR 7360 CNRS—UHA, 15 rue Jean Starcky, BP 2488, 68057 Mulhouse CEDEX, France; camelia.ghimbeu@uha.fr
* Correspondence: lauris.evariste@ensat.fr; Tel.: +33-534323936

Received: 5 March 2019; Accepted: 8 April 2019; Published: 9 April 2019

Abstract: The worldwide increase of graphene family materials raises the question of the potential consequences resulting from their release in the environment and future consequences on ecosystem health, especially in the aquatic environment in which they are likely to accumulate. Thus, there is a need to evaluate the biological and ecological risk but also to find innovative solutions leading to the production of safer materials. This work focuses on the evaluation of functional group-safety relationships regarding to graphene oxide (GO) in vivo genotoxic potential toward *X. laevis* tadpoles. For this purpose, thermal treatments in H_2 atmosphere were applied to produce reduced graphene oxide (rGOs) with different surface group compositions. Analysis performed indicated that GO induced disturbances in erythrocyte cell cycle leading to accumulation of cells in G0/G1 phase. Significant genotoxicity due to oxidative stress was observed in larvae exposed to low GO concentration (0.1 mg·L^{-1}). Reduction of GO at 200 °C and 1000 °C produced a material that was no longer genotoxic at low concentrations. X-ray photoelectron spectroscopy (XPS) analysis indicated that epoxide groups may constitute a good candidate to explain the genotoxic potential of the most oxidized form of the material. Thermal reduction of GO may constitute an appropriate "safer-by-design" strategy for the development of a safer material for environment.

Keywords: graphene oxide; reduced graphene oxide; micronucleus; oxidative stress; safer-by-design

1. Introduction

Carbon-based nanomaterials (CBMs) and especially 2D materials related to graphene [1] possess unique properties [2,3], triggering high expectations for the development of new technological applications and are forecasted to be produced at industrial-scale [4]. Among these graphene-based materials (GBMs), graphene derivatives such as graphene oxide (GO) and reduced graphene oxide (rGO) appear as very attractive due to their high stability after dispersion in various solvents, facilitating handling and processing of graphene-containing nanocomposites [5,6]. To ensure the safe and sustainable development of this innovative technology, evaluation of its biological and ecological risk, as well as finding innovative solutions to mitigate the hazard potential, are essential [7–9]. The increasing GBMs production raises concerns over their release into the environment, where it is likely to occur at any stage of the material life cycle [10–12]. However, compared to the increasing number of studies dealing with GBMs synthesis processes or application development advances, relatively few are devoted to studying their toxicity, and even less to their ecotoxicity. Due to its hydrophilic properties associated with the presence of oxygen-containing functional groups at their surface, GO and rGO could potentially be highly reactive towards multiple components of the environment [13]. Moreover, different physico-chemical behaviours between GO and rGO can be expected in the environment [14], associated with changes occurring in surface functional groups during the reduction process [15].

Most of the GBMs toxicological data available were obtained through in vitro experiments focusing on cytotoxicity towards mammalian cells [16–18]. For instance, some studies demonstrated that oxidized graphene-based nanoparticles exerted higher toxicity compared to their reduced counterparts [19–21], while others obtained contradictory results, indicating higher toxicity exerted by the reduced form of GO [22,23]. Among possible toxic effects, genotoxicity may have non-negligible consequences because unrepaired and/or improperly repaired DNA damage may in turn cause cellular dysfunctions and tumor formation, leading to the death of organisms [24] and further decline of a population [25]. However, it was pointed out that in vivo genotoxic potential of GBMs is still relatively poorly investigated [16,26,27]. In vivo experiments focusing on genotoxicity were mainly performed in rodents microinjected with nanomaterials [28–30] and data are remaining scarce particularly for aquatic species. A study performed using the comet assay in zebrafish failed to highlight genotoxic effects into fish gills after short-term exposure to GO [31]. Since the data available are contradictory, there is a need to clarify in vivo genotoxic potential and toxicological mechanisms associated to GO and rGO exposure, in order to fill persisting knowledge gaps concerning their eco-genotoxicity [32]. Amphibians are widely used for ecotoxicological studies and are recognized as sensitive organisms to genotoxic compounds, especially at the larval stage [33,34]. Tadpoles of the African clawed frog, *Xenopus laevis*, have previously been used for assessment of raw carbon-based nanoparticles ecotoxicity [35–38] and adverse effects on larval growth were previously reported after GO exposure [39].

The aim of the present work is to assess the in vivo genotoxic potential of GO in *X. laevis* as well as understanding toxicological pathways involved in the genotoxic response after exposure to a commercial form of the material. To determine the implication of the oxidation degree and surface functions in the toxicological response, thermal treatments in H_2 atmosphere were applied at two temperatures (200 °C and 1000 °C) to produce rGO exhibiting different surface functions. The complete characterization of the tested materials was performed to identify the role of functional groups in the genotoxic response.

2. Materials and Methods

2.1. Synthesis and Characterization of Graphene Oxide and Reduced Graphene Oxide

Graphene oxide was provided by Antolin Group and prepared by oxidation of Grupo Antolin Carbon Nanofibers (GANF®)(Grupo Antolín, Burgos, Spain) using the Hummer's method [40,41]. Tested rGO resulted from reduction of this GO in H_2 atmosphere with a hydrogen flow rate of 5 L·h^{-1} at 200 °C (rGO200) or 1000 °C (rGO1000). Reduction was performed under controlled conditions to modify the oxidation level with minimal impact on material morphology, lateral size, and number of layers (Figure 1). Reduction produced rGO samples with closely related physico-chemical characteristics compared to the starting GO material, except for their surface chemistry and their wetting properties. Physico-chemical characteristics of the tested materials are detailed in Table 1. Reduction at 200 °C was only partial and allowed keeping most of the oxygen in the material, while the reduction at 1000 °C almost completely removed the oxygen.

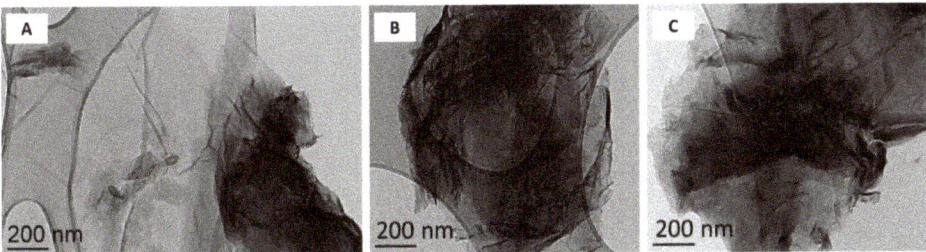

Figure 1. Transmission electron microscopy micrographs of (**A**) Graphene oxide, (**B**) reduced graphene oxide at 200 °C, (**C**) reduced graphene oxide at 1000 °C.

Table 1. Physico-chemical characteristics of graphene oxide (GO); reduced graphene oxide (rGO)200 and rGO1000. TEM: transmission electron microscope; HRTEM: high resolution TEM; BET: Brunauer-Emett-Teller; at. %: atomic %; GANF®: Grupo Antolin carbon nanofibers.

	GO	rGO200	rGO1000
Synthesis/production	GANF® processed by Hummers' method	Thermal treatment in hydrogen (5 L·h^{-1}) at 200 °C (2 h)	Thermal treatment in hydrogen (5 L·h^{-1}) at 1000 °C (2 h)
Catalyst	Ni, Fe, Co, Mn	None	None
Carbon content	69 ± 0.4 at. %	83.8 ± 0.5 at. %	98.5 ± 0.5 at. %
Oxygen content	31 ± 0.4 at. %	16.2 ± 0.3 at. %	1.5 ± 0.3 at. %
Number of layers (HRTEM)	1–5 [42,43]	1–5 [42,43]	1–5 [42,43]
Lateral size (TEM)	0.2 to 8 µm	0.2 to 8 µm	0.2 to 8 µm
Specific surface area (BET)	228 ± 6.8 m^2·g^{-1}	16 ± 0.5 m^2·g^{-1}	175 ± 5.2 m^2·g^{-1}

Elemental analysis (percentage of O and C atoms) was obtained by X-ray photoelectron spectroscopy (XPS). X-ray photoelectron spectroscopy (XPS) spectra were recorded with a VG SCIENTA SES-2002 spectrometer (Scienta Omicron, Taunusstein, Germany) equipped with a concentric hemispherical analyzer. Specific surface area was determined by N$_2$ adsorption according to the Brunauer, Emett and Teller's theory (BET) on dry powdered samples using a Micrometrics Flow Sorb II 2300 (Micromeritics, Norcross, GA, USA). The dispersion behavior of the two nanomaterials was analyzed in the exposure medium using a Turbiscan™ LAB Stability Analyzer (Formulaction SA, Toulouse, France). Transmission and backscattering of the near infrared light source (880 nm) was measured every 40 µm of the sample height. In order to ensure the detection of the nanoparticles, the concentration of 10 mg·L^{-1} of GO and rGO was selected for dispersion monitoring.

2.2. Metals and Polycyclic Aromatic Hydrocarbons (PAHs) Concentration Analysis in Graphene Oxide

GO from Grupo Antolin was prepared by oxidation of GANF® (grupo Antolin carbon nanofibers) which synthesis involve Ni, Co, Fe and Mn as metal catalysts. In addition, PAHs could be associated with GO because of their possible generation during GANF and GO synthesis and may be released by desorption from carbon nanomaterials in water [44]. The possible presence of these compounds was checked to avoid misanalysis of toxicity-related results [44]. Quantification of metal residues in mineralized GO powder was performed as described by Ayouni-Derouiche et al. [45] using ICP AES, iCAPTM 6300 analyzer (Thermo Fisher Scientific, Germany) (Crealins, Lyon, France). 32 PAHs compounds were analysed from GO dispersion in deionized water using gas chromatography-mass spectrometry (GC-MS) according to the normalized procedure NF ISO 28,540 (MicroPolluants Technologie S.A., Saint-Julien-lès-Metz, France).

2.3. Xenopus Rearing, Breeding and Exposure Conditions

Xenopus rearing and breeding were described in previous works [35,36]. Briefly, spawning of sexually mature *Xenopus* was induced by injection of pregnant mare's gonadotropin. Fecundated eggs obtained were bred in active charcoal filtered tap water at 22 ± 2 °C and fed with ground aquarium fish food (TetraPhyll®, Tetra, Melle, Germany) until they reach stage 50 according to Nieuwkoop & Faber development table [46]. Groups of 20 larvae were exposed for 12 days under semi-static conditions with daily feeding and exposure media renewal following the international standard ISO 21427-1 procedure. Negative control (NC) condition was composed of reconstituted water (RW; 294 mg·L^{-1} CaCl$_2$·2H$_2$O; 123.25 mg·L^{-1} MgSO$_4$·7H$_2$O; 64.75 mg·L^{-1} NaHCO$_3$; 5.75 mg·L^{-1} KCl) and cyclophosphamide monohydrate ([6055-19-2], Sigma-Aldrich Chimie, Saint-Quentin Fallavier, France) at 20 mg·L^{-1} in RW was used as genotoxic positive control (PC). GO tested concentration ranged from 0.1 to 50 mg·L^{-1}. Due to significant genotoxic effects induced by GO at the concentration of 0.1 mg·L^{-1}, this concentration was chosen to further determine toxicological pathways involved as well as to determine the consequences of thermal reduction on toxicity. Thus, rGO200 and rGO1000 were only tested at 0.1 mg·L^{-1}.

2.4. Micronucleus Test and Cell Cycle Analysis

After 12 days of exposure, blood samples were obtained by cardiac puncture in *Xenopus* larvae anaesthetized by immersion in MS222 solution at 0.1 g·L^{-1}. For micronuclei assay, smears were prepared from blood samples, fixed in methanol for 10 min before performing hematoxylin and eosin staining. The number of micronucleated erythrocytes (MNE) over a total of 1000 erythrocytes (MNE ‰) was counted under the optical microscope Olympus CX41 (oil immersion lens, ×1500) (Olympus, Tokyo, Japan). Blood sub-samples were fixed using cold ethanol (70% v/v) and stored at −20 °C until use. Prior to the flow cytometric analysis, cells were rinsed using PBS and labelled with FxCycle™ PI/RNase Staining Solution (Thermo Fisher Scientific, Bremen, Germany) according to manufacturer's recommendations. Propidium iodide fluorescence was measured using MACSQuant analyzer 10 (Miltenyi Biotec, San Diego, CA, USA) equipped with a 488-nm excitation laser. For each sample, 10,000 events were acquired in a region corresponding to erythrocytes after removal of cell doublets. For gating strategy, see Figure S1.

2.5. Gene Expression Analysis in the Livers

As the liver constitute the main organ of erythropoiesis and is implied in multiple metabolic functions in *X. laevis* [47], this organ was chosen to determine toxicological mechanisms involved in the genotoxic response at low GBMs concentration (0.1 mg·L^{-1}). For this purpose, analysis of the expression of 15 genes encoding for proteins involved in oxidative stress response (gpx1, cat, sod (Cu/Zn), sod(Mn)), inflammation processes (pparγ, cox1, cox2, lta4, 5-lox), detoxification (cyp1a1, tap, gst) and DNA repair (rad51, mutl, odc) was performed. Total RNA were extracted from 15 to 25 mg of liver samples using the SV Total Isolation System kit (Promega, Madison, WI, USA) according to manufacturer's instructions. Reverse transcription was carried out from 1 µg of total RNA using the GoScriptTM Reverse Transcription System kit (Promega) according to manufacturer's recommendations. Nnucleotide sequences of the primers were obtained from the online NCBI Nucleotide database and primer pairs were determined using the Primer3Plus software. All the primer pairs used are reported in Table S1.

Real-time qPCR was carried out using GoTaq® qPCR Master Mix kit (Promega, Madison, WI, USA) on five samples per condition. PCR reactions contained 17 µL of a mixture of Nuclease-Free Water and GoTaq® qPCR Master Mix containing the SyberGreen fluorescent dye, 2 µL of specific primer pairs mix (200 µM each) and 1µL of cDNA. Real-time quantitative PCR reactions were performed in a Mx3000P® qPCR System (Stratagene, La Jolla, CA, USA). The amplification program consisted in one cycle at 95 °C for 10 min, then 45 amplification cycles at 95 °C for 30 s, 60 °C for 30 s and 72 °C for 30 s. Specificity was determined for each reaction from the dissociation curve of the PCR product. This dissociation curve was obtained by following the SYBR Green fluorescence level during a gradual heating of the PCR products from 60 to 95 °C.

Cycle thresholds (Ct) were obtained from MxProTM qPCR software for each gene. Relative quantification of each gene expression level was normalized according to the mean Ct value of two stable reference genes (β actin, gapdh) according to the 2ΔCt methods described by Livak and Schmittgen [48]. Induction factors, compared to control group, were then determined as previously described [49].

2.6. Statistical Analysis

Data of micronucleus frequencies from three repeated experiments were analyzed using McGill non-parametric test [50] on median values of each group of larvae. This test consists in comparing medians of samples of size n (where n ≥ 7) and in determining their 95% confidence intervals (95% CI). 95% CI are expressed by M ± 1.57 × IQR/√n, where M is the median and IQR is the inter-quartile range [50]. The difference between the medians of the test groups and the median of the NC group is significant with 95% certainty if there is no overlap. For cell-cycle data, normality was assessed with Kolmogorov-Smirnov test and homogeneity of variances with Levene's test. One-way analysis of variance (ANOVA) followed by Tukey test were used to compare cell-cycle phase distribution among conditions. One-way ANOVA on ranks and Tukey post-hoc test ($p < 0.05$) were used to statistically compare differential gene expression levels.

3. Results and Discussion

3.1. Surface Chemistry and Dispersion Behavior

Surface chemistry of GO and rGOs evaluated by high resolution X-ray photoelectron spectroscopy (XPS) allowed identification of oxygen-containing groups present in the materials (Figure 2, Table 2).

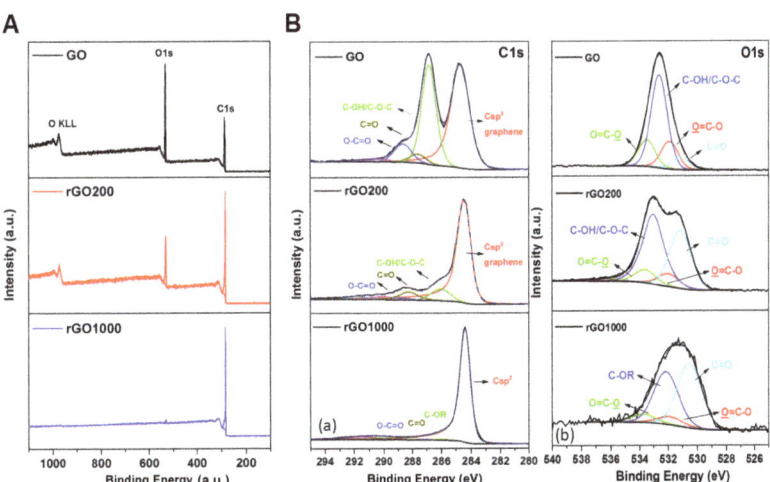

Figure 2. X-ray photoelectron spectroscopy (XPS) survey spectra of GO, rGO200 and rGO1000 materials (**A**); C1s and O1s deconvoluted XPS spectra for GO, rGO200 and rGO1000 (**B**).

For GO, the C1s spectrum obtained by XPS exhibits two main peaks at 284.6 eV and 286.8 eV (Figure 2B), which are correlated with the sp2 carbon (Csp2) of the graphene and oxygen functional groups, respectively. The 286.8 eV signal is deconvoluted into several peaks located at 286.8 eV, 288.6 eV and 287.61 eV. The most intense one is the 286.8 eV peak (24.7 at. %, Table 2), which corresponds to the carbon involved in hydroxyl groups (C-OH), ether and particularly epoxide groups (C–O–C) [51,52].

Table 2. Assignments of C1s XPS peaks for GO, rGO200 and rGO1000. Csp^2: sp^2 carbon; Sat.: shake-up satellites (π to π^* transitions).

GO		rGO200		rGO1000	
Peak Assignment	at. %	Peak Assignment	at. %	Peak Assignment	at. %
Csp2 graphene	35.5	Csp2 graphene	64.5	Csp2 graphene	89.7
C–OH/C–O–C	24.7	C–OH/C–O–C	7.8	C–OH/C–O–C	0.6
C=O	2.5	C=O	5.8	C=O	0.5
O=C–O	5.3	O=C–O	1.3	O=C–O	0.1
Sat.	1.4	Sat.	4.5	Sat.	7.7

The two other peaks are related to carbonyl (C=O) and carboxylic (O=C–O) groups and account for 2.5 and 5.3 at. %, respectively. Thermal reduction induced modifications of the chemical composition of GO. After annealing GO at 200 °C, the C1s spectra exhibited mainly one peak at 284.6 eV, corresponding to the sp2 carbon in graphene. This peak was narrower compared to that of GO, suggesting an increase in the graphitization level. The intense peak of the epoxide groups (286.8 nm) present on GO was removed by this treatment, leaving two shoulders associated with the hydroxyl groups and, to a lesser extent, with the ethers/epoxide (C–OH/C–O–C), C=O and O=C–O oxygen-containing functional groups. In agreement with previous work from Jung et al. [51], the use of temperature programmed desorption coupled with mass spectrometry (TPD-MS) indicated that removal of epoxide groups at 200 °C was accompanied by the release of CO, CO2 and H2O gases (data not shown). A dual path mechanism which proceeded by the release of solely molecular oxygen via a cycloaddition reaction from epoxide–epoxide pairs was proposed for the reduction of oxidized graphene [52]. Formation of ether–epoxide pairs at high O coverage further promoted the elimination of oxygen functional groups by releasing CO/CO2 mixtures, along with H$_2$O formation. Stronger reduction conditions (1000 °C) resulted in a material containing poorly oxygenated surface groups (Table 2), and a total oxygen content of 1.5 at. %. Details about the nature of the oxygen groups can also be seen in the O1s spectrum (Figure 2B).

The dispersion over time of GO and rGO200 in the medium of exposure (reconstituted water composed of deionized water added with salts) and in absence of Xenopus larvae is shown in Figure 3.

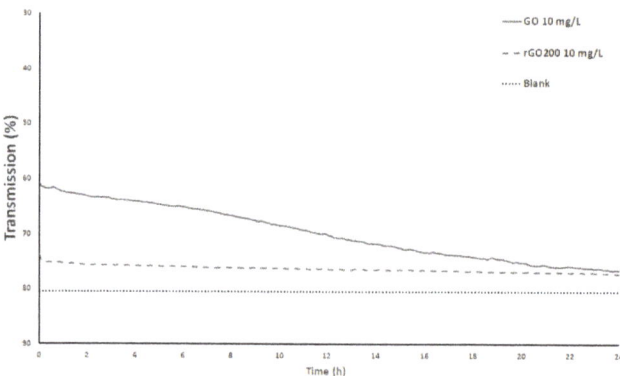

Figure 3. Monitoring of the stability of GO and rGO200 dispersion in the water column of exposure medium over 24 h (in absence of *Xenopus* larvae), expressed by the percentage of transmission detected after the light goes through the sample. Blank: medium without nanoparticles.

The results indicate a slight decrease in transmission over 24 h for the GO while this was not observed for rGO. Dispersion of these two materials was previously studied and a good dispersion capacity of both materials was observed in distilled water, with a better stability in the case of GO [53,54]. However, it was indicated that the presence of CaCl$_2$ reduced the GO stability due to adsorption of Ca^{2+} ions on the negatively charged functional groups, leading to reduced surface charge. In addition, rGO stability was less influenced by these ions due to the lower amount of functional groups, limiting Ca^{2+} adsorption [55]. As our exposure medium contains NaCl and CaCl$_2$, results from Chowdhury and collaborators [55] are consistent with our observations. Nonetheless, the dispersion state of the nanoparticles is strongly affected in presence of Xenopus larvae. As active filter feeders, it was previously observed that the water column is completely filtered in less than 24 h, resulting in nanoparticle accumulation in feces [39].

3.2. Metals and PAHs Contamination

Results of metallic residue quantifications are expressed in milligrams of metal per liter of exposure medium (Table 3).

Table 3. Concentration of metals (Ni: nickel; Co: cobalt; Fe: iron; Mn: manganese) and polycyclic aromatic hydrocarbons (PAHs) released in the exposure medium at 10 mg·L^{-1} of GO. Among the 32 analyzed PAHs, only those with a concentration over the detection limit are listed.

Metals Concentrations in the Medium (mg·L^{-1})		PAHs Concentrations in the Medium (µg·L^{-1})	
Ni	35.5	Naphtalene	3.5×10^{-4}
Co	24.7	Acenaphtene	2.5×10^{-4}
Fe	2.5	Phenanthrene	3.2×10^{-4}
Mn	5.3	Fluoranthene	2.4×10^{-4}
		Benzo(a)anthracene	2.4×10^{-4}
		Chrysene	2.5×10^{-4}
		Benzo(b+j)fluoranthene	2.5×10^{-4}
		2-Methyl Naphtalene	5.8×10^{-4}

According to these results, at 10 mg·L^{-1} of GO dispersed in medium, the concentration of metals was 6.9×10^{-4}, $<2.3 \times 10^{-4}$, $<6.0 \times 10^{-4}$ and 149.8×10^{-4} mg·L^{-1} for Ni, Co, Fe and Mn, respectively. However, a recovery efficiency of 91 ± 5% was measured from the certified reference material leading to a slight under-estimation of metal quantities in GO due to the complexity to perform metal analysis in a nanocarbon matrix. Among 32 PAHs compounds investigated in the exposure medium contaminated with GO at 10 mg·L^{-1}, 24 were below detection limit (<20 ng·L^{-1}). PAHs concentrations ranged from 2.4×10^{-4} µg·L^{-1} for Fluoranthene and Benzo(a)anthracene to 5.8×10^{-4} µg·L^{-1} for 2-Methyl Naphtalene (Table 3). After 12 days of exposure to such GO concentration, the total amount of contaminants potentially bioavailable for Xenopus larvae would be 16.6×10^{-3}, $<5.52 \times 10^{-3}$, $<14.4 \times 10^{-3}$ and 359.52×10^{-3} µg of Ni, Co, Fe and Mn, respectively and a total amount of 5.95×10^{-2} µg of PAHs. Metal ions such as Mn^{2+} and Fe^{2+} were shown to induce DNA scission when associated to GO [56] and PAHs constitute hazardous contaminants for humans and wildlife [57,58] that are known to exert genotoxicity towards amphibians [59,60]. However, total concentrations detected were too low to induce significant toxicity in larvae [61]. Thus, we can state that results obtained from bioassays performed in our study could be fully attributed to GO exposure.

3.3. Cell-cycle Analysis

Flow cytometry measurement of erythrocyte cell cycle highlighted an overall significant decrease in G2/M and S-phase cells (ANOVA, S-phase: $p < 0.001$; G2/M: $p < 0.001$) as well as an increase in G0/G1 cells (ANOVA, $p < 0.001$) with increasing concentration of GO (Figure 4).

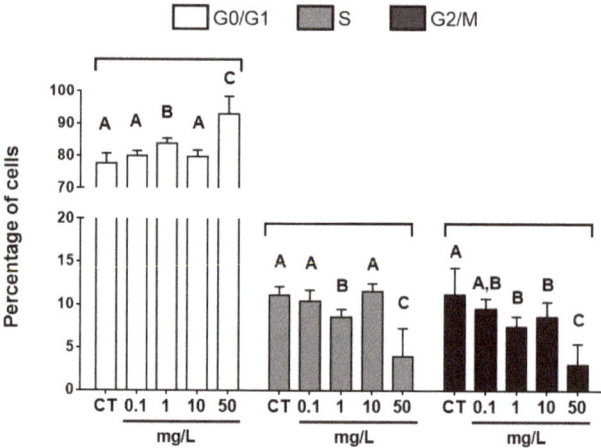

Figure 4. Cell-cycle distribution in G0/G1, S and G2/M phase analyzed from circulating erythrocytes of *Xenopus laevis* exposed to increasing concentrations of GO for 12 days. NC: negative control, N = 13, analysis of variance (ANOVA) $p < 0.001$ followed by Tukey test. Letters indicate significant differences between concentrations tested for each phase of the cell cycle.

The lowest concentration inducing significant changes in erythrocyte cell cycle was observed at 1 mg·L^{-1} of GO, resulting in significantly decreased G2/M and S-phase compared to the control group, while results obtained from organisms exposed at 0.1 mg·L^{-1} of GO were similar to the control group. After 12 days of exposure at the concentration of 50 mg·L^{-1}, erythrocyte accumulated in the G0/G1 phase of cell-cycle with a concomitant strong decrease in G2/M and S-phase percentage. According to data from the literature, almost all studies focusing on effects of GO on cell-cycle-related endpoints were performed in vitro. However, exposures to pristine or functionalized graphene oxide were shown to disturb cell-cycle progression, leading to accumulations of cells in early phases [62–65] that is consistent with our results. Petibone and collaborators [64] highlighted the key role of the p53 protein in cell cycle arrest after GO exposure, leading to cell accumulation in G0/G1 phase while p53-deficient cell line accumulated in S-phase. p53 is known to be involved in DNA damage response signaling pathway, driving to cell cycle arrest following genotoxic stress [66,67]. Upregulation of p53 expression was previously highlighted in mouse embryonic stem cells after exposure to other carbon-based nanoparticles such as carbon nanotubes and nanodiamonds [68,69]. In addition, a downregulation of protein S-phase kinase-associated protein involved in the control of the progression from G1 phase to S-phase during mitosis process was observed in human liver cancer HepG2 cells exposed to graphene oxide [70]. As the liver constitutes the main organ of erythropoiesis in *X. laevis* [47], a closely related mechanism could explain results obtained in our study. Thereby we can suggest that disturbances of erythrocyte cell-cycle observed in vivo in *X. laevis* tadpoles under our experimental conditions could be associated to modulations of gene expression and activities of proteins involved in cell-cycle regulation. However, further studies are needed to confirm these hypotheses.

Cell division constitutes a sine qua non-condition to produce a micronucleus after chromosome breakage (clastogenesis) or/and disturbance of chromosome segregation machinery (aneugenesis) [71,72]. As the majority of cells were blocked at the G0/G1 stage in larvae exposed to GO at concentrations ranging from 1 to 50 mg·L^{-1}, the decrease in erythrocyte mitotic rates measured would lead to inconsistent results in the evaluation of micronuclei induction at these concentrations.

3.4. Genotoxicity

In accordance with ISO/FDIS 21427-1 standards, as mitotic rates were significantly lower in the 1, 10 and 50 mg·L^{-1} of GO compared to the control group, micronuclei were not accounted in these conditions. In addition, in all experimental groups, larvae exposed to PC (cyclophosphamide at 20 mg·L^{-1}) exhibited significantly higher median values of micronucleated erythrocytes (MNE ‰) compared to their respective NC group, validating the results of the micronucleus tests. A significant increase in micronucleus occurrence was observed in erythrocytes of larvae exposed to the 0.1 mg·L^{-1} concentration of GO compared to the NC group (Figure 5). Contrary to the results obtained with the most oxidized form of the material, exposure to 0.1 mg·L^{-1} of rGO did not induce an increase in micronucleated erythrocyte occurrence compared to the control group, regardless of the reduction temperature performed (200 °C or 1000 °C, Figure 5).

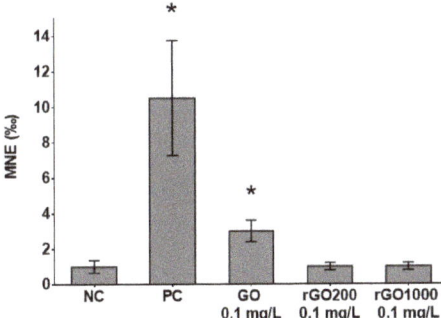

Figure 5. Micronucleus induction measured in erythrocytes of *Xenopus laevis* larvae exposed for 12 days to GO or rGO (rGO200 or rGO1000). MNE: micronucleated erythrocytes; NC: negative control; PC: positive control; *: significant difference compared to the NC (McGill test).

The results obtained demonstrated that GO is able to induce the formation of nuclear abnormalities in vivo at low concentrations in amphibian larvae. Induction of genotoxic effects through increase of micronuclei occurrence as well as DNA fragmentation or chromosome aberration were previously observed in vivo in rodents [28,29,73–75]. Thus, these data from the literature are consistent with our results. On the contrary, no genotoxicity using comet assay was found in the gills of zebrafish exposed to GO concentrations from 2 to 20 mg·L^{-1} during 72 h [31]. However, despite the differences in exposure duration and conditions, micronucleus and comet assays are not devoted to highlighting similar genotoxic pathways and mechanisms [76]. This also suggests that GO exposure induces breaks at chromosomal level rather than chromatic level [71]. It was highlighted that GO strongly interacted with DNA in vitro, causing interferences with DNA segregation during cell-cycle and generated mutagenic effects [29,77]. In addition, according to molecular dynamics simulations, the driving force of interactions between nucleotides and carbon-based nanosurfaces is the π stacking noncovalent interaction between aromatic rings, which may lead to self-assembly between DNA and graphene potentially causing DNA deformation and breakage [78]. However, this assumption is unlikely due to more limited direct interactions between GO and erythroid progenitors or circulating erythrocytes using in vivo exposure. Thus, it is more likely that mutagenic effects observed were associated to DNA damages generated by reactive oxygen species (ROS) that are described as being mainly implied in DNA fragmentation, as they are involved as secondary messengers in many intracellular signaling cascades and can damage cellular macromolecules [79].

3.5. Genes Expressions in the Livers of Larvae Exposed to GO and rGO

Analysis of the relative gene expression levels after 12 days of exposure reveals a significant induction of most of the studied genes in the liver of larvae exposed to GO at 0.1 mg·L^{-1} (Table 4). Some genes involved in oxidative stress response and inflammation (gpx1, sod(Cu/Zn), sod(Mn), ppary, 5-lox and cox1) were significantly induced from 2.6 to 5.84 times more than the negative control. Finally, some detoxification processes occurred as shown by the induction of cyp1a1 and tap. On the contrary, no significant modulation of gene expressions was noticed in rGO conditions (Table 4).

Table 4. Differential gene expression in *Xenopus larvae* liver (n = 5) after 12 days of exposure to GO, rGO200 and rGO1000 at 0.1 mg·L^{-1}. For each condition, results are given as induction (>1) or repression (<1) factors compared to the negative control. Only statistically significant values are given; "-" indicates factors similar to control levels.

Functions	Genes	Genes Relative Expression		
		GO 0.1 mg·L^{-1}	rGO200 0.1 mg·L^{-1}	rGO1000 0.1 mg·L^{-1}
Oxidative Stress Response	gpx1	5.84 ± 0.54	-	-
	cat	-	-	-
	sod(Cu/Zn)	2.76 ± 0.21	-	-
	sod(Mn)	2.48 ± 0.15	-	-
Inflammation processes	ppary	5.71 ± 0.37	-	-
	cox1	3.65 ± 0.2	-	-
	cox2	-	-	-
	lta4	-	-	-
	5-lox	2.60 ± 0.17	-	-
DNA repair	rad51	-	-	-
	mut	-	-	-
	odc	-	-	-
Detoxification	cyp1a1	4.99 ± 0.53	-	-
	tap	19.09 ± 0.95	-	-
	gst	-	-	-

Upregulation of gene expression related to cytoplasmic and mitochondrial super-oxide dismutase (sod(Cu/Zn) and sod(Mn)) indicates that exposure to 0.1 mg·L^{-1} of GO induce oxidative stress. Furthermore, contrary to RNA expression level of the catalase gene, significant upregulation of gpx1 suggest that hydrogen peroxide produced is mainly eliminated through glutathione pathway [80,81]. Capacity of GO to induce oxidative stress in vivo was observed in a wide range of biological models such as rodents [28], fish [82], nematodes [83] or paramecium [84]. In the case of carbon nanotube exposure, an interdependent relationship between ROS production and inflammatory response was evidenced [85]. Similarly, inflammatory responses were frequently observed in vivo in rodents after GO exposure [86–89] and to a lesser extent after rGO exposure [21,90]. This corroborate with our results and confirm previous hypothesis suggesting that observed genotoxicity result from oxidative stress and inflammation process in the liver [91], constituting the erythropoietic organ in *X. laevis* tadpoles. Thus, oxidative stress affecting erythrocyte progenitors associated to an absence of upregulation of DNA repair-related genes result in the release of micronucleated erythrocytes in the circulation.

Thermal reduction under a hydrogen atmosphere produced material that no longer exerted oxidative stress, inflammatory response, disturbance of erythrocyte cell cycle (data not shown) as well as genotoxicity at low concentration. Genotoxic potential of GO in vitro was previously shown to be related to material lateral size [92]. However, in our study conditions, GO and rGOs tested were of similar range of lateral size suggesting that differences observed between the two types of GBMs were not correlated to this material characteristic. The main difference between tested GO and rGOs was the oxygen content (C/O ratio) and by extension surface chemistry including the nature of oxygen-containing functionalities. This parameter appears to be a good candidate to explain differences observed in genotoxic potential of these nanomaterials. Indeed, some studies demonstrated that oxidized carbon-based nanoparticles exerted higher genotoxicity compared to their non-oxidized counterparts [20,93]. However, other studies obtained contradictory results, indicated that the reduced form of GO exerted higher toxicity compared to the oxidized material. It was observed for cytotoxicity in cell lines [22,23], bacterial growth inhibition [94] or in impairment of embryo-larval development of zebrafish [95]. However, a recent study indicated that rGO toxicity depended on the reduction pathway used to produce the material [96]. Studies previously cited highlighting a higher toxicity of rGO were performed using materials produced from acidification or using reducing agents such as hydrazine or ascorbic acid. In our case, it appears that thermal reduction in a H_2 atmosphere of GO produced safer material with lower genotoxic potential. Initially, GO is composed of several oxygen-containing functional groups such as epoxy, hydroxyl and carboxyl groups, regardless of the production process [97]. XPS analysis performed on different materials produced allowed changes in the chemical surface composition of GO during reduction process. Therefore, functional groups such as epoxides were removed after annealing GO at 200 °C. These functions could clearly be responsible for the GO-induced genotoxic effects. Indeed, these epoxide functions are also produced in the liver by Benzo[a]pyrene metabolization and are well-known for being responsible for DNA adducts and damage induction [98]. Thus, contradictory results from the literature concerning the hazard potential of GBMs may possibly be explained by differences in the surface functions of the tested materials from one study to another. In our study, the fully-reduced GO produced after thermal reduction at 1000 °C led to a material with very few residuals of oxygenated surface groups and with a C/O ratio value comparable to the few layer graphene that was shown to be non-genotoxic towards *X. laevis* under similar experimental conditions [38], which is consistent with our observations and hypotheses.

4. Conclusions

According to results obtained in this work, we showed the importance of the nature of oxygen-containing functions of GBMs, especially the epoxide groups, in their hazard potential toward aquatic species. Indeed, GO is able to induce oxidative stress and inflammatory response at low concentrations, leading to mutagenic effects in vivo in *Xenopus laevis* tadpoles. At higher concentrations, the toxicity is reflected by disturbances in erythrocytic mitosis, resulting in accumulation of cells in G0/G1 phase. Thermal reduction of GO into rGO under our study conditions produced material that no longer induced oxidative stress, inflammation and genotoxic effects at low concentration. According to data from the literature, it appears that the reduction process used to produce rGO may determine the hazard potential of the reduced material. Thereby, although the thermal treatment of GO performed at 200 °C decreased the toxic potential of GO, reduction of material oxygen content through the methodology used in our study conditions appears to constitute a good strategy to produce a safer material for aquatic species [99].

Supplementary Materials: The following are available online at http://www.mdpi.com/2079-4991/9/4/584/s1, Figure S1: Gating strategy used in flow cytometry for analysis of erythrocyte cell cycle of *Xenopus laevis* tadpoles. Cells were gated to exclude debris (A). Single cells were gated using width and area parameters of IP fluorescence (B). Analysis of cells in G0/G1, S or G2/M phase was performed (C), Table S1: Accession numbers, functions and primer pairs (aUpstream primer; bForward primer) for the 25 *X. laevis* genes studied.

Author Contributions: Conceptualization, P.G.; F.M. and E.P.; methodology, S.C. and C.M.G.; formal analysis, L.E.; L.L.; A.M.; P.L.; G.D.; G.C.; C.S.; E.O.; A.-M.G. and C.M.G.; investigation, L.E. and L.L.; resources, S.C.; writing—original draft preparation, L.E.; writing—review and editing, A.M.; supervision, P.G.; F.M.; E.P. and L.G.; project administration, F.M.; E.F. and L.G.; funding acquisition, F.M.; E.P.; E.F. and L.G.

Funding: This project has received funding from the European Union's Horizon 2020 research and innovation programme under grant agreement No 696656. This research was also supported by the French Ministry of National Education, Higher Education and Research.

Acknowledgments: Samar Hajjar is acknowledged for the help provided with the XPS measurements obtained through the use of the IS2M technical platform. Linda Ayouni-Derouiche and Inès Guizani are acknowledged for metallic impurities measurement at the Crealins laboratory.

Conflicts of Interest: The authors declare no conflict of interest.

References

1. Bianco, A.; Cheng, H.-M.; Enoki, T.; Gogotsi, Y.; Hurt, R.H.; Koratkar, N.; Kyotani, T.; Monthioux, M.; Park, C.R.; Tascon, J.M. All in the Graphene Family–A Recommended Nomenclature for Two-Dimensional Carbon Materials. *Carbon* **2013**, *65*, 1–6. [CrossRef]
2. Geim, A.K.; Novoselov, K.S. The rise of graphene. *Nat. Mater.* **2007**, *6*, 183. [CrossRef]
3. Geim, A.K. Graphene: Status and prospects. *Science* **2009**, *324*, 1530–1534. [CrossRef] [PubMed]
4. Zhu, Y.; Ji, H.; Cheng, H.-M.; Ruoff, R.S. Mass production and industrial applications of graphene materials. *Nat. Sci. Rev.* **2018**, *5*, 90–101. [CrossRef]
5. Paredes, J.I.; Villar-Rodil, S.; Martínez-Alonso, A.; Tascon, J.M.D. Graphene oxide dispersions in organic solvents. *Langmuir* **2008**, *24*, 10560–10564. [CrossRef] [PubMed]
6. Kim, H.M.; Kim, S.G.; Lee, H.S. Dispersions of partially reduced graphene oxide in various organic solvents and polymers. *Carbon Lett.* **2017**, *23*, 55–62.
7. Bianco, A.; Prato, M. Safety concerns on graphene and 2D materials: A Flagship perspective. *2D Mater.* **2015**, *2*, 030201. [CrossRef]
8. Guiney, L.M.; Wang, X.; Xia, T.; Nel, A.E.; Hersam, M.C. Assessing and Mitigating the Hazard Potential of Two-Dimensional Materials. *ACS Nano* **2018**, *12*, 6360–6377. [CrossRef] [PubMed]
9. Kraegeloh, A.; Suarez-Merino, B.; Sluijters, T.; Micheletti, C. Implementation of Safe-by-Design for Nanomaterial Development and Safe Innovation: Why We Need a Comprehensive Approach. *Nanomaterials* **2018**, *8*, 239. [CrossRef]
10. Park, M.V.D.Z.; Bleeker, E.A.J.; Brand, W.; Cassee, F.R.; van Elk, M.; Gosens, I.; de Jong, W.H.; Meesters, J.A.J.; Peijnenburg, W.J.G.M.; Quik, J.T.K.; et al. Considerations for Safe Innovation: The Case of Graphene. *ACS Nano* **2017**, *11*, 9574–9593. [CrossRef]
11. Goodwin, D.G.; Adeleye, A.S.; Sung, L.; Ho, K.T.; Burgess, R.M.; Petersen, E.J. Detection and Quantification of Graphene-Family Nanomaterials in the Environment. *Environ. Sci. Technol.* **2018**, *52*, 4491–4513. [CrossRef] [PubMed]
12. Mottier, A.; Mouchet, F.; Pinelli, É.; Gauthier, L.; Flahaut, E. Environmental impact of engineered carbon nanoparticles: From releases to effects on the aquatic biota. *Curr. Opin. Biotechnol.* **2017**, *46*, 1–6. [CrossRef] [PubMed]
13. Zhao, J.; Wang, Z.; White, J.C.; Xing, B. Graphene in the Aquatic Environment: Adsorption, Dispersion, Toxicity and Transformation. *Environ. Sci. Technol.* **2014**, *48*, 9995–10009. [CrossRef] [PubMed]
14. Ersan, G.; Apul, O.G.; Perreault, F.; Karanfil, T. Adsorption of organic contaminants by graphene nanosheets: A review. *Water Res.* **2017**, *126*, 385–398. [CrossRef]
15. Haubner, K.; Murawski, J.; Olk, P.; Eng, L.M.; Ziegler, C.; Adolphi, B.; Jaehne, E. The Route to Functional Graphene Oxide. *ChemPhysChem* **2010**, *11*, 2131–2139. [CrossRef] [PubMed]
16. Guo, X.; Mei, N. Assessment of the toxic potential of graphene family nanomaterials. *J. Food Drug Anal.* **2014**, *22*, 105–115. [CrossRef] [PubMed]
17. Ou, L.; Song, B.; Liang, H.; Liu, J.; Feng, X.; Deng, B.; Sun, T.; Shao, L. Toxicity of graphene-family nanoparticles: A general review of the origins and mechanisms. *Part. Fibre Toxicol.* **2016**, *13*, 57. [CrossRef]
18. Fadeel, B.; Bussy, C.; Merino, S.; Vázquez, E.; Flahaut, E.; Mouchet, F.; Evariste, L.; Gauthier, L.; Koivisto, A.J.; Vogel, U.; et al. Safety Assessment of Graphene-Based Materials: Focus on Human Health and the Environment. *ACS Nano* **2018**, *12*, 10582–10620. [CrossRef]
19. Das, S.; Singh, S.; Singh, V.; Joung, D.; Dowding, J.M.; Reid, D.; Anderson, J.; Zhai, L.; Khondaker, S.I.; Self, W.T.; et al. Oxygenated Functional Group Density on Graphene Oxide: Its Effect on Cell Toxicity. *Part. Part. Syst. Charact.* **2013**, *30*, 148–157. [CrossRef]
20. Hashemi, E.; Akhavan, O.; Shamsara, M.; Daliri, M.; Dashtizad, M.; Farmany, A. Synthesis and cyto-genotoxicity evaluation of graphene on mice spermatogonial stem cells. *Colloids Surf. B Biointerfaces* **2016**, *146*, 770–776. [CrossRef]
21. Li, R.; Guiney, L.M.; Chang, C.H.; Mansukhani, N.D.; Ji, Z.; Wang, X.; Liao, Y.-P.; Jiang, W.; Sun, B.; Hersam, M.C.; et al. Surface Oxidation of Graphene Oxide Determines Membrane Damage, Lipid

Peroxidation, and Cytotoxicity in Macrophages in a Pulmonary Toxicity Model. *ACS Nano* **2018**, *12*, 1390–1402. [CrossRef] [PubMed]
22. Jaworski, S.; Sawosz, E.; Kutwin, M.; Wierzbicki, M.; Hinzmann, M.; Grodzik, M.; Winnicka, A.; Lipinska, L.; Wlodyga, K.; Chwalibog, A. In vitro and in vivo effects of graphene oxide and reduced graphene oxide on glioblastoma. *Int. J. Nanomed.* **2015**, *10*, 1585–1596.
23. Contreras-Torres, F.F.; Rodríguez-Galván, A.; Guerrero-Beltrán, C.E.; Martínez-Lorán, E.; Vázquez-Garza, E.; Ornelas-Soto, N.; García-Rivas, G. Differential cytotoxicity and internalization of graphene family nanomaterials in myocardial cells. *Mater. Sci. Eng. C* **2017**, *73*, 633–642. [CrossRef]
24. Jackson, S.P.; Bartek, J. The DNA-damage response in human biology and disease. *Nature* **2009**, *461*, 1071–1078. [CrossRef] [PubMed]
25. Sukumaran, S.; Grant, A. Effects of genotoxicity and its consequences at the population level in sexual and asexual Artemia assessed by analysis of inter-simple sequence repeats (ISSR). *Mutat. Res. Toxicol. Environ. Mutagen.* **2013**, *757*, 8–14. [CrossRef] [PubMed]
26. Seabra, A.B.; Paula, A.J.; de Lima, R.; Alves, O.L.; Durán, N. Nanotoxicity of Graphene and Graphene Oxide. *Chem. Res. Toxicol.* **2014**, *27*, 159–168. [CrossRef]
27. Ema, M.; Gamo, M.; Honda, K. A review of toxicity studies on graphene-based nanomaterials in laboratory animals. *Regul. Toxicol. Pharmacol.* **2017**, *85*, 7–24. [CrossRef]
28. El-Yamany, N.A.; Mohamed, F.F.; Salaheldin, T.A.; Tohamy, A.A.; Abd El-Mohsen, W.N.; Amin, A.S. Graphene oxide nanosheets induced genotoxicity and pulmonary injury in mice. *Exp. Toxicol. Pathol.* **2017**, *69*, 383–392. [CrossRef]
29. Liu, Y.; Luo, Y.; Wu, J.; Wang, Y.; Yang, X.; Yang, R.; Wang, B.; Yang, J.; Zhang, N. Graphene oxide can induce in vitro and in vivo mutagenesis. *Sci. Rep.* **2013**, *3*, 3469. [CrossRef]
30. Mendonça, M.C.P.; Soares, E.S.; de Jesus, M.B.; Ceragioli, H.J.; Irazusta, S.P.; Batista, Â.G.; Vinolo, M.A.R.; Maróstica Júnior, M.R.; da Cruz-Höfling, M.A. Reduced graphene oxide: Nanotoxicological profile in rats. *J. Nanobiotechnol.* **2016**, *14*, 53. [CrossRef]
31. Souza, J.P.; Baretta, J.F.; Santos, F.; Paino, I.M.M.; Zucolotto, V. Toxicological effects of graphene oxide on adult zebrafish (Danio rerio). *Aquat. Toxicol.* **2017**, *186*, 11–18. [CrossRef] [PubMed]
32. Montagner, A.; Bosi, S.; Tenori, E.; Bidussi, M.; Alshatwi, A.A.; Tretiach, M.; Prato, M.; Syrgiannis, Z. Ecotoxicological effects of graphene-based materials. *2D Mater.* **2016**, *4*, 012001. [CrossRef]
33. de Lapuente, J.; Lourenço, J.; Mendo, S.A.; Borràs, M.; Martins, M.G.; Costa, P.M.; Pacheco, M. The Comet Assay and its applications in the field of ecotoxicology: A mature tool that continues to expand its perspectives. *Front. Genet.* **2015**, *6*, 180. [CrossRef] [PubMed]
34. Mouchet, F.; Gauthier, L. Genotoxicity of Contaminants: Amphibian Micronucleus Assays. In *Encyclopedia of Aquatic Ecotoxicology*; Férard, J.-F., Blaise, C., Eds.; Springer: Dordrecht, The Netherlands, 2013; pp. 547–558. ISBN 978-94-007-5704-2.
35. Mouchet, F.; Landois, P.; Sarremejean, E.; Bernard, G.; Puech, P.; Pinelli, E.; Flahaut, E.; Gauthier, L. Characterisation and in vivo ecotoxicity evaluation of double-wall carbon nanotubes in larvae of the amphibian Xenopus laevis. *Aquat. Toxicol.* **2008**, *87*, 127–137. [CrossRef] [PubMed]
36. Mouchet, F.; Landois, P.; Puech, P.; Pinelli, E.; Flahaut, E.; Gauthier, L. Carbon nanotube ecotoxicity in amphibians: Assessment of multiwalled carbon nanotubes and comparison with double-walled carbon nanotubes. *Nanomedicine* **2010**, *5*, 963–974. [CrossRef]
37. Mottier, A.; Mouchet, F.; Laplanche, C.; Cadarsi, S.; Lagier, L.; Arnault, J.-C.; Girard, H.A.; León, V.; Vázquez, E.; Sarrieu, C.; et al. Surface Area of Carbon Nanoparticles: A Dose Metric for a More Realistic Ecotoxicological Assessment. *Nano Lett.* **2016**, *16*, 3514–3518. [CrossRef]
38. Muzi, L.; Mouchet, F.; Cadarsi, S.; Janowska, I.; Russier, J.; Ménard-Moyon, C.; Risuleo, G.; Soula, B.; Galibert, A.-M.; Flahaut, E.; et al. Examining the impact of multi-layer graphene using cellular and amphibian models. *2D Mater.* **2016**, *3*, 025009. [CrossRef]
39. Lagier, L.; Mouchet, F.; Laplanche, C.; Mottier, A.; Cadarsi, S.; Evariste, L.; Sarrieu, C.; Lonchambon, P.; Pinelli, E.; Flahaut, E.; et al. Surface area of carbon-based nanoparticles prevails on dispersion for growth inhibition in amphibians. *Carbon* **2017**, *119*, 72–81. [CrossRef]
40. Hummers, W.S., Jr.; Offeman, R.E. Preparation of graphitic oxide. *J. Am. Chem. Soc.* **1958**, *80*, 1339. [CrossRef]
41. Lobato, B.; Merino, C.; Barranco, V.; Centeno, T.A. Large-scale conversion of helical-ribbon carbon nanofibers to a variety of graphene-related materials. *RSC Adv.* **2016**, *6*, 57514–57520. [CrossRef]

42. Tabet, L.; Bussy, C.; Amara, N.; Setyan, A.; Grodet, A.; Rossi, M.J.; Pairon, J.-C.; Boczkowski, J.; Lanone, S. Adverse Effects of Industrial Multiwalled Carbon Nanotubes on Human Pulmonary Cells. *J. Toxicol. Environ. Health A* **2008**, *72*, 60–73. [CrossRef]
43. Agence Nationale de Sécurité Sanitaire de L'alimentation de L'environnement et du Travail (Anses) AVIS Relatif à « L'évaluation des Risques Liés au GRAPHISTRENGTH C100 Réalisée dans le Cadre du Programme Genesis ». Available online: https://www.anses.fr/fr/system/files/AP2007sa0417-4.pdf (accessed on 8 April 2019).
44. Petersen, E.J.; Henry, T.B.; Zhao, J.; MacCuspie, R.I.; Kirschling, T.L.; Dobrovolskaia, M.A.; Hackley, V.; Xing, B.; White, J.C. Identification and Avoidance of Potential Artifacts and Misinterpretations in Nanomaterial Ecotoxicity Measurements. *Environ. Sci. Technol.* **2014**, *48*, 4226–4246. [CrossRef] [PubMed]
45. Ayouni-Derouiche, L.; Méjean, M.; Gay, P.; Milliand, M.-L.; Lantéri, P.; Gauthier, L.; Flahaut, E. Development of efficient digestion procedures for quantitative determination of cobalt and molybdenum catalyst residues in carbon nanotubes. *Carbon* **2014**, *80*, 59–67. [CrossRef]
46. Nieuwkoop, P.D.; Faber, J. Normal Table of Xenopus Laevis (Daudin). A Systematical and Chronological Survey of the Development from the Fertilized Egg Till the End of Metamorphosis. *Q. Rev. Biol.* **1958**, *33*, 85.
47. Tsiftsoglou, A.S.; Vizirianakis, I.S.; Strouboulis, J. Erythropoiesis: Model systems, molecular regulators, and developmental programs. *IUBMB Life* **2009**, *61*, 800–830. [CrossRef] [PubMed]
48. Livak, K.J.; Schmittgen, T.D. Analysis of Relative Gene Expression Data Using Real-Time Quantitative PCR and the 2−ΔΔCT Method. *Methods* **2001**, *25*, 402–408. [CrossRef] [PubMed]
49. Barjhoux, I.; Gonzalez, P.; Baudrimont, M.; Cachot, J. Molecular and phenotypic responses of Japanese medaka (Oryzias latipes) early life stages to environmental concentrations of cadmium in sediment. *Environ. Sci. Pollut. Res.* **2016**, *23*, 17969–17981. [CrossRef] [PubMed]
50. Mcgill, R.; Tukey, J.W.; Larsen, W.A. Variations of Box Plots. *Am. Stat.* **1978**, *32*, 12–16.
51. Jung, I.; Field, D.A.; Clark, N.J.; Zhu, Y.; Yang, D.; Piner, R.D.; Stankovich, S.; Dikin, D.A.; Geisler, H.; Ventrice, C.A.; et al. Reduction Kinetics of Graphene Oxide Determined by Electrical Transport Measurements and Temperature Programmed Desorption. *J. Phys. Chem. C* **2009**, *113*, 18480–18486. [CrossRef]
52. Larciprete, R.; Fabris, S.; Sun, T.; Lacovig, P.; Baraldi, A.; Lizzit, S. Dual Path Mechanism in the Thermal Reduction of Graphene Oxide. *J. Am. Chem. Soc.* **2011**, *133*, 17315–17321. [CrossRef]
53. Konios, D.; Stylianakis, M.M.; Stratakis, E.; Kymakis, E. Dispersion behaviour of graphene oxide and reduced graphene oxide. *J. Colloid Interface Sci.* **2014**, *430*, 108–112. [CrossRef]
54. Song, M.Y.; Yun, Y.S.; Kim, N.R.; Jin, H.-J. Dispersion stability of chemically reduced graphene oxide nanoribbons in organic solvents. *RSC Adv.* **2016**, *6*, 19389–19393. [CrossRef]
55. Chowdhury, I.; Mansukhani, N.D.; Guiney, L.M.; Hersam, M.C.; Bouchard, D. Aggregation and Stability of Reduced Graphene Oxide: Complex Roles of Divalent Cations, pH, and Natural Organic Matter. *Environ. Sci. Technol.* **2015**, *49*, 10886–10893. [CrossRef] [PubMed]
56. Ren, H.; Wang, C.; Zhang, J.; Zhou, X.; Xu, D.; Zheng, J.; Guo, S.; Zhang, J. DNA Cleavage System of Nanosized Graphene Oxide Sheets and Copper Ions. *ACS Nano* **2010**, *4*, 7169–7174. [CrossRef]
57. Rengarajan, T.; Rajendran, P.; Nandakumar, N.; Lokeshkumar, B.; Rajendran, P.; Nishigaki, I. Exposure to polycyclic aromatic hydrocarbons with special focus on cancer. *Asian Pac. J. Trop. Biomed.* **2015**, *5*, 182–189. [CrossRef]
58. Abdel-Shafy, H.I.; Mansour, M.S.M. A review on polycyclic aromatic hydrocarbons: Source, environmental impact, effect on human health and remediation. *Egypt. J. Pet.* **2016**, *25*, 107–123. [CrossRef]
59. Gauthier, L.; Tardy, E.; Mouchet, F.; Marty, J. Biomonitoring of the genotoxic potential (micronucleus assay) and detoxifying activity (EROD induction) in the River Dadou (France), using the amphibian Xenopus laevis. *Sci. Total Environ.* **2004**, *323*, 47–61. [CrossRef]
60. Mouchet, F.; Gauthier, L.; Mailhes, C.; Ferrier, V.; Devaux, A. Comparative study of the comet assay and the micronucleus test in amphibian larvae (Xenopus laevis) using benzo(a)pyrene, ethyl methanesulfonate, and methyl methanesulfonate: Establishment of a positive control in the amphibian comet assay. *Environ. Toxicol.* **2005**, *20*, 74–84. [CrossRef] [PubMed]
61. Wang, Y.; Wang, J.; Mu, J.; Wang, Z.; Cong, Y.; Yao, Z.; Lin, Z. Aquatic predicted no-effect concentrations of 16 polycyclic aromatic hydrocarbons and their ecological risks in surface seawater of Liaodong Bay, China: Aquatic PNECs of 16 PAHs and their ecological risks. *Environ. Toxicol. Chem.* **2016**, *35*, 1587–1593. [CrossRef]

62. Matesanz, M.-C.; Vila, M.; Feito, M.-J.; Linares, J.; Gonçalves, G.; Vallet-Regi, M.; Marques, P.-A.A.P.; Portolés, M.-T. The effects of graphene oxide nanosheets localized on F-actin filaments on cell-cycle alterations. *Biomaterials* **2013**, *34*, 1562–1569. [CrossRef]
63. Kang, Y.; Liu, J.; Wu, J.; Yin, Q.; Liang, H.; Chen, A.; Shao, L. Graphene oxide and reduced graphene oxide induced neural pheochromocytoma-derived PC12 cell lines apoptosis and cell cycle alterations via the ERK signaling pathways. *Int. J. Nanomed.* **2017**, *12*, 5501–5510. [CrossRef]
64. Petibone, D.M.; Mustafa, T.; Bourdo, S.E.; Lafont, A.; Ding, W.; Karmakar, A.; Nima, Z.A.; Watanabe, F.; Casciano, D.; Morris, S.M.; et al. p53-competent cells and p53-deficient cells display different susceptibility to oxygen functionalized graphene cytotoxicity and genotoxicity: p53 function in oxygen functionalized graphene toxicity. *J. Appl. Toxicol.* **2017**, *37*, 1333–1345. [CrossRef] [PubMed]
65. Wang, Y.; Xu, J.; Xu, L.; Tan, X.; Feng, L.; Luo, Y.; Liu, J.; Liu, Z.; Peng, R. Functionalized graphene oxide triggers cell cycle checkpoint control through both the ATM and the ATR signaling pathways. *Carbon* **2018**, *129*, 495–503. [CrossRef]
66. Helton, E.S.; Chen, X. p53 modulation of the DNA damage response. *J. Cell. Biochem.* **2007**, *100*, 883–896. [CrossRef] [PubMed]
67. Kastenhuber, E.R.; Lowe, S.W. Putting p53 in Context. *Cell* **2017**, *170*, 1062–1078. [CrossRef] [PubMed]
68. Zhu, L.; Chang, D.W.; Dai, L.; Hong, Y. DNA Damage Induced by Multiwalled Carbon Nanotubes in Mouse Embryonic Stem Cells. *Nano Lett.* **2007**, *7*, 3592–3597. [CrossRef]
69. Xing, Y.; Xiong, W.; Zhu, L.; Ōsawa, E.; Hussin, S.; Dai, L. DNA Damage in Embryonic Stem Cells Caused by Nanodiamonds. *ACS Nano* **2011**, *5*, 2376–2384. [CrossRef] [PubMed]
70. Yuan, J.; Gao, H.; Sui, J.; Duan, H.; Chen, W.N.; Ching, C.B. Cytotoxicity Evaluation of Oxidized Single-Walled Carbon Nanotubes and Graphene Oxide on Human Hepatoma HepG2 cells: An iTRAQ-Coupled 2D LC-MS/MS Proteome Analysis. *Toxicol. Sci.* **2012**, *126*, 149–161. [CrossRef]
71. Araldi, R.P.; de Melo, T.C.; Mendes, T.B.; de Sá Júnior, P.L.; Nozima, B.H.N.; Ito, E.T.; de Carvalho, R.F.; de Souza, E.B.; de Cassia Stocco, R. Using the comet and micronucleus assays for genotoxicity studies: A review. *Biomed. Pharmacother.* **2015**, *72*, 74–82. [CrossRef]
72. Fenech, M.; Kirsch-Volders, M.; Natarajan, A.T.; Surralles, J.; Crott, J.W.; Parry, J.; Norppa, H.; Eastmond, D.A.; Tucker, J.D.; Thomas, P. Molecular mechanisms of micronucleus, nucleoplasmic bridge and nuclear bud formation in mammalian and human cells. *Mutagenesis* **2011**, *26*, 125–132. [CrossRef]
73. Akhavan, O.; Ghaderi, E.; Hashemi, E.; Akbari, E. Dose-dependent effects of nanoscale graphene oxide on reproduction capability of mammals. *Carbon* **2015**, *95*, 309–317. [CrossRef]
74. Durán, M.; Durán, N.; Fávaro, W.J. In vivo nanotoxicological profile of graphene oxide. *J. Phys. Conf. Ser.* **2017**, *838*, 012026. [CrossRef]
75. Lu, C.-J.; Jiang, X.-F.; Junaid, M.; Ma, Y.-B.; Jia, P.-P.; Wang, H.-B.; Pei, D.-S. Graphene oxide nanosheets induce DNA damage and activate the base excision repair (BER) signaling pathway both in vitro and in vivo. *Chemosphere* **2017**, *184*, 795–805. [CrossRef]
76. Maluf, S.W. Monitoring DNA damage following radiation exposure using cytokinesis–block micronucleus method and alkaline single-cell gel electrophoresis. *Clin. Chim. Acta* **2004**, *347*, 15–24. [CrossRef]
77. Ivask, A.; Voelcker, N.H.; Seabrook, S.A.; Hor, M.; Kirby, J.K.; Fenech, M.; Davis, T.P.; Ke, P.C. DNA Melting and Genotoxicity Induced by Silver Nanoparticles and Graphene. *Chem. Res. Toxicol.* **2015**, *28*, 1023–1035. [CrossRef]
78. Zhao, X. Self-Assembly of DNA Segments on Graphene and Carbon Nanotube Arrays in Aqueous Solution: A Molecular Simulation Study. *J. Phys. Chem. C* **2011**, *115*, 6181–6189. [CrossRef]
79. Petersen, E.J.; Nelson, B.C. Mechanisms and measurements of nanomaterial-induced oxidative damage to DNA. *Anal. Bioanal. Chem.* **2010**, *398*, 613–650. [CrossRef]
80. Ribas, V.; García-Ruiz, C.; Fernández-Checa, J.C. Glutathione and mitochondria. *Front. Pharmacol.* **2014**, *5*, 151. [CrossRef]
81. Ighodaro, O.M.; Akinloye, O.A. First line defence antioxidants-superoxide dismutase (SOD), catalase (CAT) and glutathione peroxidase (GPX): Their fundamental role in the entire antioxidant defence grid. *Alex. J. Med.* **2017**, *54*, 4. [CrossRef]
82. Chen, M.; Yin, J.; Liang, Y.; Yuan, S.; Wang, F.; Song, M.; Wang, H. Oxidative stress and immunotoxicity induced by graphene oxide in zebrafish. *Aquat. Toxicol.* **2016**, *174*, 54–60. [CrossRef]

83. Zhang, W.; Wang, C.; Li, Z.; Lu, Z.; Li, Y.; Yin, J.-J.; Zhou, Y.-T.; Gao, X.; Fang, Y.; Nie, G.; et al. Unraveling Stress-Induced Toxicity Properties of Graphene Oxide and the Underlying Mechanism. *Adv. Mater.* **2012**, *24*, 5391–5397. [CrossRef]
84. Kryuchkova, M.; Danilushkina, A.; Lvov, Y.; Fakhrullin, R. Evaluation of toxicity of nanoclays and graphene oxide in vivo: A Paramecium caudatum study. *Environ. Sci. Nano* **2016**, *3*, 442–452. [CrossRef]
85. Manke, A.; Wang, L.; Rojanasakul, Y. Mechanisms of Nanoparticle-Induced Oxidative Stress and Toxicity. *BioMed Res. Int.* **2013**, *2013*, 1–15. [CrossRef]
86. Zhang, X.; Yin, J.; Peng, C.; Hu, W.; Zhu, Z.; Li, W.; Fan, C.; Huang, Q. Distribution and biocompatibility studies of graphene oxide in mice after intravenous administration. *Carbon* **2011**, *49*, 986–995. [CrossRef]
87. Sydlik, S.A.; Jhunjhunwala, S.; Webber, M.J.; Anderson, D.G.; Langer, R. In Vivo Compatibility of Graphene Oxide with Differing Oxidation States. *ACS Nano* **2015**, *9*, 3866–3874. [CrossRef]
88. Ma, J.; Liu, R.; Wang, X.; Liu, Q.; Chen, Y.; Valle, R.P.; Zuo, Y.Y.; Xia, T.; Liu, S. Crucial Role of Lateral Size for Graphene Oxide in Activating Macrophages and Stimulating Pro-inflammatory Responses in Cells and Animals. *ACS Nano* **2015**, *9*, 10498–10515. [CrossRef]
89. Xu, M.; Zhu, J.; Wang, F.; Xiong, Y.; Wu, Y.; Wang, Q.; Weng, J.; Zhang, Z.; Chen, W.; Liu, S. Improved In Vitro and In Vivo Biocompatibility of Graphene Oxide through Surface Modification: Poly(Acrylic Acid)-Functionalization is Superior to PEGylation. *ACS Nano* **2016**, *10*, 3267–3281. [CrossRef]
90. Bengtson, S.; Kling, K.; Madsen, A.M.; Noergaard, A.W.; Jacobsen, N.R.; Clausen, P.A.; Alonso, B.; Pesquera, A.; Zurutuza, A.; Ramos, R.; et al. No cytotoxicity or genotoxicity of graphene and graphene oxide in murine lung epithelial FE1 cells in vitro: Graphene and Graphene Oxide in Vitro. *Environ. Mol. Mutagen.* **2016**, *57*, 469–482. [CrossRef]
91. Magdolenova, Z.; Collins, A.; Kumar, A.; Dhawan, A.; Stone, V.; Dusinska, M. Mechanisms of genotoxicity. A review of in vitro and in vivo studies with engineered nanoparticles. *Nanotoxicology* **2014**, *8*, 233–278. [CrossRef]
92. De Marzi, L.; Ottaviano, L.; Perrozzi, F.; Nardone, M.; Santucci, S.; de Lapuente, J.; Borras, M.; Treossi, E.; Palermo, V.; Poma, A. Flake size-dependent cyto and genotoxic evaluation of graphene oxide on in vitro A549, CaCo2 and Vero cell lines. *J. Biol. Regul. Homeost Agents* **2014**, *28*, 281–289.
93. Ursini, C.L.; Cavallo, D.; Fresegna, A.M.; Ciervo, A.; Maiello, R.; Buresti, G.; Casciardi, S.; Tombolini, F.; Bellucci, S.; Iavicoli, S. Comparative cyto-genotoxicity assessment of functionalized and pristine multiwalled carbon nanotubes on human lung epithelial cells. *Toxicol. In Vitro* **2012**, *26*, 831–840. [CrossRef]
94. Guo, Z.; Xie, C.; Zhang, P.; Zhang, J.; Wang, G.; He, X.; Ma, Y.; Zhao, B.; Zhang, Z. Toxicity and transformation of graphene oxide and reduced graphene oxide in bacteria biofilm. *Sci. Total Environ.* **2017**, *580*, 1300–1308. [CrossRef]
95. Liu, X.T.; MU, X.Y.; WU, X.L.; Meng, L.X.; Guan, W.B.; Qiang, Y.; Hua, S.U.N.; Wang, C.J.; LI, X.F. Toxicity of multi-walled carbon nanotubes, graphene oxide, and reduced graphene oxide to zebrafish embryos. *Biomed. Environ. Sci.* **2014**, *27*, 676–683.
96. Zhang, Q.; Liu, X.; Meng, H.; Liu, S.; Zhang, C. Reduction pathway-dependent cytotoxicity of reduced graphene oxide. *Environ. Sci. Nano* **2018**, *5*, 1361–1371. [CrossRef]
97. Compton, O.C.; Nguyen, S.T. Graphene oxide, highly reduced graphene oxide, and graphene: Versatile building blocks for carbon-based materials. *Small* **2010**, *6*, 711–723. [CrossRef]
98. Xue, W.; Warshawsky, D. Metabolic activation of polycyclic and heterocyclic aromatic hydrocarbons and DNA damage: A review. *Toxicol. Appl. Pharmacol.* **2005**, *206*, 73–93. [CrossRef] [PubMed]
99. Cobaleda-Siles, M.; Guillamon, A.P.; Delpivo, C.; Vázquez-Campos, S.; Puntes, V.F. Safer by design strategies. *J. Phys. Conf. Ser.* **2017**, *838*, 012016. [CrossRef]

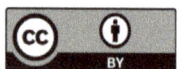

© 2019 by the authors. Licensee MDPI, Basel, Switzerland. This article is an open access article distributed under the terms and conditions of the Creative Commons Attribution (CC BY) license (http://creativecommons.org/licenses/by/4.0/).

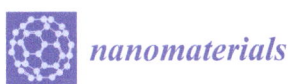

Article

ToxTracker Reporter Cell Lines as a Tool for Mechanism-Based (Geno)Toxicity Screening of Nanoparticles—Metals, Oxides and Quantum Dots

Sarah McCarrick [1], Francesca Cappellini [1], Amanda Kessler [2], Nynke Moelijker [3], Remco Derr [3], Jonas Hedberg [2], Susanna Wold [2], Eva Blomberg [2,4], Inger Odnevall Wallinder [2], Giel Hendriks [3] and Hanna L. Karlsson [1,*]

1. Institute of Environmental Medicine, Karolinska Institutet, 171 77 Stockholm, Sweden
2. KTH Royal Institute of Technology, Division of Surface and Corrosion Science, Department of Chemistry, 100 44 Stockholm, Sweden
3. Toxys, 2333 CG Leiden, The Netherlands
4. Division Bioscience and Materials, RISE Research Institutes of Sweden, 111 21 Stockholm, Sweden
* Correspondence: hanna.l.karlsson@ki.se

Received: 28 November 2019; Accepted: 25 December 2019; Published: 6 January 2020

Abstract: The increased use of nanoparticles (NPs) requires efficient testing of their potential toxic effects. A promising approach is to use reporter cell lines to quickly assess the activation of cellular stress response pathways. This study aimed to use the ToxTracker reporter cell lines to investigate (geno)toxicity of various metal- or metal oxide NPs and draw general conclusions on NP-induced effects, in combination with our previous findings. The NPs tested in this study ($n = 18$) also included quantum dots (QDs) in different sizes. The results showed a large variation in cytotoxicity of the NPs tested. Furthermore, whereas many induced oxidative stress only few activated reporters related to DNA damage. NPs of manganese (Mn and Mn_3O_4) induced the most remarkable ToxTracker response with activation of reporters for oxidative stress, DNA damage, protein unfolding and p53-related stress. The QDs (CdTe) were highly toxic showing clearly size-dependent effects and calculations suggest surface area as the most relevant dose metric. Of all NPs investigated in this and previous studies the following induce the DNA damage reporter; CuO, Co, CoO, CdTe QDs, Mn, Mn_3O_4, V_2O_5, and welding NPs. We suggest that these NPs are of particular concern when considering genotoxicity induced by metal- and metal oxide NPs.

Keywords: nanotoxicology; genotoxicity; DNA damage; metal oxides; high throughput screening

1. Introduction

The use of nanoparticles (NPs) is increasing worldwide in various applications, resulting in a need to more rapidly evaluate their potential toxicity. The genotoxic potential is a crucial part in the risk and safety evaluation of NPs and currently this is most often evaluated by a battery of established methods including the comet assay and the micronucleus assay [1–3]. However, these methods are relatively time-consuming and there is consequently a great demand for efficient and more high throughput assays for screening of the genotoxicity of NPs [4]. As reviewed by Nelson et al. [5], some of the established genotoxicity assays have been modified and optimized to give increased sample capacity and throughput such as flow cytometry based micronucleus assay as well as comet on a chip.

An alternative approach with great potential is the use of reporter cell lines, which are designed to fluorescence upon activation of specific signaling pathways. In the field of genotoxicity there are some validated reporter assays available such as the GreenScreen HC assay [6] and the luminescence-based reporter assay Bluescreen HC [7]. Both assays target $GADD45\alpha$, which is induced upon various cellular stresses including genotoxic stress. A combination of several reporter cell lines is required to provide a more mechanistic evaluation of the genotoxic potential. The ToxTracker reporter assay consists of a panel of six mouse embryonic stem (mES) cell lines that are modified with different green fluorescent protein (GFP) tagged reporters for various cellular signaling pathways involved in carcinogenesis [8,9]. By using this set of reporter cell lines, it is possible to monitor the activation of signaling pathways associated with DNA damage, oxidative stress, general p53-dependent cellular stress as well as protein unfolding response (see Table 1). We have previously shown the ToxTracker assay to be a valid reporter assay for detecting (geno)toxic properties of NPs with results correlating to those of more conventional assays [10]. Furthermore, we have shown the applicability of these reporters for various NPs including nickel-based [11], cobalt-based [12], and welding fume NPs [13].

Table 1. ToxTracker GFP-reporters.

Biological Damage	Cellular Pathway	Biomarker Gene
Oxidative stress	NRF2 antioxidant response	Srxn1
	NRF2 independent	Blvrb
DNA damage	NF-kB signaling	Rtkn
	ATR/Chk1 DNA damage signaling	Bscl2
Protein damage	Unfolded protein response	Ddit3
Cellular stress	P53 signaling	Btg2

In the present study we focus on a variety of metal-containing NPs including quantum dots (QDs). Metal based NPs are industrially relevant nanomaterials being widely used in consumer products such as cosmetics, food products, batteries as well as in medicinal applications [14,15]. Metal oxide NPs often have semi-conductive and catalytical properties and are therefore appealing from a technical point of view and often produced in large scale at industrial settings. Therefore, the potential occupational and non-occupational exposure to metal NPs is increasing.

Quantum dots (QDs) are fluorescent semiconducting nanocrystals that, due to their small size, have distinctive optical and electronic properties resulting in bright and highly stable fluorescence. Their small sizes in combination with large specific surface areas make QDs able to target ligands for site-directed activity [16,17]. Absorption and emission of QDs are dependent on properties such as composition, crystal structure and size, which result in unique physicochemical properties for each individual type of QDs [18]. QDs have for this reason been proposed to not be considered as a uniform group of nanomaterials [16]. Cadmium-containing QDs, including cadmium telluride (CdTe) and cadmium selenide, are among the most commercially available types and considered particularly attractive for optical, bioanalytical and bio imaging applications where CdTe utilizes the infrared regions [17–19]. CdTe QDs have been shown to induce various toxic effects in vitro including cytotoxicity and generation of reactive oxygen species (ROS) [20,21].

Although a large number of studies have investigated the in vitro genotoxicity of e.g., various metal oxides, as reviewed in Golbamaki et al. [22] and Magdolenova et al. [3], the underlying mechanisms are still not clear. Furthermore, few studies have focused on comparing metal NPs and corresponding oxides as well as the importance of size for their genotoxic potency. The aim of this study was to use the ToxTracker reporter cell lines to investigate (geno)toxicity of various metal- or metal oxide NPs as well as QDs of different size. A further aim was to summarize and draw general conclusions on toxicity of NPs as well as underlying pathways using our present and previous work with the ToxTracker reporter cell lines.

2. Materials and Methods

2.1. Nanoparticles

The CdTe QDs (1.5–8.6 nm) were purchased from PlasmaChem GmbH (Berlin, Germany). Mn (20–40 nm), Mn_3O_4 (<100 nm), Cr (35–45 nm), Cr_2O_3 (10–30 nm), Sn (10–20 nm) and SnO_2 (20–40 nm) NPs were all obtained from American Elements (Los Angeles, CA, USA). V (80–100 nm) and V_2O_5 (80 nm) NPs were purchased from Nanoshel (Wilmington, DE, USA), Sb NPs (N/A) from Campine NV (Beerse, Belgium) and Sb_2O_3 NPs (150 nm) from Sigma Aldrich (Ramstadt, Germany). Au, Ag and Pt NPs (5 nm) were obtained from nanoComposix (San Diego, CA, USA) in the form of stock dispersions (1 mg/mL) in aqueous 2 mM citrate (Ag and Pt) and in ultrapure water (milli-Q) (Au).

For the NPs in dry powder form, NP suspensions of 1 mg/mL in cell medium were sonicated for 2×10 min in an ultrasonic water bath alternated by 10 s vortexing. The particle suspensions were freshly prepared for every experiment and further diluted to desired concentrations in cell media immediately before the cell exposure.

2.2. Particle Morphology

Transmission electron microscopy (TEM) was employed to study the primary size and shape of the NPs received as powders. Three drops of a particle suspension of 1 mg/mL ethanol were applied to 200 mesh TEM copper grids with formvar/carbon support films (Ted Pella, Inc., Redding, CA, USA). The suspension was sonicated for 15 min and vortexed before applied onto the grid. Drying was made at ambient laboratory conditions. Imaging was conducted using a HT7700 TEM (Hitachi, Tokyo, Japan) instrument operating at 100 kV.

TEM images of the Au, Ag and Pt NPs are reported elsewhere [23]. No TEM imaging was made on the CdTe QDs.

2.3. Characterization of Particle Agglomeration

PCCS (Photon cross correlation spectroscopy) was used to study changes in size distribution of the particles, agglomeration and concentration (possible reduction due to sedimentation) over time in the cell medium. Particle suspensions of 1 mg/mL medium were prepared by ultrasonication for 2×10 min alternated by 10 s vortexing at 37 °C. The samples were prepared in disposable single sealed cuvettes, LOTG17501P (Eppendorf AG, Hamburg, Germany) at a concentration of 0.1 mg/mL. The samples were stored at 37 °C and measured in triplicates after 0, 2 and 24 h using the NANOPHOX 90–250 V (Sympatec GmbH, Claustahl-Zellerfeld, Germany) instrument. Windox 5, the PCCS software (version 10, SympatecGmbH, Claustahl-Zellerfeld, Germany), was used to fit the size distribution data for each measurement. Measurements of standard latex particles (100 nm) and non-particle containing media were performed to ensure high quality data. The samples were measured after 24 h. Measurements were performed on the metal and metal oxide NPs as well as the QDs.

Particle size measurements of the Au, Ag and Pt NPs were determined using NTA (Nanoparticle Tracking Analysis) as described in Lebedova et al. [23].

2.4. Cell Culture and Reagents

mES cells were cultured as previously described [9]. In short, the cells were maintained in the presence of irradiated mouse embryonic fibroblasts as feeder cells in knockout DMEM supplemented with 10% FBS, 2 mM GlutaMAX, 1 mM sodium pyruvate, 100 mM b-mercaptoethanol and leukemia inhibitory factor (LIF). Prior to exposure, cells were seeded at a density of 4×10^4 cells per well on gelatin-coated 96-well plates in complete mES cell medium in the absence of feeder cells for 24 h.

2.5. ToxTracker Assay (mES Cells)

An initial screening of the cytotoxicity of the NPs was performed in non-modified mES cells at increasing concentrations of the NPs (0–100 µg/mL) at 24 h. Based on this, the doses for GFP reporter analysis were determined so that the highest dose caused 50–75% cytotoxicity. Four additional doses in two-fold dilution steps from the highest dose were then selected. In cases of no observed cytotoxicity, the NPs were tested up to 100 µg/mL. Thus, some of the NPs were not tested up to cytotoxic concentrations. Following exposure, cells were washed and trypsinized. Induction of GFP was determined using a Guava easyCyte 8HT flow cytometer (Millipore, Burlington, MA, USA) in intact single cells as described previously [9]. Mean GFP fluorescence was used to calculate GFP reporter induction compared to vehicle control exposure. Cytotoxicity was assessed by cell count after 24 h exposure using flow cytometry and expressed as percent of intact cells compared to vehicle control exposure. Possible autofluorescence was recorded for the NPs tested, and in the case of CdTe QDs subtracted for in the GFP-reporter values. Presented results are based on at least three independent experiments and error bars represent standard error of the mean. The GFP response is considered positive if exceeding a 2-fold increase, which is based on previous validations [8,9]. All the GFP-reporters were tested with the positive controls cisplatin (2.5–10 µM), diethyl maleate (62.5–250 µM) and tunicamycin (1–4 µM). Similar as to what was reported by Hendriks et al. [8], cisplatin resulted in an induction of the reporters Bscl2, Rtkn, Btg2, Srxn1 and Blvrb, diethyl maleate induced both of the oxidative stress reporters Srxn1 and Blvrb while tunicamycin induced solely the Ddit3 GFP-reporter.

2.6. Dose Metric Modelling Analysis

Firstly, the number of particles per unit of volume was calculated for each concentration used, based on information from the supplier. The dose-response data for all reporter cells was analyzed with the PROAST software (version 38.9, National Institute for Public Health and the Environment (RIVM), Bilthoven, the Netherlands) to find the number of QDs needed to induce a 20% decrease in viability. The relationship among these equi-response doses was used to identify the appropriate dose metric as described in Delmaar et al. [24]. Briefly, the equi-response doses were plotted as a point in the plane spanned by the 10log of the diameter and the 10log of the number of particles. If the administered surface area or volume or number of particles is the appropriate metric, then the resulting curve should be a straight line, mathematically described as:

$$\log(N) = m \times \log(d) + q \tag{1}$$

where N is the number of particles and d is the diameter of the NPs. The slope of this curve describes the correct metric: surface area has a slope equal to −2, volume equal to −3 and number of particles equal to 0. If the slope is equal to none of these numbers, then the dose metric is:

$$10^q = N \times d^{-m} \tag{2}$$

2.7. Statistical Analysis

Results are expressed as mean values of at least three independent experiments ($n = 3$) ± standard error of the mean (SEM), except for PCCS data expressed as mean values ± standard deviation. LD50 (lethal dose in 50%) values were estimated by dose-response modeling assuming Hills slope (slope = 1). LD50 values as well as linear regression for dosimetry were calculated using GraphPad Prism 5.02 statistical software (GraphPad Inc., La Jolla, CA, USA).

3. Results

3.1. Particle Characterization

TEM observations revealed a majority of the metal and metal oxide particles to be approximately spherical with primary sizes ranging from 10 to 250 nm, Figure 1 and Table 2. Main outliers in primary size were observed for NPs of Mn_3O_4, V, V_2O_5, Sb and SnO_2. The Mn_3O_4 NPs comprised smaller cubic particles (similar to observations for the other NPs) and long rods with a length scale up to 8 µm. Rods (nm-sized) were the predominating shape for the V NPs. The V_2O_5 and the Sb NPs had irregular shapes and primary particle sizes up to 1.2 µm. The SnO_2 NPs formed aggregates of individual particles sized 2–3 nm. Compositional information of the outermost surface (oxide particles) and surface oxide (metal particles) of the NPs is given in Table 2 based on XRD, Raman, and XPS findings based on [25–34] (see supporting information, Figures S1–S3). The main surface oxides observed for the metallic NPs were in general similar to observations for the corresponding bulk metal oxide with the exception for the Mn NPs (Table 2).

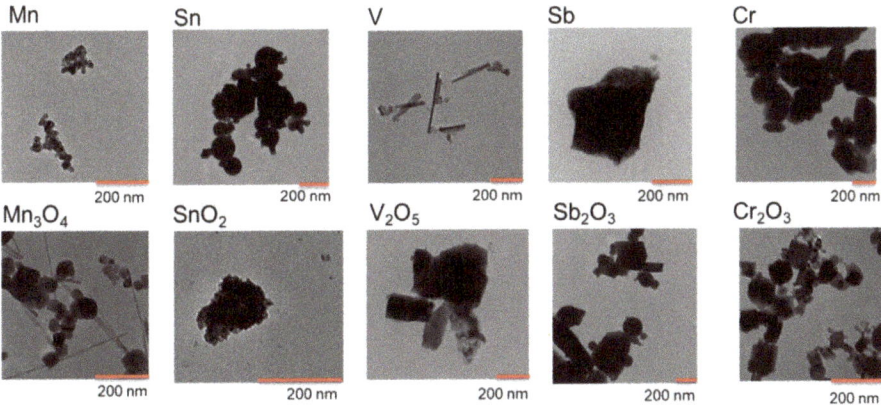

Figure 1. TEM images of the metal and metal oxide NPs.

Table 2. Summary of primary particle size, approximated particle morphology and main surface oxide composition of the metal and metal oxide NPs based on XRD, Raman and XPS measurements. See Figures S1–S3 and supporting information for surface analytical findings supporting the compositional analysis of the outermost surface oxide.

Particle	Primary Size (TEM)/nm	Oxide Composition
Ag	Spherical, 5.2 ± 1.1 [a]	N/A
Au	Spherical, 5.2 ± 0.9 [a]	N/A
CdTe QDs	Spherical, 1.6, 2.6, 4.5, 6.5, 8.6 [b]	N/A
Cr	Cubic and spherical, 10–115	Cr */Cr_2O_3
Cr_2O_3	Oval, 90–460	Cr_2O_3
Mn	Spherical, 15–50	Mn */MnO/MnO_2/Mn_2O_3/Mn_3O_4
Mn_3O_4	Cubic 20–180, rods 8000 × 400	Mn_3O_4/MnO
Pt	Spherical, 4.8 ± 0.8 [a]	N/A
Sb	Irregular, 90–1200	Sb */Sb_2O_3
Sb_2O_3	Spherical, 70–250	Sb_2O_3
Sn	Spherical, 20–250	Sn */SnO/SnO_2
SnO_2	Spherical, 2–3 (as aggregates)	SnO_2
V	Rods 20 × 20 to 400 × 40	V_2O_5/VO_2
V_2O_5	Irregular 40–450	V_2O_5/VO_2

* metallic signal implies a thin surface oxide, <5–10 nm. N/A not analyzed. [a] from Lebedova et al. [23], [b] based on supplier information.

The primary size of Au, Ag and Pt NPs were previously confirmed to be 5 nm [23]. Primary particle sizes of the CdTe QDs are reported in Table 2 based on supplier information. No compositional analyses were performed.

Changes in scattered light intensities of the NPs over time in the ToxTracker cell medium is presented in Figure 2 together with parallel measurements for the blank solution (cell medium without NPs). Agglomeration of cell medium constituents (no NPs) with time was evident (increased light intensities with time). Observations with similar count rates between blank solutions (no NPs) and the NP-containing solutions indicate NP sedimentation. If no changes in intensities are observed with time and sedimentation of the NPs has taken place, measured count rates relate to agglomerated medium constituents. Low count rates observed already at time 0 h imply rapid sedimentation taking place before any measurements have been made (<5 min) (i.e., during dispersion preparation as indicated by low particle concentration in solution).

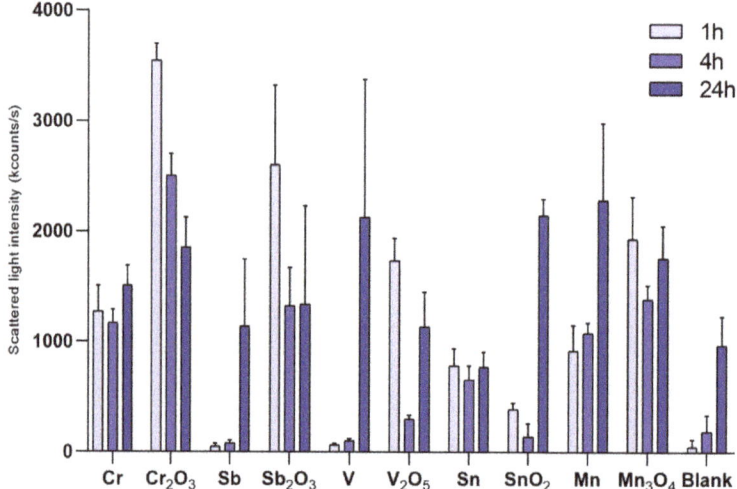

Figure 2. Changes in scattered light intensities for the different metal and metal oxide NPs after 0, 2, and 24 h of exposure in cell medium recorded by means of PCCS. Particle loading: 100 µg/mL; Blank cell medium only without any NPs. The error bars represent the standard deviation based on three independent samples.

Most NPs showed evident signs of sedimentation over time (most notable after 24 h), except for the Mn NPs and to some extent the SnO_2 NPs (reduced intensities or similar intensities with time compared to findings for the blank solution). The Mn NPs seemed to have a higher ability to remain dispersed in solution over time (increased intensities with prolonged exposure). The SnO_2 NPs showed signs of sedimentation already at time 0 h and after 2 h (reduced light intensity), but increased intensities after 24 h. This effect could possibly be related to agglomeration of cell medium constituents. Almost complete sedimentation was observed for Sb and V NPs immediately upon sample preparation (similar intensities as the blank at time 0 h).

As a result of extensive particle sedimentation due to formation of large agglomerates, any estimate of particle size distributions in solution become very approximate and hence not reported.

Sizes of the QDs were not possible to discern by means of PCCS in the cell media due to their small size and similar size range as the cell media components only. Time dependent measurements implied no evident agglomeration of the QDs up to 24 h.

3.2. Nontoxic NPs—Several NPs Cause No Toxicity or ToxTracker Activation

Several of the metal-containing NPs investigated did not cause any major changes in cell viability at doses up to 80–100 μg/mL at 24 h exposure, including Ag, Au, Cr, Cr_2O_3, Pt, (data not shown) SnO_2 and V (Figure 3). Furthermore, these NPs did not cause activation of any of the six GFP-markers, except for Ag NPs which resulted in a minor increase in one of the oxidative stress markers at the highest dose level (Supplement Table S1 and Figure 4). Furthermore, Cr_2O_3 caused a weak activation of one of the oxidative stress reporters (Srxn-1) and one of the DNA damage reporters (Rtkn). The absence of activation of any of the GFP-reporters has previously been observed in response to other NPs including TiO_2, Fe_3O_4 and Co_3O_4 [10,12].

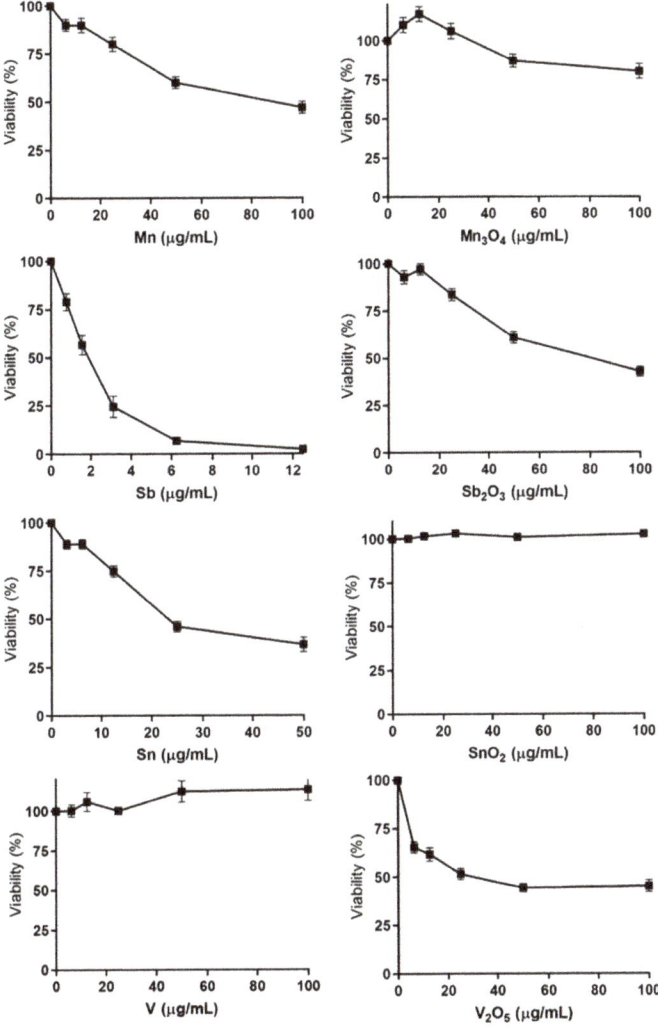

Figure 3. Cytotoxicity in mES cells following 24 h exposure to metal and metal oxide NPs. Cytotoxicity was determined by measuring the fraction of intact cells following exposure using flow cytometry. The results are presented as mean ± standard error of the mean of three or four independent experiments (*n* = 3–4).

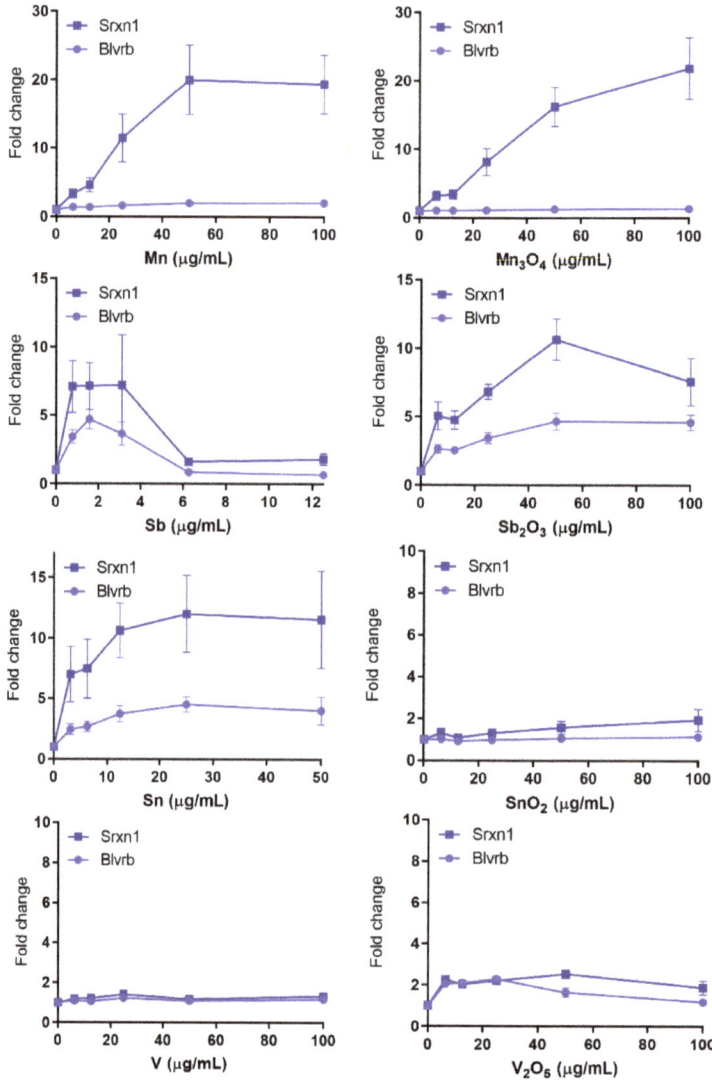

Figure 4. Oxidative stress GFP-reporter activation in response to metal and metal oxide NPs. ToxTracker reporter activation in live cells was measured as GFP-fluorescence using flow cytometry. The Srxn1-GFP reporter is Nrf2-associated, while the Blvrb is Nrf2-independent. The results are presented as mean ± standard error of the mean of three or four independent experiments (n = 3–4).

3.3. Cytotoxicity—Several NPs and QDs Affect Cell Viability

In contrast to the non-cytotoxic NPs, several other NPs caused effects on viability at various doses (Figure 3 and Figure S4). The most toxic NPs were the Sb NPs with a LD50 already at 1.53 µg/mL (Figure 3). This was comparable to the cytotoxic effect induced by the smallest (1.4 nm) QDs (LD50 1.1 µg Cd/mL) (Supplementary Figure S4). The Sb NPs were more cytotoxic compared to the Sb_2O_3 NPs (LD50 90 µg/mL). Similarly, the Mn (LD50 86 µg/mL) and the Sn NPs (LD50 29 µg/mL) were more toxic compared to their corresponding oxides (Mn_3O_4 and SnO_2; LD50 > 100 µg/mL). In contrast, the V_2O_5 NPs (LD50 31 µg/mL) were more cytotoxic than the metal V NPs (LD50 > 100 µg/mL).

The results on cytotoxicity showed large variances between the differently sized CdTe QDs, demonstrating smaller size of QDs to be toxic at considerably lower doses compared to the larger sized particles (Supplementary Figure S4). The LD50 values for QDs of primary sizes of 1.5, 2.6, 4.5, 6.5 and 8.6 nm were approximately 1, 2, 4, 8.7 and 15.8 μg Cd/mL, respectively. A soluble salt of Cd (CdCl2) was found to be most toxic, with an LD50 of 0.69 μg Cd/mL.

3.4. Oxidative Stress—Many NPs and All QDs Induce Reporters Related to Oxidative Stress

The most frequently activated reporter was the Srxn1-GFP reporter. The Srxn1 protein is involved in the reduction of hyperoxidized peroxiredoxin and regulated by the nuclear factor (erythroid derived 2)- like 2 (NRF2) transcription factor, which plays a key role in the oxidative stress response and regulation of various antioxidant gene networks [8,9]. Of the NPs tested, Mn and Mn_3O_4 NPs caused by far the largest activation of the Srxn1-GFP reporter resulting in around 20-fold maximum increase compared with control (Figure 4). The Sn, Sb_2O_3 and Sb NPs were also active, inducing approximately a 7–10 fold increase (Figure 4), which is comparable to previous observations for Ni and NiO NPs [11], and for Co and CoO NPs [12]. Some induction (2.5 and 2.7-fold) was also observed for the V_2O_5 and Ag NPs, respectively (Figure 4 and Supplementary Table S1).

A strong induction of the oxidative stress related Srxn1-GFP reporter was observed for all QDs (Figure 5). The induction started at similarly low doses for the 3 smallest sizes and at somewhat higher doses for slightly larger particles sized 6.5 and 8.6 nm. CdTe QDs of 1.5 and 2.6 nm seemed to be most potent reaching up to a 5-fold increase compared to control. An increase was also observed for Srxn1 in response to the soluble $CdCl_2$ salt starting at a lower dose of Cd compared to the QDs and reaching a maximum of 9-fold increase.

Fewer NPs activated the second oxidative stress marker Blvrb. This marker has been shown to play an important role in heme metabolism and has been associated with cellular antioxidant response. However it does not contain any NRF2 binding motif and thus does not overlap with the signaling pathways associated with Srxn1-GFP reporter [8]. Exposure to the Sn, Sb_2O_3, Sb and Mn NPs resulted in a maximum increase of approximately 4.5, 4.5, 3.5 and 2-fold, respectively (Figure 4). In addition, a weaker yet positive (or borderline) induction was observed for the QDs of sizes 2.6, 6.5 and 8.6 nm while the soluble $CdCl_2$ salt resulted in a 3.5-fold increase (Figure 5). None of the previously studied NPs has been found to activate this marker [11–13].

3.5. DNA Damage—Few NPs Induce Reporters Related to DNA Damage

In general, few NPs induced reporters related to DNA damage (Figure 6). The Rtkn-GFP marker is associated with the NF-Kb cytokine signaling pathway, which further has been associated with activation of the ATM DNA damage kinase [8]. ATM is rapidly activated upon induction of DNA-double strand breaks and directly phosphorylates both CHK2 checkpoint kinase and p53 tumor suppressor resulting in inhibition of cell cycle progression, activation of DNA repair or inducing apoptosis. The Mn and Mn_3O_4 NPs were found to induce Rtkn at all doses tested (6.25–100 μg/mL) with a maximum increase corresponding to 3.5 and 3.3-fold, respectively (Figure 6). A marginal increase was also observed in response to V_2O_5 NPs, although at rather cytotoxic doses (40–50%), whereas no induction was observed for the V NPs (Figure 6). In our previous studies, CuO (unpublished), Co, and CoO NPs [12] as well as welding fume NPs [13] have activated the Rtkn reporter at magnitudes ranging from 2 to 3-fold increase. A slight increase (above 1.5-fold) was also observed for Cr_2O_3 NPs, as also previously observed for Ni and NiO NPs [11].

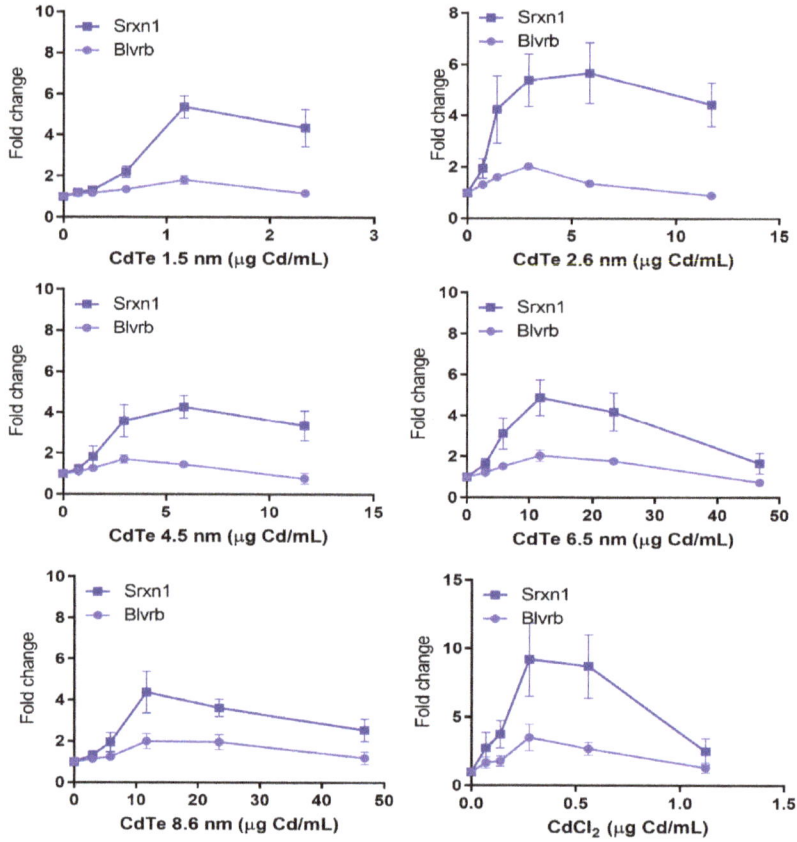

Figure 5. Oxidative stress GFP-reporter activation in response to CdTe QDs of various sizes and CdCl$_2$. ToxTracker reporter activation in live cells was measured as GFP-fluorescence using flow cytometry. The Srxn1-GFP reporter is Nrf2-associated, while the Blvrb is Nrf2-independent. The results are presented as mean ± standard error of the mean of three or four independent experiments (n = 3–4).

The second DNA damage reporter Bscl2 is associated with DNA replication and activation of the ATR (ataxia telangiectasia and Rad3-related) DNA damage signalling pathway [9]. Exposure to the Mn NPs resulted in an activation of the Bscl2 just above the 2-fold threshold (Figure 6). As of now, none of the other NPs investigated in this or previous studies, in total 32 different NPs [10–13] has clearly induced the Bscl2 reporter. This indicates that most likely none of the tested NPs, or released metal species, could bind directly to DNA and cause stalled replication forks.

None of the QDs or CdCl$_2$ had an effect on the DNA damage markers Rtkn or Bscl2 (Supplementary Table S1), except for a borderline increase of Rtkn in response to the 2.6 nm sized QDs.

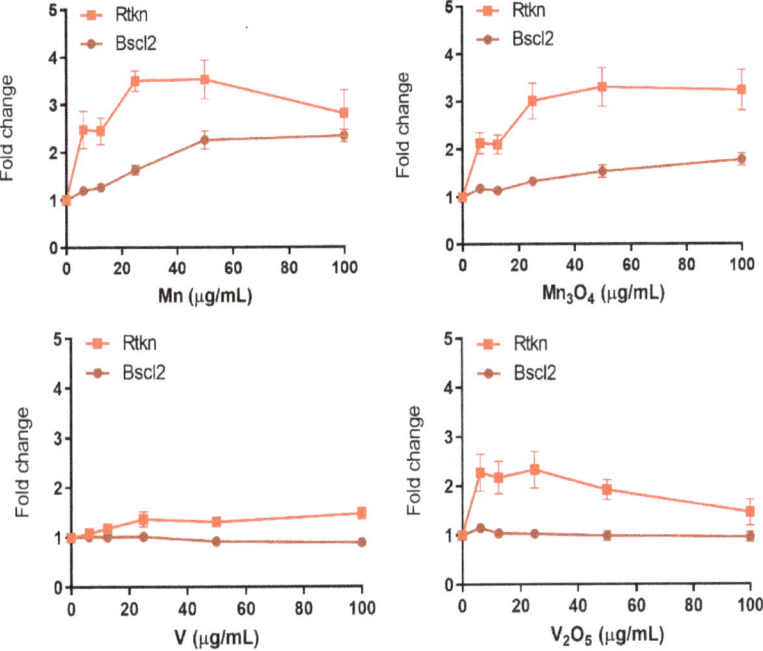

Figure 6. DNA damage GFP-reporter activation in response to metal and metal oxide NPs. ToxTracker reporter activation in live cells was measured as GFP-fluorescence using flow cytometry. The Bscl2-GFP and Rtkn-GFP report on DNA damage associated with ATR/Chk1 or NF-kB signaling, respectively. The results are presented as mean ± standard error of the mean of three or four independent experiments (n = 3–4).

3.6. Protein Unfolding and p53 Related Stress—Few NPs and QDs Induce These Reporters

The unfolded protein response (UPR) is an additional pathway associated with carcinogenicity. Ddit3 (DNA damage-inducible transcript 3) is a transcriptional factor associated with multiple functions such as cell cycle arrest, apoptosis and endoplasmic reticulum (ER) stress. It further encodes the transcription factor CHOP, which has a vital role in the response to a wide variety of cell stressors following ER stress [8]. The Mn NPs revealed the strongest induction of the Ddit3-GFP reporter, with a maximum of almost 8-fold increase (Figure 7). This is equivalent to the maximum fold induction of Ddit3-GFP historically observed for ToxTracker [8]. This high increase was followed by the Mn_3O_4 and Sb_2O_3 NPs, both inducing a 4-fold increase, as well as the Sn NPs with an increase marginally exceeding the 2-fold threshold (Figure 7). No increase was observed in response to the SnO_2 NPs (Figure 7). Exposure to Sb NPs further resulted in an increase of the Ddit3-GFP reporter, reaching a 2 to 5-fold increase, although results exceeding the 2-fold level were observed at viability levels less than 25% (Figure 7).

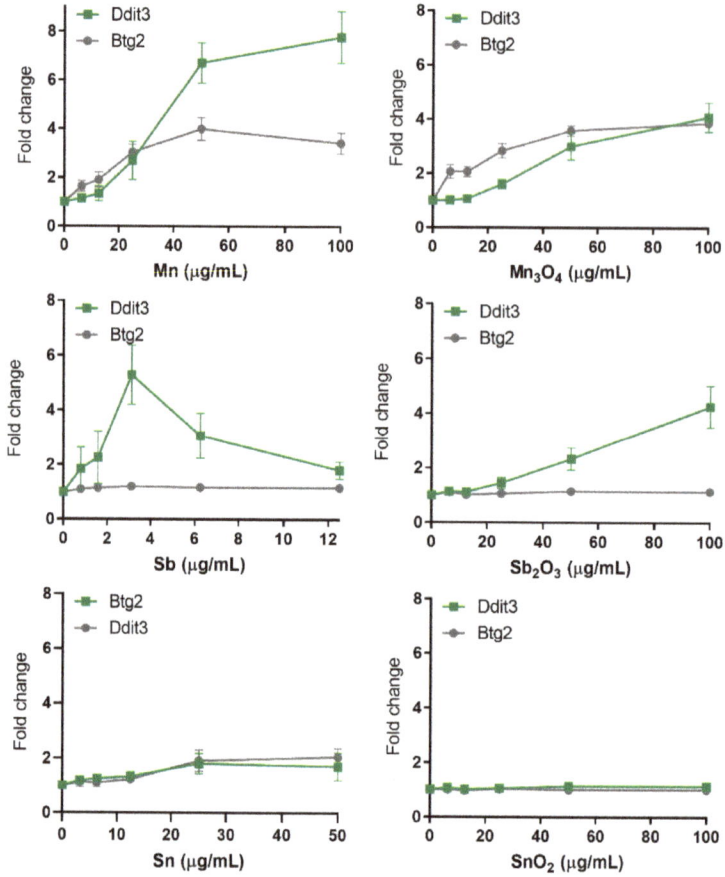

Figure 7. Protein and general cellular stress GFP-reporter activation in response to metal and metal oxide NPs. ToxTracker reporter activation in live cells was measured as GFP-fluorescence using flow cytometry. The Ddit3-GFP and Btg2-GFP indicate unfolded protein response or p53-associated cellular stress, respectively. The results are presented as mean ± standard error of the mean of three or four independent experiments (n = 3–4).

A clear induction of the protein stress UPR-marker Ddit3 was observed for all QDs, where the induction started at lower doses for the 3 smallest sized QDs compared to the larger sized ones (Figure 8). CdTe QDs sized 2.6 nm was the most potent, inducing up to 6.5-fold increase, although this was observed at a viability level less than 25%. Noteworthy is that the QDs sized 1.5 and 6.5 nm only resulted in an induction of Ddit3 at a viability level less than 25%. The soluble $CdCl_2$ salt caused an approximately 2-fold increase.

In general, very few of the investigated NPs resulted in an activation of the p53-dependent Btg2-GFP reporter. Only the Mn and Mn_3O_4 NPs induced the reporter with approximately a 4-fold increase (Figure 7). No effect was observed on the p53-responsive Btg2-GFP reporter for either QDs or soluble $CdCl_2$ (Figure 8). These findings can be compared to previous studies, where welding fume NPs were the only NPs that resulted in an activation at comparable levels, approximately 4-fold [13]. In addition, NiO NPs were seen to induce the Btg2-GFP reporter in the first study by Karlsson et al. [10]. However, the same effect was not observed in a later study by Akerlund et al. [11].

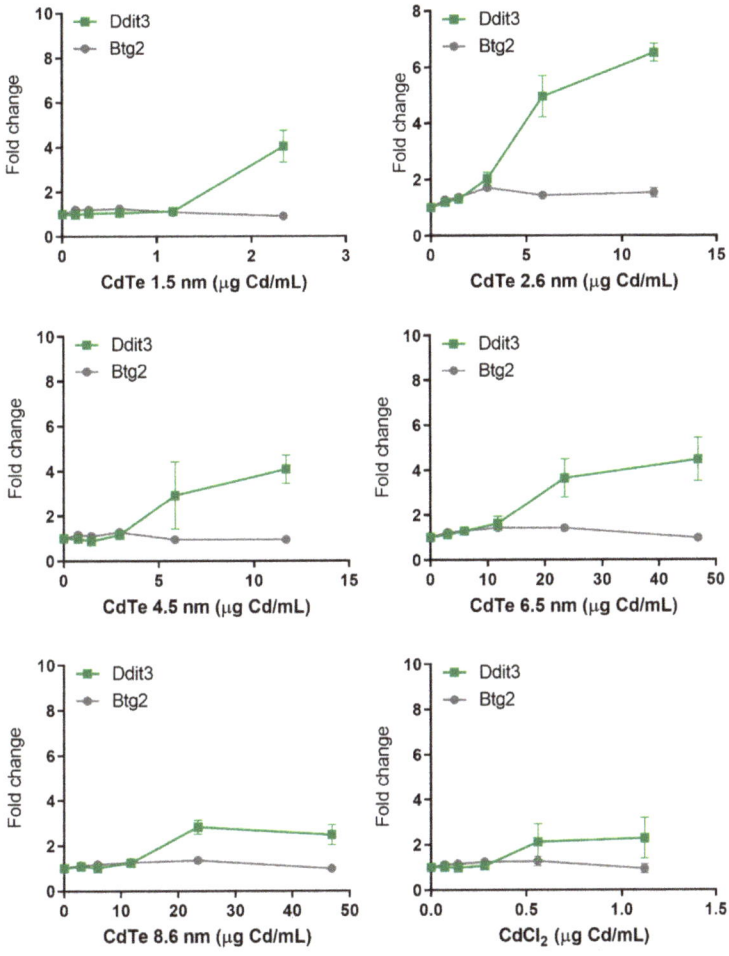

Figure 8. Protein and general cellular stress GFP-reporter activation in response to CdTe QDs of various sizes and CdCl$_2$. ToxTracker reporter activation in live cells was measured as GFP-fluorescence using flow cytometry. The Ddit3-GFP and Btg2-GFP indicate unfolded protein response or p53-associated cellular stress, respectively. The results are presented as mean ± standard error of the mean of three or four independent experiments (n = 3–4).

3.7. Dose Metric: Surface Area Appears to be the Most Suitable Dose Metric for CdTe QD Toxicity

Since the metal- and metal oxide NPs of this study were not investigated in different sizes, these results cannot be used to further investigate the appropriate dose metric. For the QDs, however, five different particle sizes ranging from 1.5 to 8.6 nm were investigated. To assess the most appropriate dose metric for cytotoxicity induced by the CdTe QDs, we used the approach suggested by Delmaar et al. [24]. Consequently, the equi-response doses representing 20% decrease in cytotoxicity were plotted as a point in the plane spanned by the 10log of the diameter and the 10log of the number of particles (Figure 9 and Supplementary Figure S5). The results showed that the slopes of the calculated curves (ranging between −1.4 to −1.7) were closest to the value of −2 for all reporter cell lines, which suggests that the surface area [24] is the most appropriate dose metric (i.e., the total surface area of NPs causes similar toxicity no matter the size of the NPs).

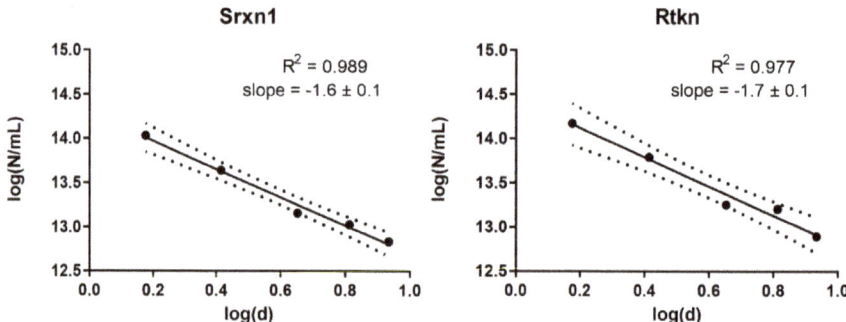

Figure 9. Equi-response curves for CdTe QDs (1.5, 2.6, 4.5, 6.5, 8.6 nm) representing a 20% reduction in cell viability compared to control for Srxn1 and Rtkn reporter. Slopes are plotted according to the model proposed by Delmaar et al. [24] where N denotes the number of particles and d the diameter of the particle.

Further, the exposure dose (µg/mL) of the QDs was converted to surface area (cm^2/mL), based on supplier's information, which was plotted against viability for all 5 sizes of QDs (Figure 10). The results showed similar and somewhat overlapping curves for the two largest sized particles (8.6 and 6.5 nm), and similarly the curves of the QDs with size of 4.5 and 2.6 nm, respectively, were comparable. The smallest QDs tested resulted in a somewhat steeper curve compared to the larger sizes. These results support the conclusion of surface area being a good dose metric for QDs, but also indicates that the smallest QDs (1.5 nm) could have additional toxic effects not entirely explained by the larger surface area.

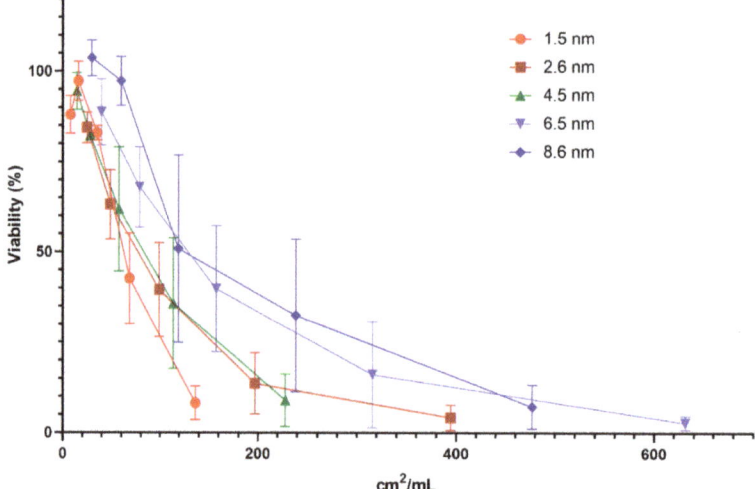

Figure 10. Viability in mES cells following 24 h exposure to CdTe QDs of varying sizes at doses expressed as surface area (cm^2/mL). Cytotoxicity was determined by measuring the fraction of intact cells following exposure using flow cytometry. The results are presented as mean ± standard error of the mean of three or four independent experiments ($n = 3$–4).

4. Discussion

The increasing manufacturing and usage of NPs require faster and more efficient testing of their potential toxic effects. Traditional in vitro genotoxicity assays are often time-consuming and have the limitations that they frequently lack the ability to provide mechanistic insight. One alternative approach, as employed in this study, is to assess the cellular stress response pathways that are activated after exposure to NPs using ToxTracker assay. The results from this study show that whereas many NPs induce oxidative stress, few of them induce DNA damage reporters. The NPs with most remarkable response in the ToxTracker assay were the Mn and Mn_3O_4 NPs causing massive oxidative stress, induction of reporters for DNA damage, protein unfolding and p53-related stress. This study also highlights the clear particle size dependent toxicity of CdTe QDs.

Our present study supports the general notion that ROS generation and oxidative stress is one of the main mechanisms behind the toxicity of NPs, of which the Mn-containing NPs clearly were the most active. Similar findings have been observed in other studies. Mn_3O_4 NPs have been shown to induce the highest ROS level among four different metal oxides tested (Mn_3O_4, TiO_2, Fe_2O_3 and Co_3O_4) in A549 cells [35] as well as in rat macrophage cell lines [36]. In addition, Mn_3O_4 NPs induced the highest amount of acellular ROS out of 11 metal oxides tested [37]. The Mn-based NPs also caused induction of the DNA damage reporter Rtkn. The Rtkn reporter is activated upon induction of DNA double strand breaks and likely, high levels of ROS production caused by the Mn NPs can result in high levels of DNA single strand breaks that in turn will lead to DNA double strand breaks during DNA replication. The Mn NPs were further the only NPs investigated so far (in total 33 different NPs) that caused a clear induction of the DNA damage reporter Bscl2, indicating DNA damage that result in interference of replication. The literature seems scarce on the genotoxic effects of Mn NPs. However, Alarifi et al. [38] reported MnO_2 NPs to induce DNA damage in human neuronal SH-SY5Y cells. In another study, MnO_2 NPs were found to cause genotoxicity in vivo with a significant increase in DNA damage in leukocytes as well as micronuclei and chromosomal aberrations in bone marrow cells after oral exposure [39]. Based on the ToxTracker reporter response in this study, it appears somewhat surprising that the Mn-based NPs only showed minor cytotoxicity.

Another response clearly observed for the Mn-based NPs was the protein unfolding response (Ddit3-reporter) related to ER stress. As stated in the review by Cao et al. [40], ER stress has been proposed as a possible mechanism for NP induced toxicity and several metal NPs have been found to induce ER stress in various test systems in vitro such as Ag [41], Au [42], SiO_2 [43] and ZnO NPs [44]. In our study, we observed this effect only for the Mn and Mn_3O_4 NPs as well as for the QDs. Mn ionic species (from $MnCl_2$) have previously been shown to induce ER stress in neuronal cells that is proposed to be closely linked to their neurodegenerative effect [45].

Five QDs of different size were investigated in the present study allowing for exploration of size-dependent effects. The cytotoxicity observed after exposure to the six different reporter cell lines clearly demonstrate that QDs of smaller size are more cytotoxic compared to their larger sizes. Our calculations suggest that surface area is a more appropriate dose metric for the QDs measured, while the results also indicate that the smallest sized QDs may have additional toxic effects other than that explained by increased surface area. This is in line with previous studies reporting the same size dependent trend in BEAS-2B [46], L929 mouse fibroblasts [47] and Rat pheochromocytoma PC12 cells [20]. The generation of ROS and oxidative stress in response to CdTe QDs has previously been shown in various cell types [21,47–49]. Furthermore, the addition of the antioxidant NAC has been reported to reduce CdTe QD cytotoxicity and preserve mitochondrial morphology [20,21]. The activation of UPR observed in response to CdTe QDs in this study is in line with findings of Jiang et al. [50], demonstrating low concentrations of CdTe QDs to be distributed at ER, resulting in ER expansion and UPR activation in HEK kidney cells. These findings were further confirmed in the kidneys of mice exposed to CdTe QDs, demonstrating that UPR mediates the toxicity of CdTe QDs both in vitro and in vivo [50]. CdTe QDs have also been shown to target endothelial ER in human umbilical vein endothelial cells (HUVECs) by causing ER stress, activating the UPR pathway and all of the three downstream ER stress-mediated apoptosis pathways, and ultimately triggered ER stress-induced apoptotic cell death [51].

When comparing effects observed in ToxTracker between the QDs and the soluble $CdCl_2$ salt, based on Cd-content, $CdCl_2$ induced cytotoxicity at a lower concentration of Cd compared to that of CdTe QDs sized 1.5 nm. This is somewhat in conflict with previous findings demonstrating CdTe QDs to be more cytotoxic compared to $CdCl_2$ at similar concentrations of Cd in HepG2 [52] and HEK cells [50]. Cho et al. [53] report no dose-dependent correlation between cell viability and intracellular $[Cd^{2+}]$ following exposure to CdTe QDs, implying the cytotoxicity observed in MCF-7 cell not solely to be related to free Cd ions or Cd-complexes in solution. In the present study, $CdCl_2$ was further found to induce the Srxn1 as well as the Ddit3-GFP markers at a lower dose and greater magnitude compared to the smallest sized CdTe QDs (1.5 nm).

In this study, several metallic NPs were compared with their corresponding bulk oxides. Mn-based NPs (Mn, Mn_3O_4) were shown to have a very similar potency indicating that they may be grouped together for risk assessment. This may be related to the similar composition of the outermost surface for the metal and the oxide, the actual interface between the particles and the cells, and highlights its importance for the cytotoxic potency. In both cases of the Sb- and Sn-based NPs, the metallic form (metal core with surface oxides) was found to be more toxic and reactive compared to their corresponding bulk oxides (Sb_2O_3 and SnO_2), despite the fact that these oxide NPs had a lower primary size (Figure 1). Sedimentation of the Sb NPs was faster compared with its corresponding oxide (Sb_2O_3 NPs, Figure 2), which resulted in a higher cellular dose that may influence the toxicity. This was, however, not the case for the Sn NPs. The V NPs showed rapid sedimentation but were still less toxic than the corresponding oxide (V_2O_5 NPs). Thus, it seems difficult to draw any general conclusions regarding the role of surface oxide composition, particle shape/morphology, and sedimentation rate for the toxic potency of metal NPs vs. their corresponding bulk oxide NPs.

One general concern when studying toxicity of NPs is their possible interaction with the different assays, as has been suggested for genotoxicity assays such as comet assay, micronucleus assay and Ames test [54–56]. One possible concern could be lack of cell uptake in the mES cells. This is unlikely since we previously showed clear uptake of the NPs [10]. Another problem may be if the NPs emit fluorescence causing a risk of false positive results. By always testing the non-modified mES cells in a dose finding study such an increase in fluorescence can be corrected for, as we did for the QDs in this study. Taken together, assay interaction appears not to be a problem if possible fluorescence of the NPs is corrected for.

Taken together with previous data published on ToxTracker findings, the results on the different NPs (n = 33) show a great diversity in activation of GFP-markers as well as in magnitudes of induction, as visualized in Figure 11. This indicates that ToxTracker is a sensitive method for mechanistic screening of NPs and thus able to distinguish differences in toxic effects between various NPs tested. It is evident that the oxidative stress related reporters are the most frequently induced with 20 out of 33 different NPs investigated inducing the Srxn1-GFP reporter. The following NPs clearly induced (exceeding the 2-fold threshold) the Rtkn DNA damage reporter: CuO, Co, CoO, CdTe QDs, Mn, Mn_3O_4, V_2O_5, and welding NPs. Some induction (>1.5-fold, but less than 2-fold) of the Rtkn reporter was also observed with the Ni, NiO and Cr_2O_3 NPs. We suggest that the NPs activating Rtkn reporter are of particular concern when considering genotoxicity of metal- and metal oxide NPs. Ten of the investigated NPs (CdTe QDs, Mn, Mn_3O_4, Sb, Sb_2O_3 and Sn) also induced the Ddit3-GFP reporter, supporting protein stress as a possible mechanism behind their toxicity.

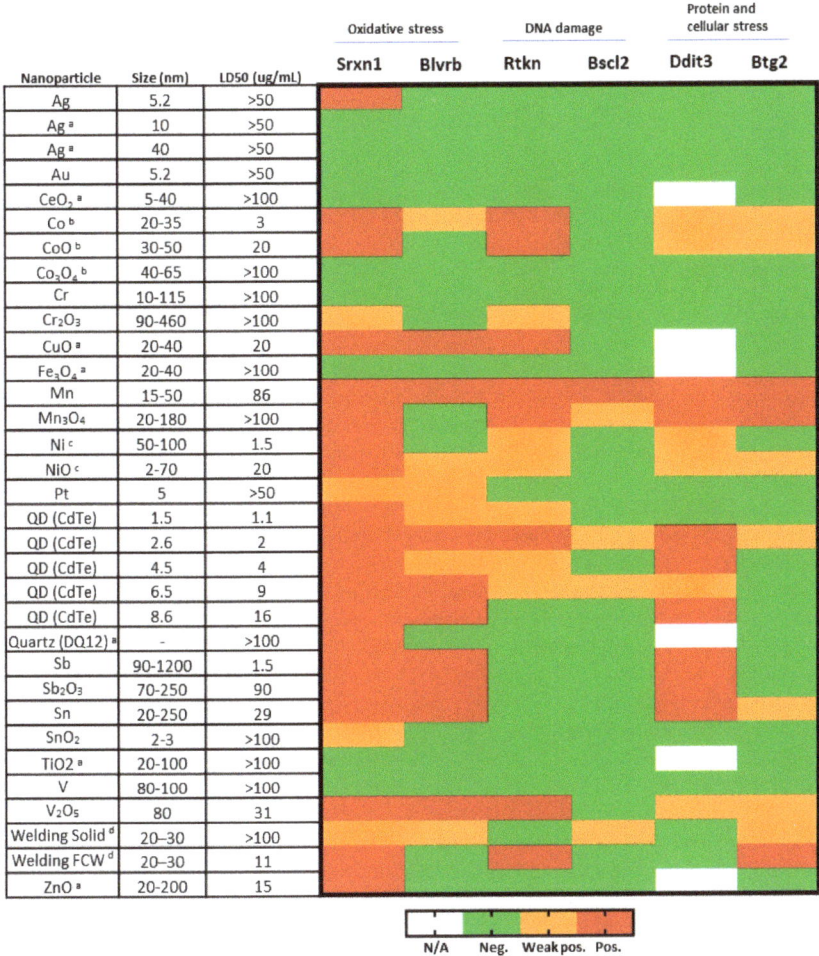

Figure 11. Heatmap of ToxTracker activation of all NPs tested. Size is approximate and based on information from the supplier or TEM imaging. LD50 corresponds to 50% decrease in viability and is based on viability in Srxn1 reporter cells. Weak positive corresponds to >1.5 but <2 fold increase, while positive corresponds to > 2 fold increase at viability levels above 25%. [a] Karlsson et al. [10], [b] Cappellini et al. [12], [c] Akerlund et al. [11], [d] McCarrick et al. [13]; welded using solid or flux cored wire, respectively.

5. Conclusions

In conclusion, we have shown the applicability of using the ToxTracker assay for rapid screening of genotoxic properties of NPs of different size and characteristics, and its suitability as a tool for read-across and for assessing possible toxic mechanisms for further in-depth investigations.

Supplementary Materials: The following are available online at http://www.mdpi.com/2079-4991/10/1/110/s1, Methods for Raman spectroscopy, X-ray photoelectron spectroscopy, X-ray diffraction, Results for oxide characterization including Figure S1: XRD spectra of Mn NPs and Mn_3O_4 NPs, Figure S2: XRD results for SN and SnO_2 NPs, Figure S3: Raman spectra of Sb and Sb_2O_3 NPs as well as Figure S4: Viability of CdTe QDs, Figure S5: Equi-response curves for CdTe QDs and Table S1: Maximum ToxTracker activation.

Author Contributions: Conceptualization: H.L.K., I.O.W. and G.H.; Investigation: S.M. and F.C. (treatment of cells and ToxTracker analysis), A.K. and J.H. (nanoparticle characterization), F.C. and S.W. (dose metric calculations);

Supervision: N.M., R.D. and G.H. (ToxTracker), I.O.W. and E.B. (particle characterization); Figure preparations: S.M.; Writing—Original Draft Preparation: S.M., A.K., I.O.W. and H.L.K.; Writing—Review and Editing: all authors; Funding Acquisition: H.L.K. and I.O.W. All authors have read and agreed to the published version of the manuscript.

Funding: This research was funded by the Swedish Research Council (VR), projects grant numbers 2014-4598 and 2017-03931.

Conflicts of Interest: N.M., R.D. and G.H. are employed by Toxys, a Dutch company that offers ToxTracker as a commercial service. The funders had no role in the design of the study; in the collection, analyses, or interpretation of data; in the writing of the manuscript, or in the decision to publish the results.

References and Notes

1. Karlsson, H.L. The comet assay in nanotoxicology research. *Anal. Bioanal. Chem.* **2010**, *398*, 651–666. [CrossRef] [PubMed]
2. Gonzalez, L.; Sanderson, B.J.; Kirsch-Volders, M. Adaptations of the in vitro MN assay for the genotoxicity assessment of nanomaterials. *Mutagenesis* **2011**, *26*, 185–191. [CrossRef] [PubMed]
3. Magdolenova, Z.; Collins, A.; Kumar, A.; Dhawan, A.; Stone, V.; Dusinska, M. Mechanisms of genotoxicity. A review of in vitro and in vivo studies with engineered nanoparticles. *Nanotoxicology* **2014**, *8*, 233–278. [CrossRef] [PubMed]
4. Nel, A.; Xia, T.; Meng, H.; Wang, X.; Lin, S.; Ji, Z.; Zhang, H. Nanomaterial toxicity testing in the 21st century: Use of a predictive toxicological approach and high-throughput screening. *Acc. Chem. Res.* **2013**, *46*, 607–621. [CrossRef] [PubMed]
5. Nelson, B.C.; Wright, C.W.; Ibuki, Y.; Moreno-Villanueva, M.; Karlsson, H.L.; Hendriks, G.; Sims, C.M.; Singh, N.; Doak, S.H. Emerging metrology for high-throughput nanomaterial genotoxicology. *Mutagenesis* **2017**, *32*, 215–232. [CrossRef] [PubMed]
6. Hastwell, P.W.; Chai, L.L.; Roberts, K.J.; Webster, T.W.; Harvey, J.S.; Rees, R.W.; Walmsley, R.M. High-specificity and high-sensitivity genotoxicity assessment in a human cell line: Validation of the GreenScreen HC GADD45a-GFP genotoxicity assay. *Mutat. Res.* **2006**, *607*, 160–175. [CrossRef]
7. Hughes, C.; Rabinowitz, A.; Tate, M.; Birrell, L.; Allsup, J.; Billinton, N.; Walmsley, R.M. Development of a high-throughput Gaussia luciferase reporter assay for the activation of the GADD45a gene by mutagens, promutagens, clastogens, and aneugens. *J. Biomol. Screen.* **2012**, *17*, 1302–1315. [CrossRef]
8. Hendriks, G.; Derr, R.S.; Misovic, B.; Morolli, B.; Calleja, F.M.; Vrieling, H. The extended ToxTracker assay discriminates between induction of DNA damage, oxidative stress, and protein misfolding. *Toxicol. Sci.* **2016**, *150*, 190–203. [CrossRef]
9. Hendriks, G.; Atallah, M.; Morolli, B.; Calleja, F.; Ras-Verloop, N.; Huijskens, I.; Raamsman, M.; van de Water, B.; Vrieling, H. The ToxTracker assay: Novel GFP reporter systems that provide mechanistic insight into the genotoxic properties of chemicals. *Toxicol. Sci.* **2012**, *125*, 285–298. [CrossRef]
10. Karlsson, H.L.; Gliga, A.R.; Calléja, F.M.; Gonçalves, C.S.; Odnevall Wallinder, I.; Vrieling, H.; Fadeel, B.; Hendriks, G. Mechanism-based genotoxicity screening of metal oxide nanoparticles using the ToxTracker panel of reporter cell lines. *Part. Fibre Toxicol.* **2014**, *11*, 41. [CrossRef]
11. Akerlund, E.; Cappellini, F.; Di Bucchianico, S.; Islam, S.; Skoglund, S.; Derr, R.; Odnevall Wallinder, I.; Hendriks, G.; Karlsson, H.L. Genotoxic and mutagenic properties of Ni and NiO nanoparticles investigated by comet assay, gamma-H2AX staining, Hprt mutation assay and ToxTracker reporter cell lines. *Environ. Mol. Mutagenesis* **2018**, *59*, 211–222. [CrossRef] [PubMed]
12. Cappellini, F.; Hedberg, Y.; McCarrick, S.; Hedberg, J.; Derr, R.; Hendriks, G.; Odnevall Wallinder, I.; Karlsson, H.L. Mechanistic insight into reactivity and (geno)toxicity of well-characterized nanoparticles of cobalt metal and oxides. *Nanotoxicology* **2018**, *12*, 602–620. [CrossRef]
13. McCarrick, S.; Wei, Z.; Moelijker, N.; Derr, R.; Persson, K.-A.; Hendriks, G.; Odnevall Wallinder, I.; Hedberg, Y.; Karlsson, H.L. High variability in toxicity of welding fume nanoparticles from stainless steel in lung cells and reporter cell lines: The role of particle reactivity and solubility. *Nanotoxicology* **2019**, 1–17. [CrossRef] [PubMed]
14. Stark, W.J.; Stoessel, P.R.; Wohlleben, W.; Hafner, A. Industrial applications of nanoparticles. *Chem. Soc. Rev.* **2015**, *44*, 5793–5805. [CrossRef] [PubMed]

15. Klebowski, B.; Depciuch, J.; Parlinska-Wojtan, M.; Baran, J. Applications of noble metal-based nanoparticles in medicine. *Int. J. Mol. Sci.* **2018**, *19*, 4031. [CrossRef] [PubMed]
16. Michalet, X.; Pinaud, F.F.; Bentolila, L.A.; Tsay, J.M.; Doose, S.; Li, J.J.; Sundaresan, G.; Wu, A.M.; Gambhir, S.S.; Weiss, S. Quantum dots for live cells, in vivo imaging, and diagnostics. *Science* **2005**, *307*, 538–544. [CrossRef]
17. Rzigalinski, B.A.; Strobl, J.S. Cadmium-containing nanoparticles: Perspectives on pharmacology and toxicology of quantum dots. *Toxicol. Appl. Pharmacol.* **2009**, *238*, 280–288. [CrossRef]
18. Hardman, R. A toxicologic review of quantum dots: Toxicity depends on physicochemical and environmental factors. *Environ. Health Perspect.* **2006**, *114*, 165–172. [CrossRef]
19. Wang, F.; Shu, L.; Wang, J.; Pan, X.; Huang, R.; Lin, Y.; Cai, X. Perspectives on the toxicology of cadmium-based quantum dots. *Curr. Drug Metab.* **2013**, *14*, 847–856. [CrossRef]
20. Lovric, J.; Bazzi, H.S.; Cuie, Y.; Fortin, G.R.; Winnik, F.M.; Maysinger, D. Differences in subcellular distribution and toxicity of green and red emitting CdTe quantum dots. *J. Mol. Med.* **2005**, *83*, 377–385. [CrossRef]
21. Lovric, J.; Cho, S.J.; Winnik, F.M.; Maysinger, D. Unmodified cadmium telluride quantum dots induce reactive oxygen species formation leading to multiple organelle damage and cell death. *Chem. Biol.* **2005**, *12*, 1227–1234. [CrossRef]
22. Golbamaki, N.; Rasulev, B.; Cassano, A.; Marchese Robinson, R.L.; Benfenati, E.; Leszczynski, J.; Cronin, M.T. Genotoxicity of metal oxide nanomaterials: Review of recent data and discussion of possible mechanisms. *Nanoscale* **2015**, *7*, 2154–2198. [CrossRef] [PubMed]
23. Lebedova, J.; Hedberg, Y.S.; Odnevall Wallinder, I.; Karlsson, H.L. Size-dependent genotoxicity of silver, gold and platinum nanoparticles studied using the mini-gel comet assay and micronucleus scoring with flow cytometry. *Mutagenesis* **2018**, *33*, 77–85. [CrossRef] [PubMed]
24. Delmaar, C.J.; Peijnenburg, W.J.; Oomen, A.G.; Chen, J.; de Jong, W.H.; Sips, A.J.; Wang, Z.; Park, M.V. A practical approach to determine dose metrics for nanomaterials. *Environ. Toxicol. Chem.* **2015**, *34*, 1015–1022. [CrossRef] [PubMed]
25. Zahn, D.; Buciuman, F.; Patcas, F.; Craciun, R. Vibrational spectroscopy of bulk and supported manganese oxides. *Phys. Chem. Chem. Phys.* **1999**, *1*, 185–190.
26. Hedberg, Y.S.; Pradhan, S.; Cappellini, F.; Karlsson, M.E.; Blomberg, E.; Karlsson, H.L.; Odnevall Wallinder, I.; Hedberg, J.F. Electrochemical surface oxide characteristics of metal nanoparticles (Mn, Cu and Al) and the relation to toxicity. *Electrochim. Acta* **2016**, *212*, 360–371. [CrossRef]
27. Lin, A.W.C.; Armstrong, N.R.; Kuwana, T. X-ray photoelectron/Auger electron spectroscopic studies of tin and indium metal foils and oxides. *Anal. Chem.* **1977**, *49*, 1228–1235. [CrossRef]
28. Silversmit, G.; Depla, D.; Poelman, H.; Marin, G.B.; De Gryse, R. Determination of the V2p XPS binding energies for different vanadium oxidation states (V5+ to V0+). *J. Electron. Spectrosc. Relat. Phenom.* **2004**, *135*, 167–175. [CrossRef]
29. Biesinger, M.C.; Payne, B.P.; Grosvenor, A.P.; Lau, L.W.M.; Gerson, A.R.; Smart, R.S.C. Resolving surface chemical states in XPS analysis of first row transition metals, oxides and hydroxides: Cr, Mn, Fe, Co and Ni. *Appl. Surf. Sci.* **2011**, *257*, 2717–2730. [CrossRef]
30. ICDD. JCPDS no 35-732.
31. ICDD. JCPDS card No. 11-689.
32. Pereira, A.L.J.; Gracia, L.; Santamaría-Pérez, D.; Vilaplana, R.; Manjón, F.J.; Errandonea, D.; Nalin, M.; Beltrán, A. Structural and vibrational study of cubic Sb_2O_3 under high pressure. *Phys. Rev. B* **2012**, *85*, 174108. [CrossRef]
33. Pérez, O.E.L.; Sánchez, M.D.; López Teijelo, M. Characterization of growth of anodic antimony oxide films by ellipsometry and XPS. *J. Electroanal. Chem.* **2010**, *645*, 143–148. [CrossRef]
34. Spanier, J.E.; Robinson, R.D.; Zhang, F.; Chan, S.-W.; Herman, I.P. Size-dependent properties of CeO_{2-y} nanoparticles as studied by Raman scattering. *Phys. Rev. B* **2001**, *64*, 245407. [CrossRef]
35. Limbach, L.K.; Wick, P.; Manser, P.; Grass, R.N.; Bruinink, A.; Stark, W.J. Exposure of engineered nanoparticles to human lung epithelial cells: Influence of chemical composition and catalytic activity on oxidative stress. *Environ. Sci. Technol.* **2007**, *41*, 4158–4163. [CrossRef] [PubMed]

36. Urner, M.; Schlicker, A.; Z'Graggen, B.R.; Stepuk, A.; Booy, C.; Buehler, K.P.; Limbach, L.; Chmiel, C.; Stark, W.J.; Beck-Schimmer, B. Inflammatory response of lung macrophages and epithelial cells after exposure to redox active nanoparticles: Effect of solubility and antioxidant treatment. *Environ. Sci. Technol.* **2014**, *48*, 13960–13968. [CrossRef]
37. Ivask, A.; Titma, T.; Visnapuu, M.; Vija, H.; Kakinen, A.; Sihtmae, M.; Pokhrel, S.; Madler, L.; Heinlaan, M.; Kisand, V.; et al. Toxicity of 11 metal oxide nanoparticles to three mammalian cell types in vitro. *Curr. Top. Med. Chem.* **2015**, *15*, 1914–1929. [CrossRef]
38. Alarifi, S.; Ali, D.; Alkahtani, S. Oxidative stress-induced DNA damage by manganese dioxide nanoparticles in human neuronal cells. *Biomed. Res. Int.* **2017**, *2017*, 5478790. [CrossRef]
39. Singh, S.P.; Kumari, M.; Kumari, S.I.; Rahman, M.F.; Mahboob, M.; Grover, P. Toxicity assessment of manganese oxide micro and nanoparticles in Wistar rats after 28 days of repeated oral exposure. *J. Appl. Toxicol.* **2013**, *33*, 1165–1179. [CrossRef]
40. Cao, Y.; Long, J.; Liu, L.; He, T.; Jiang, L.; Zhao, C.; Li, Z. A review of endoplasmic reticulum (ER) stress and nanoparticle (NP) exposure. *Life Sci.* **2017**, *186*, 33–42. [CrossRef]
41. Simard, J.-C.; Durocher, I.; Girard, D. Silver nanoparticles induce irremediable endoplasmic reticulum stress leading to unfolded protein response dependent apoptosis in breast cancer cells. *Apoptosis* **2016**, *21*, 1279–1290. [CrossRef]
42. Noel, C.; Simard, J.C.; Girard, D. Gold nanoparticles induce apoptosis, endoplasmic reticulum stress events and cleavage of cytoskeletal proteins in human neutrophils. *Toxicol. Vitr.* **2016**, *31*, 12–22. [CrossRef]
43. Christen, V.; Fent, K. Silica nanoparticles induce endoplasmic reticulum stress response and activate mitogen activated kinase (MAPK) signalling. *Toxicol. Rep.* **2016**, *3*, 832–840. [CrossRef] [PubMed]
44. Chen, R.; Huo, L.; Shi, X.; Bai, R.; Zhang, Z.; Zhao, Y.; Chang, Y.; Chen, C. Endoplasmic reticulum stress induced by zinc oxide nanoparticles is an earlier biomarker for nanotoxicological evaluation. *ACS Nano* **2014**, *8*, 2562–2574. [CrossRef] [PubMed]
45. Chun, H.S.; Lee, H.; Son, J.H. Manganese induces endoplasmic reticulum (ER) stress and activates multiple caspases in nigral dopaminergic neuronal cells, SN4741. *Neurosci. Lett.* **2001**, *316*, 5–8. [CrossRef]
46. Zheng, W.; Xu, Y.M.; Wu, D.D.; Yao, Y.; Liang, Z.L.; Tan, H.W.; Lau, A.T.Y. Acute and chronic cadmium telluride quantum dots-exposed human bronchial epithelial cells: The effects of particle sizes on their cytotoxicity and carcinogenicity. *Biochem. Biophys. Res. Commun.* **2018**, *495*, 899–903. [CrossRef]
47. Zhang, T.; Wang, Y.; Kong, L.; Xue, Y.; Tang, M. Threshold dose of three types of quantum dots (QDs) induces oxidative stress triggers DNA damage and apoptosis in mouse fibroblast L929 cells. *Int. J. Environ. Res. Public Health* **2015**, *12*, 13435–13454. [CrossRef]
48. Nguyen, K.C.; Willmore, W.G.; Tayabali, A.F. Cadmium telluride quantum dots cause oxidative stress leading to extrinsic and intrinsic apoptosis in hepatocellular carcinoma HepG2 cells. *Toxicology* **2013**, *306*, 114–123. [CrossRef]
49. Katubi, K.M.; Alzahrani, F.M.; Ali, D.; Alarifi, S. Dose- and duration-dependent cytotoxicity and genotoxicity in human hepato carcinoma cells due to CdTe QDs exposure. *Hum. Exp. Toxicol.* **2019**, *38*, 914–926. [CrossRef]
50. Jiang, S.; Lin, Y.; Yao, H.; Yang, C.; Zhang, L.; Luo, B.; Lei, Z.; Cao, L.; Lin, N.; Liu, X.; et al. The role of unfolded protein response and ER-phagy in quantum dots-induced nephrotoxicity: An in vitro and in vivo study. *Arch. Toxicol.* **2018**, *92*, 1421–1434. [CrossRef]
51. Yan, M.; Zhang, Y.; Qin, H.; Liu, K.; Guo, M.; Ge, Y.; Xu, M.; Sun, Y.; Zheng, X. Cytotoxicity of CdTe quantum dots in human umbilical vein endothelial cells: The involvement of cellular uptake and induction of pro-apoptotic endoplasmic reticulum stress. *Int. J. Nanomed.* **2016**, *11*, 529–542. [CrossRef]
52. Nguyen, K.C.; Rippstein, P.; Tayabali, A.F.; Willmore, W.G. Mitochondrial toxicity of cadmium telluride quantum dot nanoparticles in mammalian hepatocytes. *Toxicol. Sci.* **2015**, *146*, 31–42. [CrossRef]
53. Cho, S.J.; Maysinger, D.; Jain, M.; Röder, B.; Hackbarth, S.; Winnik, F.M. Long-term exposure to CdTe quantum dots causes functional impairments in live cells. *Langmuir* **2007**, *23*, 1974–1980. [CrossRef] [PubMed]
54. Pfuhler, S.; Elespuru, R.; Aardema, M.J.; Doak, S.H.; Maria Donner, E.; Honma, M.; Kirsch-Volders, M.; Landsiedel, R.; Manjanatha, M.; Singer, T.; et al. Genotoxicity of nanomaterials: Refining strategies and tests for hazard identification. *Environ. Mol. Mutagenesis* **2013**, *54*, 229–239. [CrossRef] [PubMed]

55. Karlsson, H.L.; Di Bucchianico, S.; Collins, A.R.; Dusinska, M. Can the comet assay be used reliably to detect nanoparticle-induced genotoxicity? *Environ. Mol. Mutagenesis* **2015**, *56*, 82–96. [CrossRef] [PubMed]
56. Li, Y.; Doak, S.H.; Yan, J.; Chen, D.H.; Zhou, M.; Mittelstaedt, R.A.; Chen, Y.; Li, C.; Chen, T. Factors affecting the in vitro micronucleus assay for evaluation of nanomaterials. *Mutagenesis* **2017**, *32*, 151–159. [CrossRef] [PubMed]

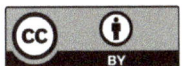

© 2020 by the authors. Licensee MDPI, Basel, Switzerland. This article is an open access article distributed under the terms and conditions of the Creative Commons Attribution (CC BY) license (http://creativecommons.org/licenses/by/4.0/).

MDPI
St. Alban-Anlage 66
4052 Basel
Switzerland
Tel. +41 61 683 77 34
Fax +41 61 302 89 18
www.mdpi.com

Nanomaterials Editorial Office
E-mail: nanomaterials@mdpi.com
www.mdpi.com/journal/nanomaterials

www.ingramcontent.com/pod-product-compliance
Lightning Source LLC
LaVergne TN
LVHW070152120526
838202LV00013BA/1025